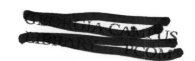

Atlas of
Osteoporosis

Third Edition

Editor

Eric S. Orwoll, MD

Professor of Medicine
Department of Medicine
Director, Oregon Clinical and Translational Research Institute
Oregon Health and Sciences University
Portland, Oregon

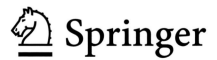 Springer

CURRENT MEDICINE GROUP LLC, PART OF SPRINGER SCIENCE+BUSINESS MEDIA LLC

400 Market Street, Suite 700 • Philadelphia, PA 19106

Senior Developmental Editor	Diana Winters
Developmental Editor	Stephanie Weidel Brown
Editorial Assistant	Juleen Deaner
Managing Editor	Megan Charlton
Design and Layout	Heather Hoch
Illustrators	Daniel Britt, Kim Broadbent, Marie Dean, Heather Hoch, Sara Krause, Wieslawa Langenfeld, Jacqueline Leonard, Maureen Looney
Production Coordinator	Carolyn Naylor
Indexer	Holly Lukens

Library of Congress Cataloging-in-Publication Data

Atlas of osteoporosis / editor, Eric S. Orwoll ; with 22 contributors. -- 3rd ed.
    p. ; cm.
  Includes bibliographical references and index.
  ISBN 978-1-57340-296-5 (alk. paper)
  1. Osteoporosis--Atlases. I. Orwoll, Eric S. II. Title.
  [DNLM: 1. Osteoporosis--Atlases. WE 17 A8806331 2008]

  RC931.O73.A856 2008
  616.7'16--dc22

                    2008032873

  ISBN 978-1-57340-296-5
  ISBN 1-57340-296-6

www.springer.com

For more information, please call 1 (800) 777-4643
or email us at orders-ny@springer.com

www.currentmedicinegroup.com

10 9 8 7 6 5 4 3 2 1

Printed in China by L. Rex Printing Company Limited

This book was printed on acid-free paper

Preface

Osteoporosis has long been known to be a major health care problem, in both individual and public health terms, but in the last two decades tremendous increases in scientific inquiry have yielded a much greater understanding of the basic biology, clinical character, and epidemiology of the condition. These advances have been translated into much more sophisticated and effective tools for clinicians to use in the prevention and treatment of the disease. These tools, initially available only to specialists in endocrinology and rheumatology, are now available to a wide range of clinicians. Appropriately, the public is also becoming more educated and it is not uncommon for clinicians to have sophisticated discussions with well-read patients about the diagnosis, prevention, and treatment of osteoporosis.

The Third Edition of the *Atlas of Osteoporosis* builds on the foundation of previous editions and once again is designed to be useful to a broad readership. In a format that makes extensive use of graphical displays of important data, the authors have encapsulated not only the well-established basics of osteoporosis but also new developments in the field.

Exciting new chapters have been added, including the histology of bone remodeling and metabolic bone disorders. A chapter on emerging therapies reflects the considerable promise of new treatment approaches. The important problem of renal bone disease is now addressed in a chapter dedicated to that issue. Moreover, topics that are well known to be important to skeletal biology and osteoporosis have been updated, and the chapters that were new in the Second Edition (*eg*, genetics and biomechanics) have been expanded. Other chapters have been extensively revised to capture recent developments. For instance, the range of bisphosphonates drugs available for prevention and therapy has grown and parathyroid hormone treatment for osteoporosis, which was new at the time of the Second Edition, is now better understood. More information about both is provided.

Although osteoporosis has been recognized for millennia, knowledge regarding this disorder continues to evolve. The sheer volume of available information, as well as its complexity, poses considerable challenges to those attempting to summarize it. To whatever extent the *Atlas* has succeeded in this endeavor, it is a tribute to the many outstanding contributors who devoted time and considerable expertise to the effort.

Eric S. Orwoll, MD

Contributors

Diana Antoniucci, MD
Assistant Clinical Professor of Medicine
Department of Medicine
University of California
San Francisco, California

Laura K. Bachrach, MD
Professor of Pediatrics
Department of Pediatrics
Division of Endocrinology
Stanford University School of Medicine
Stanford, California

Neil Binkley, MD
Associate Professor
Department of Medicine
Section of Geriatrics and Endocrinology
University of Wisconsin
Madison, Wisconsin

Jane A. Cauley, DrPH
Department of Epidemiology
Graduate School of Public Health
University of Pittsburgh
Pittsburgh, Pennsylvania

Cyrus Cooper, MD, FRCP, FMedSci
MRC Epidemiology Resource Centre
University of Southampton
Southampton, United Kingdom
Botnar Research Center
University of Oxford
Oxford, United Kingdom

Jeffrey Curtis, MD, MPH
Assistant Professor of Medicine
Division of Clinical Immunology and Rheumatology
University of Alabama at Birmingham
Director
UAB Arthritis Clinical Intervention Program
Associate Director
UAB Center for Education and Research on the Therapeutics of
  Musculoskeletal Disorders (CERTs)
Associate Scientist
UAB Center for Metabolic Bone Disease
Birmingham, Alabama

Richard Eastell, MD, FRCP, FRCPath, FMedSci
Professor of Bone Metabolism
Head of Academic Unit of Bone Metabolism
School of Medicine and Biomedical Sciences
University of Sheffield
Metabolic Bone Center
Northern General Hospital
Sheffield, United Kingdom

Sol Epstein, MD
Mount Sinai School of Medicine
New York, New York

Dina E. Green, MD
Assistant Professor of Medicine
Division of Endocrinology, Diabetes, and Bone Disease
Mount Sinai School of Medicine
New York, New York

Karl J. Jepsen, PhD
Associate Professor
Leni and Peter W. May Department of Orthopaedics
Mount Sinai School of Medicine
New York, New York

David Kendler, MD, FRCPC
Associate Professor
Department of Medicine (Endocrinology)
University of British Columbia
Vancouver, British Columbia, Canada

Robert F. Klein, MD
Professor of Medicine
Division of Endocrinology, Diabetes, and Clinical Nutrition
Oregon Health and Science University
Chief
Endocrinology and Metabolism Section
Department of Hospital and Specialty Medicine
Portland VA Medical Center
Portland, Oregon

Philipp K. Lang, MD, MBA
Director, Musculoskeletal Radiology
Department of Radiology
Brigham and Women's Hospital
Harvard Medical School
Boston, Massachusetts

Michael R. McClung, MD, FACP
Assistant Director
Medical Education
Providence Portland Medical Center
Founding Director
Oregon Osteoporosis Center
Portland, Oregon

Paul D. Miller, MD
Distinguished Clinical Professor of Medicine
University of Colorado Health Sciences Center
Medical Director
Colorado Center for Bone Research
Lakewood, Colorado

Eric S. Orwoll, MD
Professor of Medicine
Department of Medicine
Director, Oregon Clinical Translational Research Institute
Oregon Health and Sciences Center
Portland, Oregon

Susan M. Ott, MD
Associate Professor
Department of Medicine
University of Washington
Seattle, Washington

Deborah E. Sellmeyer, MD
Associate Professor of Medicine
Division of Endocrinology
Department of Medicine
The Johns Hopkins Bayview Medical Center
Baltimore, Maryland

Elsa S. Strotmeyer, PhD, MPH
Assistant Professor
Department of Epidemiology
University of Pittsburgh
Pittsburgh, Pennsylvania

Jan E. Vandevenne, MD
Department of Radiology
Ziekenhuizen Oost-Limburg
Genk, Belgium

Chaim Vanek, MD
Department of Endocrinology, Diabetes, and Clinical Nutrition
Bone and Mineral Unit
Oregon Health and Science University
Portland, Oregon

Tjeerd-Pieter van Staa, MD
Head of Research
General Practice Research Database
London, United Kingdom
Associate Professor
Department of Pharmacoepidemiology
Utrecht Institute for Pharmaceutical Sciences
Utrecht University
Utrecht, The Netherlands

Connie M. Weaver, PhD
Department Head Foods and Nutrition
Purdue University
West Lafayette, Indiana

Robert S. Weinstein, MD
Professor of Medicine
Bone Morphometry Laboratory
Division of Endocrinology and Metabolism
Center for Osteoporosis and Metabolic Bone Diseases
Department of Internal Medicine
Central Arkansas Veterans Health Care System
University of Arkansas for Medical Sciences
Little Rock, Arkansas

Carl S. Winalski, MD
Head, Musculoskeletal MRI
Department of Radiology
Brigham and Women's Hospital
Harvard Medical School
Boston, Massachusetts

Contents

The Nature of Osteoporosis

Eric S. Orwoll and Chaim Vanek

The recent emergence of osteoporosis as a major focus of investigation in fields as diverse as mechanical engineering, pediatrics, and epidemiology has led to many important advances in the understanding of and therapeutics for this disease. Whereas the topic of osteoporosis formerly occupied just a few paragraphs in standard texts, it is now the primary focus of several journals and textbooks. This volume provides current information regarding skeletal health and its disruption. Attention is given to bone acquisition during growth years, mechanisms of adult bone loss, and new developments in osteoporosis diagnostics and therapeutics. In the final analysis, osteoporosis is a condition of bone, a complex tissue that undergoes physiologic repair throughout life. This chapter introduces the reader to the "nature" of osteoporosis, the physical characteristics of healthy and fragile bone. The study of bone transcends a measurement of its amount or mineral density to encompass aspects of its geometry and material properties. Bone remodeling is a continuous renewal process. Alterations in remodeling are the basis for the changes in the amount, geometry, and quality of bone during adult life.

Osteoporotic Bone

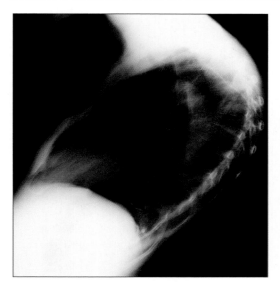

Figure 1-1. Lateral chest radiograph showing a classic spine deformity called kyphosis. Kyphosis is the end result of multiple vertebral compression fractures. *Osteoporosis* is defined as a skeletal condition of decreased bone quantity accompanied by abnormalities in the microscopic architecture of bone that renders a person more likely to sustain a fracture with little or no trauma. Osteoporosis frequently is considered in the context of specific fracture syndromes, including vertebral compression, Colles' (distal radial) fracture, and hip fracture. However, osteoporosis truly is a disease of global skeletal fragility, with increased risk of low-trauma fractures in all portions of the skeleton. (*Courtesy of* R. Marcus, MD.)

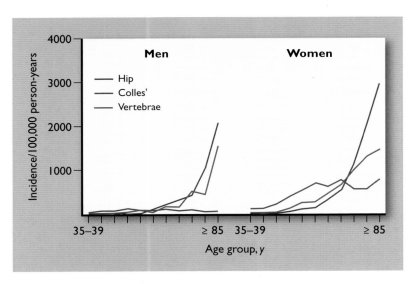

Figure 1-2. Incidence of osteoporotic fractures. The clinical consequences of bone fragility are fractures. Shown here are curves representing age-related incidences of vertebral, forearm, and hip fractures in North American men and women. The incidence of all fractures is about twice as great in women as it is in men, but osteoporosis is not exclusively a disease of women. The incidence of hip fracture increases rapidly in men older than 70 years of age. One-third of vertebral fractures result in pain sufficient to cause the patient to seek medical attention; however, many occur without obvious symptoms, becoming apparent only as there is a loss of height or development of curvature. Wrist fractures typically occur at a younger age than hip fractures. This may be explained by differences in the mechanism of the fall. Wrist fractures most commonly result when a person standing upright falls forward and attempts to break the fall by arm extension and pronation as happens in a younger subject. Older subjects commonly suffer hip fractures when they fall backwards and directly impact the femoral trochanter. Thus, the occurrence of fractures is a function not only of osteoporosis and intrinsic bone quality but also of the type and mechanism of the fall itself. (*Adapted from* Cooper and Melton [1].)

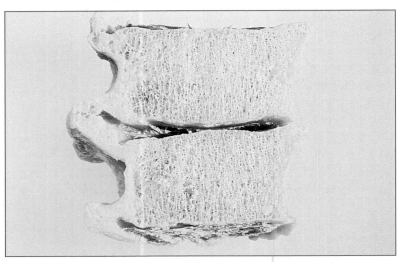

Figure 1-3. Normal vertebral bodies. Vertebral bodies are composed of a thin external cortical shell and a central honeycomb of vertical and horizontal bars, or trabeculae. Both the cortical shell and the central trabeculae contribute to the strength of the vertebrae and, thus, to its resistance to fracture. In adults, trabecular interstices of the axial (central) skeleton constitute the primary repository of red bone marrow. The trabecular surface is in proximity to the marrow cellular constituents responsible for bone turnover. Events leading to the loss of bone occur at these surfaces. Changes in bone mass occur earlier and to a greater extent in trabecular bone than they do in regions of the skeleton not adjacent to the marrow environment, such as cortical bone. (*Courtesy of* R. Marcus, MD.)

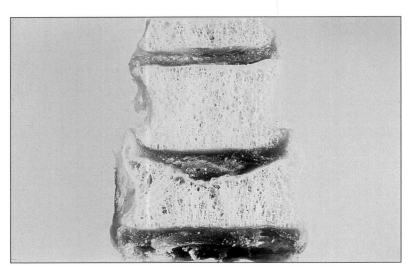

Figure 1-4. Osteoporotic vertebral bodies. Weakness of the trabecular structure results in mechanical failure, with collapse of the intervertebral disk into the underlying bony substance. This weakness reflects a decrease in the total amount of bone within the vertebral body and also a disruption of the normal trabecular microarchitecture, as is evident by the appearance of cavities where bone has been lost. A formal definition of the term *osteoporosis* is a skeletal condition characterized by low bone mass and abnormal microarchitecture, leading to increased risk of fracture with minimal trauma. (*Courtesy of* R. Marcus, MD.)

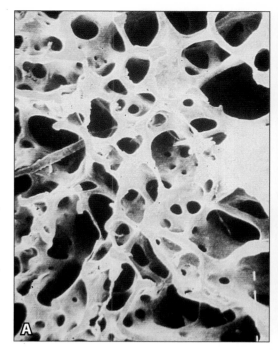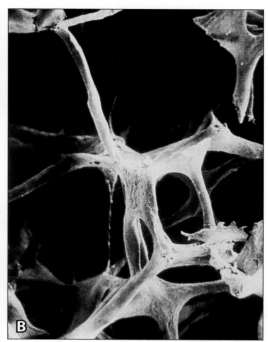

Figure 1-5. Scanning electron micrograph of normal (**A**) and osteoporotic (**B**) trabecular structures. In osteoporosis, the normal plate-like trabeculae have been replaced by thin rods. The microarchitecture and quality of the vertebral structure have been irreparably damaged by trabecular perforation resulting in loss of trabecular connectivity and continuity. (*Courtesy of* J. Kosek.)

Bone Mass Measurement

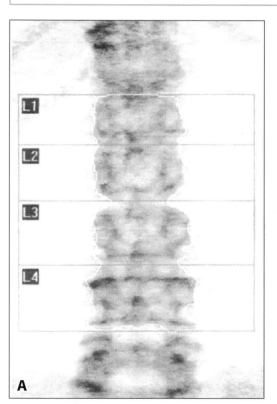

A

B

DXA Results Summary

Region	Area, cm²	BMC, g	BMD, g/cm²	T-score	Z-score
L1	11.01	8.27	0.751	−1.6	0.5
L2	12.25	8.97	0.733	−2.7	−0.3
L3	14.52	9.98	0.688	−3.6	−1.1
L4	16.47	12.64	0.768	−3.2	−0.6
Total	54.25	39.87	0.735	−2.8	−0.5

Total BMD CV 1.0%

Figure 1-6. Dual-energy x-ray absorptiometry (DXA). **A**, Printout from a lumbar spine bone density examination. Although low bone mass and architectural disruption are essential components of the diagnosis of osteoporosis, current applicable diagnostic tools provide measurements of bone mass (the amount of bone) only and do not address other aspects of bone quality that contribute to fragility, such as geometry, material properties, and microarchitecture. DXA is a technique that exploits the ability of bone mineral to attenuate the passage of x-rays through the body to provide estimates of the bone mineral density (BMD). **B**, Machine software estimates the area and mineral content of bones in the region scanned. A calculated areal BMD (measured in g/cm²) is generated for the scanned region. For clinical purposes, the scanned regions generally include the lumbar spine, proximal femur, forearm, and whole body. For research purposes, any skeletal region can be assessed. BMC—bone mineral content.

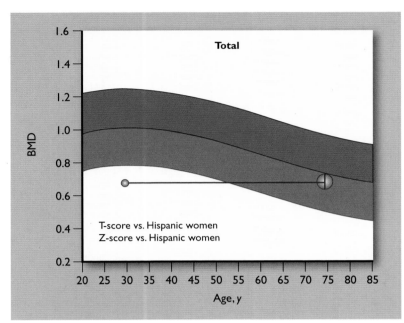

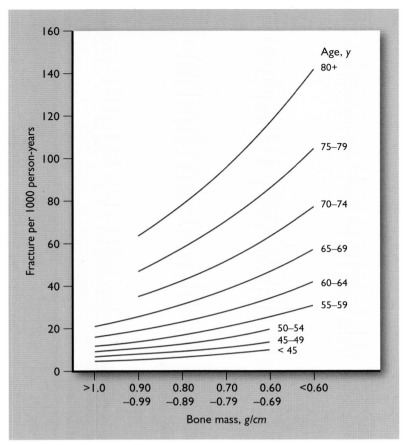

Figure 1-7. Bone mineral density (BMD) by dual-energy x-ray absorptiometry (DXA). Patient value (*cross*) is superimposed on a graph representing the mean ± 2 SD per age intervals for a healthy population. Absolute BMD results (g/cm²) are commonly expressed in terms of units of SD from population averages. When comparing a patient with his or her age-matched population, these SD units are expressed as Z-scores. When a patient is compared with the average of a young population, SD units are expressed as T-scores. In this case, the patient's value is within 2 SD of the expected value for a 74-year-old person (Z-score = –0.5) and more than 2.5 SD below the peak bone density of a person 30 years of age (T-score = –2.8). Reference data for the young adult population are currently sex specific and are race specific for some densitometers. However, in the future, reference data from young white women may be used for all populations.

Figure 1-8. Interaction of age and bone mineral density (BMD) on fracture incidence. A large cohort of women was followed over time. Fracture incidence is shown on the vertical axis and the women are stratified by bone density along the horizontal axis. In addition, women are stratified by age, represented by a family of curves. At any given BMD, fracture incidence is higher with increasing age. In fact, the slope of the relationship to fracture is steeper for age than it is for BMD, which would not be expected if BMD itself were the sole determinant of fracture risk. For the oldest women, the incidence of falls is greater and contributes to the added fracture risk. However, falls and BMD do not entirely account for the added fractures that occur at older ages. These fractures may be the result of so-called qualitative or material properties of bone that affect fragility but are not accounted for by BMD measurement or other currently available imaging modalities. (*Adapted from* Hui *et al.* [2].)

Qualitative Abnormalities in Osteoporotic Bone

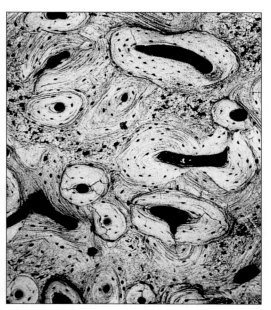

Factors That Contribute to Bone Quality
Altered mineral or matrix composition
Cement lines
Cortical porosity
Fatigue accumulation
Trabecular disruption

Figure 1-9. Factors that contribute to bone quality. This figure lists some of the qualitative properties of bone that could contribute to poor bone strength and increased fragility but are not well assessed by bone density measurements.

Figure 1-10. Micrograph of a biopsy specimen of the iliac crest showing qualitative abnormalities in bone. Cortical porosity is seen in this specimen from an 80-year-old man. Porosity is evident as large Haversian canals (*dark areas*) that result from excess resorption. Also note the high prevalence of Haversian systems, indicating active remodeling events [3].

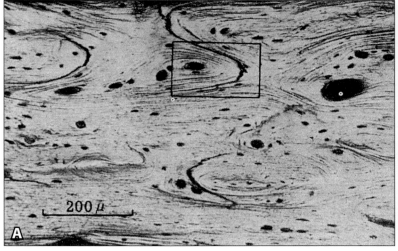

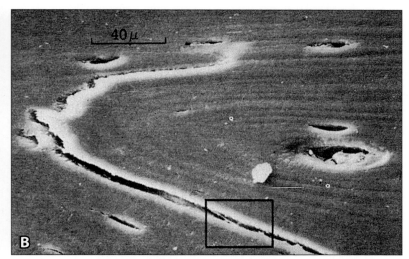

Figure 1-11. Micrograph of qualitative abnormalities in bone showing cement lines [4]. **A**, Cement lines are the residue of a previous bone resorption event. Composed of a filigree of woven, rather than dense, lamellar collagen, cement lines represent an area susceptible to structural failure. The *box* shows a Haversian system bounded by a curved cement line. **B**, Dehiscence of a cement line after application of a bending force to the whole bone. Bone breakage occurs as a propagation of fracture lines from one cement line to the next [5]. The *box* shows separation at the cement line between Haversian systems.

Bone Geometry

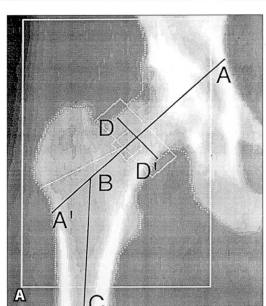

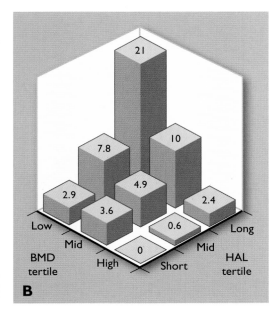

Figure 1-12. Geometric contributions to bone strength and fracture risk. Despite an undisputed relationship between bone mineral density (BMD) and fracture incidence, factors independent of BMD make important contributions to fractures. Of particular importance are bone geometry and the occurrence of falls. To illustrate the role of macroscopic bone geometry, this figure shows the important effect a measurement called the hip axial length (HAL) has on hip fracture risk. **A,** HAL is the length of a straight line connecting the inferior surface of the greater trochanter to the inner surface of the hip acetabulum (*line A-A'*). *Line D-D'* is the width of the femoral neck. **B,** Results of a large prospective observational study of elderly women showing that the incidence of hip fracture is dependent on HAL. At any level of BMD, women with longer HAL had significantly greater risk of hip fracture. Indeed, women with BMD in the lowest tertile who also had HAL in the longest tertile had a 21-fold increased relative risk of hip fracture. (**B** *adapted from* Faulkner *et al.* [6].)

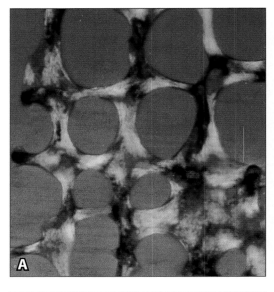

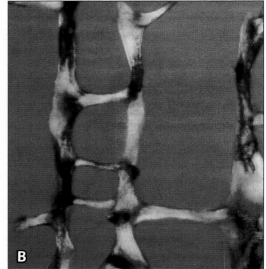

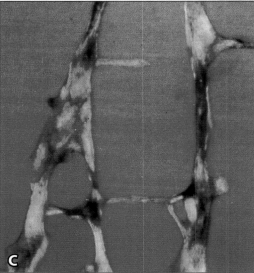

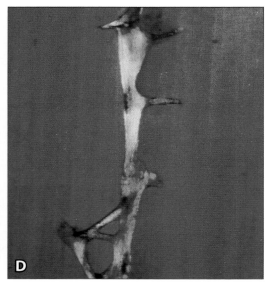

Figure 1-13. Geometric contributions to bone strength and fracture risk. During the development of osteoporosis, the loss of horizontal connections between the trabeculae is more prominent than the loss of vertical elements; this loss is a major factor in the loss of resistance to compressive forces. The microscopic architecture is shown in a 50-year-old man (**A**), a 58-year-old man (**B**), a 76-year-old man (**C**), and an 80-year-old woman (**D**) [7].

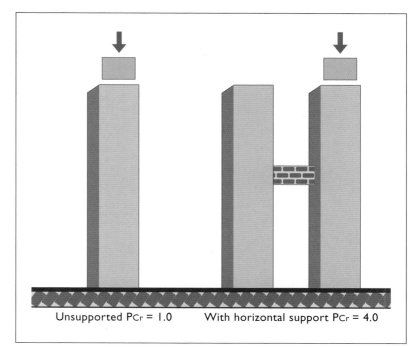

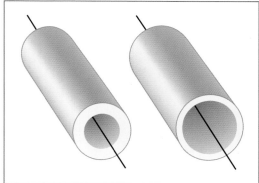

Figure 1-14. Geometric contributions to bone strength and fracture risk showing the consequences of horizontal trabecular loss. A single horizontal connecting strut increases by fourfold the maximum load (Pcr) that can be carried by a vertical bar without buckling. Thus, loss of horizontal trabeculae with age has a profound independent effect on vertebral trabecular strength. (*Adapted from* Snow-Harter and Marcus [8].)

Figure 1-15. Geometric contributions to bone strength and fracture risk showing the effect of cortical mass distribution on strength in a long bone. Assume that the two cylinders have equal mass. The one on the right has a greater distribution of mass farther from the axis of bending compared with the left; this is called the cross-sectional moment of inertia (CSMI). Despite the thinner walls of this structure, the distribution results in a substantially increased resistance to bending along the length of the cylinder. The long bones of men generally are larger and thus have larger CSMI compared with those of women. The increased CSMI confers on them relative greater protection against fracture at any given value of bone mineral density. (*Adapted from* Snow-Harter and Marcus [8].)

Role of Remodeling in Lifelong Acquisition and Loss of Bone

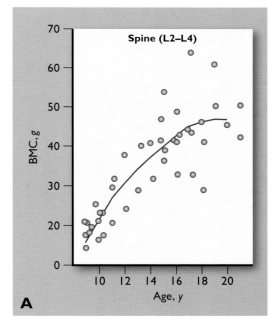

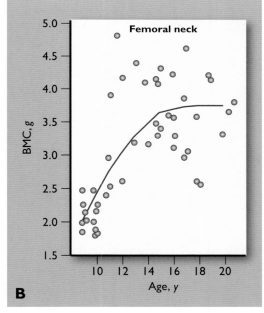

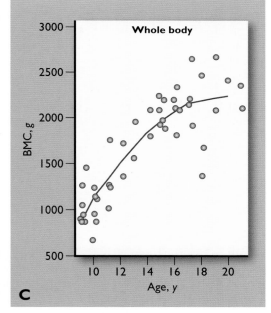

Figure 1-16. A–C, Acquisition of bone during adolescence. At any time during adult life, bone mass reflects bone that has been gained during years of growth minus bone that subsequently has been lost. Previous theories about osteoporosis have not adequately considered the role of bone acquisition in determining lifelong fracture risk. This study of healthy white girls aged 9 to 21 years shows that about 60% of final adult "peak" bone mass is acquired during the adolescent growth spurt. Only about 5% of peak bone mass is acquired after 18 years of age. Thus, adolescence constitutes a window of opportunity when genetic, dietary, hormonal, and other factors determine the magnitude of bone gain. About 80% of peak bone mass is genetically determined. Important environmental factors include dietary calcium intake, reproductive endocrine status, and habitual physical activity. However, adolescence is also a window of vulnerability when inadequate attention to these same factors can lead to low bone mass at skeletal maturity. Persons who have not gained adequate bone mass would not need to lose very much bone in adulthood to have a substantially increased risk of osteoporosis and fracture. Of particular concern are dietary calcium intake (which is generally low in American teenaged girls), a relatively sedentary lifestyle, and the high prevalence of anorexia nervosa and other eating disorders. BMC—bone mineral content. (*Adapted from* Katzman *et al.* [9].)

Delayed puberty
Immobilization or therapeutic rest
Specific disorders
  Anorexia nervosa
  Cystic fibrosis
  Intestinal or renal disease
  Marfan syndrome
  Osteogenesis imperfecta

Figure 1-17. Acquisitional osteopenia. This list includes some childhood conditions that are known to interfere with the acquisition of peak bone mass. Low peak bone mass may result in an increased risk for fractures later in life.

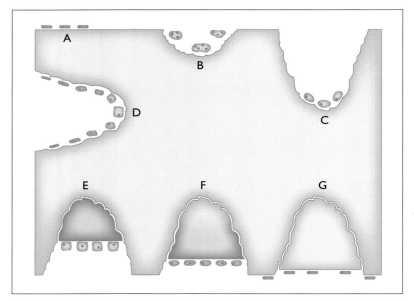

Figure 1-18. Bone remodeling. Once new bone is laid down, it is subject to a continuous process of breakdown and renewal called remodeling that continues throughout life. After linear growth stops and peak bone mass has been reached, remodeling constitutes the final common pathway by which bone mass is adjusted throughout adult life. Remodeling is carried out by thousands of individual and independent "bone remodeling units" on the surfaces of bone throughout the skeleton.

A, About 90% of bone surface is normally inactive, covered by a thin layer of lining cells. **B,** In response to physical or biochemical signals, recruitment of marrow precursor cells to a site at the bone surface results in their fusion into the characteristic multinucleated osteoclasts that resorb, or dig a cavity into, the bone. In cortical bone, resorption creates tunnels with haversian canals, whereas trabecular resorption creates scalloped areas of the bone surface called Howship lacunas. **C,** On termination of the resorption phase, a 60-μm cavity remains and is bordered at its deepest extent by a cement line, a region of loosely organized collagen fibrils. **D,** Completion of resorption is followed by ingress of preosteoblasts derived from marrow stromal stem cells into the base of the resorption cavity. **E,** These cells develop the characteristic osteoblastic phenotype and begin to replace the resorbed bone by elaborating new bone matrix constituents, such as collagen, osteocalcin, and other proteins. **F,** Once the newly formed osteoid reaches a thickness of about 20 μm, mineralization begins.

The remodeling cycle normally is completed in about 6 months (**G**). No net change in bone mass occurs as a result of remodeling when the amount of resorbed bone replaced equals the amount removed. Persistence of small bone deficits on the completion of each cycle, however, reflects an inefficiency in remodeling dynamics. The lifelong accumulation of remodeling deficits underlies the phenomenon of age-related bone loss. (*Adapted from* Marcus [10].)

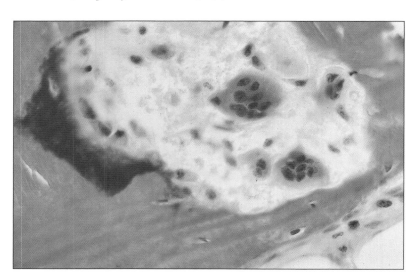

Figure 1-19. Bone biopsy specimen from the iliac crest showing the cellular participants in bone remodeling. Large multinucleated cells seen in the middle of the field are osteoclasts. Derived from a mononuclear macrophage precursor, these cells migrate to a locus on the bone surface, become adherent to the surface with the participation of a number of adherence molecules, and resorb bone (both organic matrix and mineral). The layer of cuboidal mononuclear cells at the bone surface is osteoblasts and the thick red band beneath them represents organic matrix that has not yet been mineralized (osteoid). Mineralized bone is olive in color (Goldner stain). (*Courtesy of* J. Kosek.)

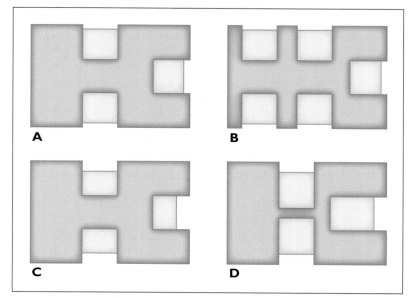

Figure 1-20. Perturbations in remodeling. Alterations in remodeling activity represent the pathway through which diverse stimuli such as dietary insufficiency, hormones, and drugs affect bone balance. A change in the whole body remodeling rate can be brought about through distinct perturbations in remodeling dynamics.

A representation of normal remodeling is shown in **A:** three areas of remodeling activity, each with identical resorption lacunae that have filled in with new bone (*shaded area*). Identical small bone deficits are shown with each remodeling area, reflecting remodeling insufficiency. **B,** Increased remodeling, as shown by five remodeling units, such as is seen in conditions that increase the activation or birthrate of new remodeling units. Examples include hyperparathyroidism, hyperthyroidism, and hypervitaminosis D. Although each remodeling unit is similar to those in **A,** the total bone mass is reduced. **C,** Exaggerated inefficiency of osteoblastic response. The number of remodeling units is similar to **A**; however, the magnitude of the bone deficit is increased due to poor osteoblastic bone formation. Such changes are typical of osteoblastic toxins such as ethanol and glucocorticoids. Progressive age may also be associated with increasing deficits in osteoblast recruitment and function. **D,** Exaggerated osteoclastic activity. A variety of conditions (eg, estrogen deficiency or immobilization) may augment osteoclastic resorptive capacity. If the resorption cavities perforate the trabeculae, no scaffold remains for new bone formation to take place. Such resorption becomes a permanent loss of bone.

At any given time, a transient deficit in bone called the remodeling space exists, which represents sites of bone resorption that have not yet been filled. In response to any stimulus that alters the birth rate of new remodeling units, the remodeling space will either increase or decrease accordingly until a new steady state is established. This adjustment is seen as an increase or decrease in bone density. (*Adapted from* Marcus [10].)

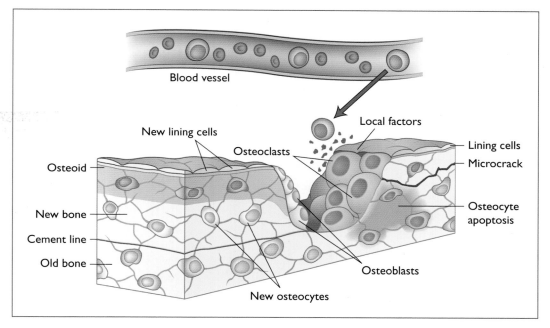

Figure 1-21. Remodeling cycle. After the completion of bone formation, osteoblasts that remain within the newly formed osteoid become osteocytes. Osteocytes have cytoplasmic processes that extend through the matrix in canaliculi. Osteocytes and their network of processes detect strain and microfractures and transmit this information to induce new bone remodeling and repair. For instance, microfractures sever osteocyte processes and initiate a cascade of growth factors and cellular migration that begets osteoclast bone resorption followed by osteoblast bone formation. (*Adapted from* Seeman and Delmas [11].)

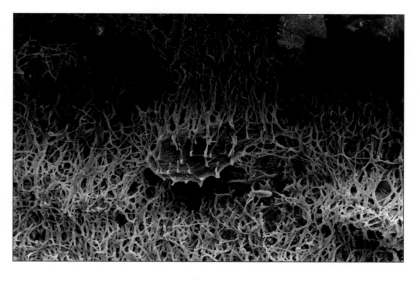

Figure 1-22. Osteocytes are the most numerous and longest living cells in bone [12]. They connect with one another and bone surfaces through a network of canalicular processes. There are approximately 10,000 osteocytes per cubic millimeter of bone with 50 processes per cell. Canalicular processes orchestrate focal bone remodeling by detecting bone strain. (*Courtesy of* L. Bonewald and J. Feng.)

Figure 1-23. Age-related bone loss. A large cross-sectional study of cortical bone mineral density (BMD) of the radius in men and women across the adult lifespan is represented. BMD remains relatively stable until about an age of 50 years when, on average, progressive bone loss occurs in men and women. Bone loss is more rapid in women aged 50 to 60 years (~2%–3%/y) compared with men (~1%/y). This difference reflects the impact of menopausal loss of estrogen production. Subsequently, age-related losses of BMD are similar for men and women [13]. Although bone loss is generally detected only by routine densitometric methods performed after 50 years of age, more sensitive methods (*eg,* computed tomography or histomorphometry) show the beginning of age-related bone loss as early as the third decade of life [7].

At any time in adult life, areal BMD is higher in men than it is in women. However, to some extent this represents an artifact of bone size, which is larger in men. If 1-cm cubes of bone from average young men and women were compared, the mineral content would be equal. It is not trivial that bone diameters in men are larger than those in women because bone strength is a function of BMD squared times the cross sectional area (*see* Figure 1-15 for a related topic). Thus, with bones of equal true BMD, larger cross-sectional areas confer relative protection against fractures in men.

Maintaining bone density throughout adult life requires meeting many challenges imposed by both physiologic and environmental factors. From the principles of bone remodeling, discussed previously, it can be seen that

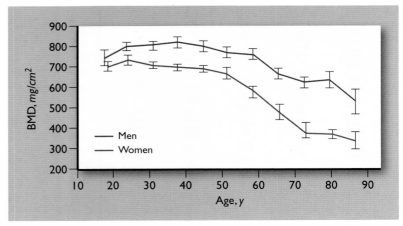

any factors that tend to increase overall bone remodeling will promote bone loss, whereas factors that reduce bone remodeling may lower the rate of bone loss. Only a few of the important factors that may promote bone remodeling and bone loss in elderly persons are listed, which include decreases in sex steroids in men and women; increases in circulating parathyroid hormone, which may reflect a decreased calcium nutritional state either from limited nutrient intake or age-imposed deficits in vitamin D status and intestinal calcium absorption efficiency; and age-related decrease in habitual physical activity and recreational exercise.

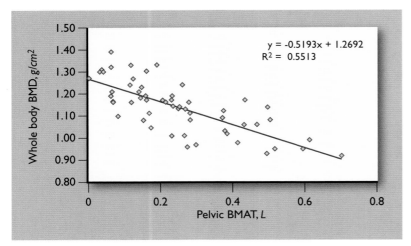

Figure 1-24. Marrow fat and aging. MRI studies show an inverse correlation between bone marrow adipose tissue (BMAT) and whole body bone mineral density (BMD). An increase in bone marrow fat occurs with aging and the amount of marrow fat is inversely related to BMD. A possible connection between the two phenomena is the mesenchymal stem cell, which is a precursor to both the preosteoblast and the preadipocyte. Various transcription factors, such as peroxisome proliferative activated receptor gamma, may increase with aging and drive the mesenchymal stem cell toward adipocyte differentiation at the expense of osteoblast formation and bone growth [14,15]. (*From* Shen *et al.* [14]; with permission.)

Requirements for Maintenance of Skeletal Integrity

Nutrient adequacy

Physical activity

Reproductive hormone status

Figure 1-25. Requirements to maintain skeletal integrity. Skeletal integrity requires adequacy of the habitual mechanical environment (physical activity), reproductive hormone status, and nutrients. Overzealous attention to any two of these factors does not suffice when the third factor is neglected. Thus, an immobilized patient loses bone even when both reproductive hormone and nutritional status are more than adequate. Similarly, a woman athlete who exercises to the point of developing amenorrhea (and low estrogen status) loses bone, despite a high mechanical environment and calcium supplementation.

References

1. Cooper C, Melton LJ III: Epidemiology of osteoporosis. *Trends Endocrinol Metab* 1992, 3:224–229.

2. Hui SL, Slemenda CW, Johnston CC Jr: Age and bone mass as predictors of fracture in a prospective study. *J Clin Invest* 1988, 81:1804–1809.

3. Grynpas M: Age and disease-related changes in the mineral of bone. *Calcif Tiss Int* 1993, 53(Suppl 1):S57–S64.

4. Marcus R: The nature of osteoporosis. In *Osteoporosis*. Edited by Marcus R, Feldman D, Kelsey J. San Diego: Academic; 1996:647–659.

5. Carter DR, Hayes WC: Compact bone fatigue damage: a microscopic examination. *Clin Orthp Rel Res* 1977, 127:265–274.

6. Faulkner K, Cummings S, Black D: Simple measurement of femoral geometry predicts hip fracture: the study of osteoporotic fractures. *J Bone Miner Res* 1993, 8:1211–1217.

7. Mosekilde L: Age-related changes in vertebral trabecular bone architecture: assessed by a new method. *Bone* 1988, 9:247–250.

8. Snow-Harter C, Marcus R: Exercise, bone density, and osteoporosis. *Exerc Sports Sci Rev* 1991, 19:351–388.

9. Katzman DK, Bachrach LK, Carter DR, Marcus R: Clinical and anthropometric correlates of bone mineral acquisition in healthy adolescent girls. *J Clin Endocrinol Metab* 1991, 73:1332–1399.

10. Marcus R: Normal and abnormal bone remodeling in man. *Annu Rev Med* 1987, 38:129–141.

11. Seeman E, Delmas PD: Bone quality: the material and structural basis of bone strength and fragility. *N Engl J Med* 2006, 354:2250–2261.

12. Seeman E: Osteocytes: martyrs for integrity of bone strength. *Osteoporos Int* 2006, 17:1443–1448.

13. Meema H, Meema S: Compact bone mineral density of the normal human radius. *Acta Radiol Oncol* 1978, 17:342–350.

14. Shen W, Chen J, Punyanitya M, *et al.*: MRI-measured bone marrow adipose tissue is inversely related to DXA measured bone mineral in Caucasian women. *Osteoporos Int* 2007, 18:641–647.

15. Rosen CJ, Bouxsein ML: Mechanisms of disease: is osteoporosis the obesity of bone? *Nat Clin Pract* 2006, 2:35–43.

Understanding Bone Histomorphometry: Sampling, Evaluation, and Interpretation

2

Robert S. Weinstein

The clinical approach to metabolic disorders of the skeleton has been considerably enhanced by developments in bone densitometry and biochemical indices of bone turnover. However, after an extensive work-up, fractures in some patients remain unexplained and, therefore, the examination of a bone biopsy specimen remains an indispensable part of the evaluation of disorders of bone and mineral metabolism. A histomorphometric examination of bone is much more than a qualitative look at the overall structure and arrangement of bone tissue. Today, the use of microprocessor-operated, stereomicroscope-guided, heavy-duty rotary microtomes; computers with drawing tubes and digitizing tablets; and digital cameras with sophisticated image-analysis software contribute speed, precision, and accuracy to the histomorphometric examination of bone whether viewed by bright-field, epifluorescence, polarized light, phase-contrast, or differential interference contrast microscopy. Furthermore, histomorphometry comprises a large repertoire of possible measurements such as cortical width and porosity; cancellous microarchitecture (trabecular width, separation, and number), osteoid area and width, and wall width (the width of newly completed packets of bone); counts of osteoblasts, osteocytes, and osteoclasts; the prevalence of bone cell apoptosis; and kinetic measurements of bone formation. Acquisition of the best possible bone specimen and determination of the best subset of measurements to address a particular question are crucial. Correct interpretation of the results requires cooperation between the clinician, biopsy operator, and histopathologist; therefore, to increase communication in this rapidly expanding field, the nomenclature, symbols, and units of bone histomorphometry have been standardized [1,2].

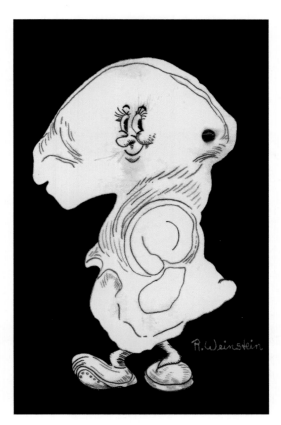

Figure 2-1. A bone biopsy for histomorphometry must be done at the same location as is used for the normal data: 2.5 cm below and behind the anterior–superior iliac spine, as indicated in the illustration by the dark hole at the upper right part of the bone. Patient tolerability of the procedure is good [3].

When to Do a Bone Biopsy

Unexplained bone loss

Borderline or inconclusive laboratory findings or a noninvasive evaluation is inadequate

Rapid progression (*eg*, "Could this much bone loss have occurred since her menopause?")

Unusually painful

Skeletal fragility with normal bone mineral density

Recognize subtle osteomalacia

Distinguish between the various forms of renal osteodystrophy

Chronic hypophosphatemia

Figure 2-2. When to do a bone biopsy. This table provides guidelines on when a bone biopsy should be performed.

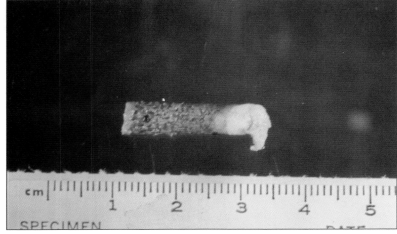

Figure 2-3. Transiliac bone biopsy specimen. A transiliac bone biopsy specimen must have two cortices with the intervening cancellous bone intact for a quantitative histologic assessment. The cortices of a well-obtained specimen usually display a parallelogram appearance. (*Adapted from* Weinstein [4].)

Limitations of Bone Biopsy

Sample of only a single, relatively small, skeletal site

The primary cause of the bone loss could be over

Transient effects from recent medications can be confusing

Main usefulness is in renal osteodystrophy or suspected occult osteomalacia

The rate of bone resorption is difficult to estimate except in diseases with extremely high bone turnover such as Paget's disease or renal hyperparathyroidism

A complete histomorphometric report may take as long as 25 d or more after the bone biopsy specimen is sent to the histomorphometer

Figure 2-4. Limitations of bone biopsy. This table provides guidelines on the limitations of bone biopsy.

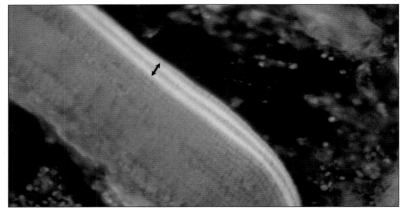

Figure 2-5. The bone biopsy procedure must be delayed for 24 days while the patient receives two time-spaced courses of oral tetracycline: the dosage is one capsule three or four times per day for 3 days, then 2 weeks without any tetracycline, and then one capsule three or four times per day for 3 more days. This is a 3-14-3 regimen. The distance between the two tetracycline labels (*double-headed arrow*) divided by the days between the oral course of tetracycline is the mineral appositional rate in micrometers per day. On the two 3-day periods that the subject receives the tetracycline, dairy products (especially milk), antacids, calcium supplements, and iron-containing medications must be avoided. An unstained section viewed with epifluorescent light, magnification ×250, is shown.

Bone Biopsy Arrangements

Learn as much as possible about the tetracycline labeling and bone biopsy procedure

Find an experienced bone biopsy operator familiar with the 7-mm biopsy trocar

Locate a specialist in bone histomorphometry

Recruit someone to fix the core and do the paperwork

Let the subject read about the biopsy before the physical examination is done. After completing the examination, tell the subject about the procedure. Caution to avoid dairy products, calcium, and antacids with the tetracycline. Highlight the steps taken to ensure the patient's comfort: prebiopsy analgesia, Novocain, and suture removal

Figure 2-6. Bone biopsy arrangements. Procedures for arranging a bone biopsy are provided in this table.

Bone Biopsy Specimen Handling Procedures

7-mm transiliac bone cores must be fixed in about 50 mL of 4°C Millonig's buffered formalin (check that the pH = 7.4)

After 20–24 h in cold Millonig's, transfer the core to a clean 20-mL glass vial filled with 70% ethanol and keep at 4°C

Put a 1 × 4-cm strip of index card with the subject's name, allocation number, and the date of biopsy written in pencil inside the vial with the specimen; tighten the cap; and seal with several wraps of labfilm

Wrap the vial with padding, surround it with mailer ice packs, and send by express mail. Include a sheet with the tetracycline regimen dates, subject's name, and the referring physician's name and fax number

Figure 2-7. Bone biopsy specimen-handling procedures. Procedures for handing bone biopsy specimens are given in this table.

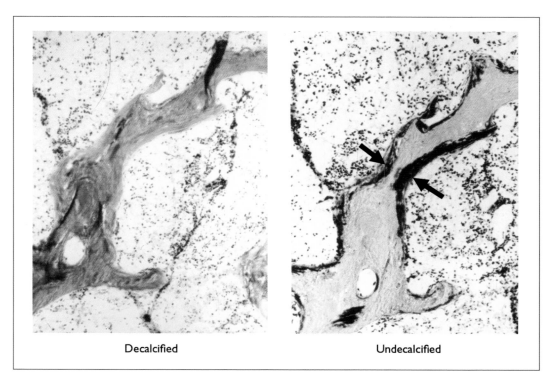

Decalcified   Undecalcified

Figure 2-8. Proper specimen handling is required to fix the tissue and avoid decalcification. Once the bone has been decalcified, no stain can adequately determine where the mineral used to be. Moreover, decalcification will eliminate the tetracycline labels. The *left* and *right panels* of this figure illustrate the same trabeculae, decalcified on the *left* and undecalcified on the *right*. Mineralized bone is shown in light gray and osteoid in black. The thick osteoid seams noted in the right panel (*arrows*) would be missed in the decalcified specimen, shown in the *left panel*. These sections were stained with Weigert's hematoxylin and eosin and viewed at ×100.

Confusing Terms

Term	Explanation
Active vs inactive	Should be more explicit. May indicate the presence of bone cells or imply their vigor.
Resorptive parameters	Precisely which measurement is used should be clearly stated. The best measure of resorption is the osteoclast number or surface.
Eroded surface	The eroded surface is composed of the osteoclast surface plus the reversal surface and is an unfaithful measure of bone resorption. Treatment with an antiresorptive agent will decrease the osteoclast surface and increase the reversal surface.
Formation parameters	Precisely which measurement is used should be clearly stated. Osteoid is not an index of bone formation because it can accumulate with increased bone formation or from delayed mineralization. The only measure of bone formation is the tetracycline-based bone formation rate.
Coupling and balance	Coupling refers to the appearance of osteoblasts at the site where osteoclasts have recently eroded bone cavities. Balance indicates that the new bone deposited by osteoblasts exactly equals the amount previously removed by osteoclasts.
Osteoblasts and osteoclasts: surface or areal referent?	Osteoblasts and osteoclasts can only be on bone surfaces. The appropriate referent is the bone surface. Only osteocytes are correctly reported per bone area.
Activation frequency	The incidence of new remodeling cycles (which usually refers to cancellous bone) can be estimated by dividing the bone formation rate by the wall width, an index of the amount of bone made by a previous team of osteoblasts.
Micro-CT histomorphometry	This is a misnomer. Micro-CT does not reveal excess osteoid, woven bone, or embedded cartilage cores, features that are easily noted with histologic assessment of the cancellous microarchitecture. The quantification of bone cells and the rate of turnover can only be done by a histologic examination.

Figure 2-9. Confusing terms. Explanations of some confusing terms related to bone biopsy are provided.

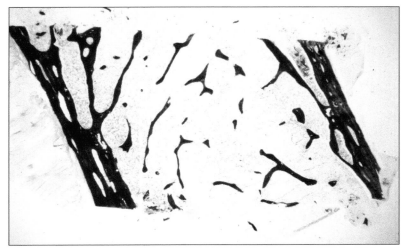

Figure 2-10. After longitudinal sectioning, this transiliac bone biopsy specimen taken from a 70-year-old patient with osteoporotic fractures shows both cortical and cancellous osteopenia: the normally continuous networks of curved trabecular plates have been transformed to a disconnected, gossamer array of thin struts. The trabecular separation is increased because the intervening trabeculae have been completely resorbed. There has been a loss of 25% of the cortical bone and 50% of the cancellous bone, sometimes referred to as "emphysema of the skeleton." The cortical bone has deep and coalescent endocortical erosions that are carving broad new "trabeculae" from the previously solid cortex in a process known as trabecularization or cancellization of the cortex. A modified Masson stain, magnification ×10, is shown. (*Adapted from* Weinstein and Manolagas [5].)

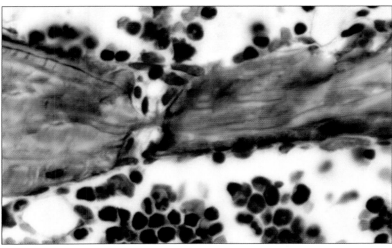

Figure 2-11. Fractures may occur even with normal amounts of cancellous bone on bone biopsy and normal bone mineral density if numerous trabecular perforations are present. Shown here are two opposing erosion bays arising from the top and bottom of the trabecular surface. Even if the trabeculae is not eventually completely penetrated, these bays represent weakened lesions called "stress risers," which are especially dangerous in load-bearing, vertically oriented, vertebral trabeculae. These sections were stained with toluidine blue, magnification ×250.

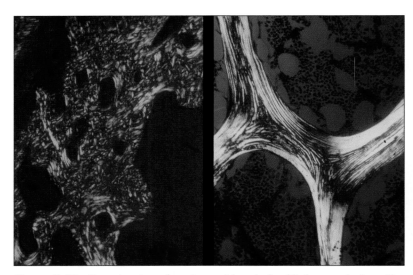

Figure 2-12. Examination of sections with polarized light reveals the collagen architecture. The haphazard, patchwork-quilt appearance of woven bone is shown in the *left panel* and the normal orderly grain of lamellar bone is shown on the *right*. Woven bone always represents pathology in adults. This image shows decalcified sections stained with Weigert's hematoxylin and eosin and viewed with polarized light at ×100.

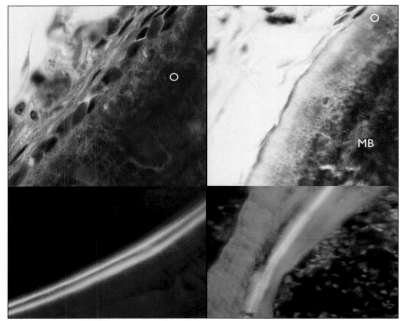

Figure 2-13. There are two ways to get increased osteoid (decreased ash content). These two ways are different from pathophysiologic mechanisms and require different therapy. On the *left side* of this figure, osteoid width is excessive but plump, cuboidal osteoblasts line the osteoid, and the widely separated double tetracycline labels shown below indicate that the mineral appositional rate is increased and that the excess osteoid is due to increased bone formation. An appropriate treatment may be efforts to reduce an elevated parathyroid hormone level. On the *right side* of the figure, excess osteoid is covered by flattened lining cells and the tetracycline labels shown below are closely spaced, indicating a defect or delay in the mineral appositional rate. An appropriate treatment may be supplementation with vitamin D, calcium, or phosphorus. MB—mineralized bone; O—osteoid. (*Adapted from* Weinstein [6].)

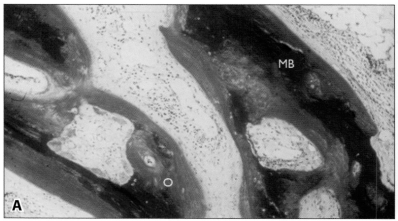

A

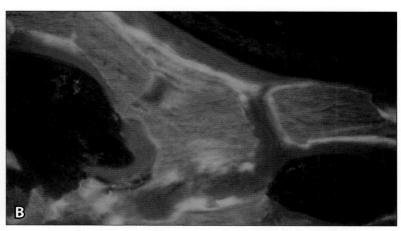

B

Figure 2-14. Osteomalacia is more than just excess osteoid. A rigorous diagnosis of osteomalacia requires the simultaneous presence of three histologic criteria. Two of these criteria are shown in **A**; osteoid is abundant (> 10% of the bone area) and this is not only due to increased osteoid-covered cancellous surface but to augmentation of the osteoid seam width (> 15 μm). **B**, Tetracycline labels appear as only a single wide band although two oral courses of tetracycline were given. This indicates that the rate of mineral apposition (μm/d) is near 0, fulfilling the third criteria, prolongation of the mineralization lag time (seam width divided by the adjusted appositional rate; > 100 days) [7]. MB—mineralized bone; O—osteoid. (*Adapted from* Weinstein [6].)

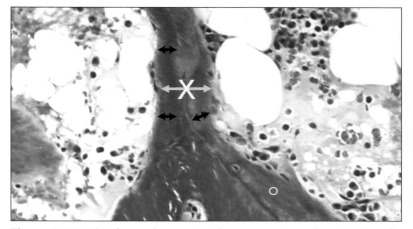

Figure 2-15. This figure shows osteoid seams on two adjacent sides of a trabeculae. The two seams represent two separate and independent events. Osteoid seam width is correctly measured, as indicated by the *black arrows*. The measurement indicated by the *yellow arrow* would incorrectly exaggerate osteoid width by adding two independent events. Modified Masson stain, magnification ×250, is shown. MB—mineralized bone; O—osteoid.

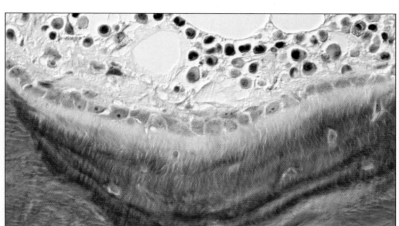

Figure 2-16. The osteoblast perimeter is characterized by palisades of plump, cuboidal osteoblasts lining a partly mineralized osteoid seam. Note the perinuclear halo of the prominent Golgi apparatus in the osteoblasts. Modified Masson stain, magnification ×250, is shown.

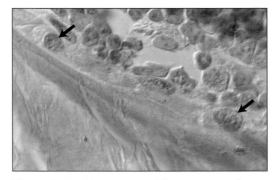

Figure 2-17. Treatment with long-term prednisone results in apoptotic osteoblasts, identified by the brown staining and nuclear condensation (*arrows*) [8]. In situ detection of DNA fragmentation, a marker of apoptosis, was done with the transferase-mediated biotin-deoxy uridine triphosphate nick-end labeling reaction. Shown here, it is counterstained with methyl green and viewed by Nomarski differential interference contrast microscopy, magnification ×250.

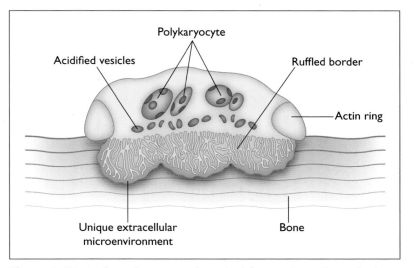

Figure 2-18. Multinucleate osteoclasts (polykaryons) attach to the bone surface with an actin ring containing integrin receptors that recognize specific bone matrix proteins. Once sealed to the bone, lysosomal enzymes, hydrogen ions, and collagenase are secreted through the ruffled border of microvilli, creating a unique extracellular microenvironment that is ideal for bone resorption. (*Adapted from* Weinstein and Manolagas [5].)

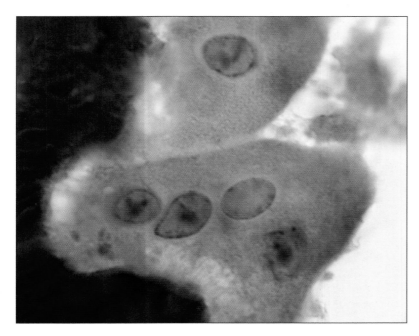

Figure 2-19. This photomicrograph shows the sealing zone and lysosomal-rich clear area of the ventral surface of a multinucleated osteoclast. Note the prominent nucleoli. Tiny fragments of blue mineralized bone can be seen inside the cell. Modified Masson stain, magnification ×1000, is shown.

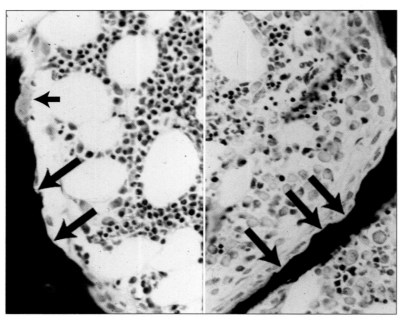

Figure 2-20. After osteoclasts finish excavating a cavity and leave the bone surface, there is a pause before osteoblasts are recruited to reconstitute the previously eroded cavity. This pause between the end of bone resorption and the beginning of bone formation is the reversal phase, when mononuclear phagocytes smooth out the jagged erosion bays. During this phase, the old bone is coated by a thin layer of a cement-like substance, a collagen- and mineral-poor matrix rich in glycosaminoglycans, glycoproteins, and acid phosphatase to which the new osteoblasts attach. New osteoblasts assemble only at sites where osteoclasts have recently been active, a phenomenon referred to as coupling. The reversal phase is, however, not a faithful indicator of bone resorption as it increases after treatment with antiresorptive drugs and accumulates with a delay in bone formation as occurs with glucocorticoid therapy [9]. The *small arrow* indicates an osteoclast in a resorption cavity and the *large arrows* show previous resorption cavities that are now empty and known as the reversal surface. The osteoclast surface plus the reversal surface equals the eroded surface. Modified Masson stain, magnification ×250, is shown.

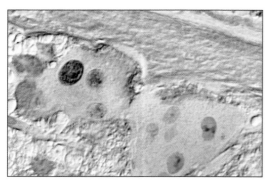

Figure 2-21. Eventually all osteoclasts die by apoptosis. With just two apoptotic nuclei (*brown staining*), this osteoclast is still attached to bone but the DNA fragmentation detected by in situ nick-end labeling allows the cell to be recognized as apoptotic. This osteoclast is counterstained with methyl green and viewed by Nomarski differential interference contrast microscopy, magnification ×400.

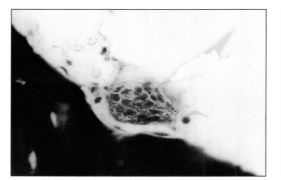

Figure 2-22. After treatment of Paget's disease of bone with alendronate, end-stage osteoclast apoptosis occurs. This osteoclast has prominent cytoplasmic blebbing and has detached from the bone surface. All the nuclei are condensed and disintegrating. These findings are rarely seen due to the fleeting existence of apoptotic osteoclasts before they are swept away by phagocytosis. Modified Masson stain, magnification ×250, is shown.

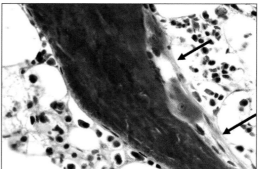

Figure 2-23. Two osteoclasts are seen resorbing cancellous bone beneath a canopy (*arrows*) of former lining cells that separates the osteoclasts from the bone marrow. Modified Masson stain, magnification ×250, is shown. (*Adapted from* Parfitt [10].)

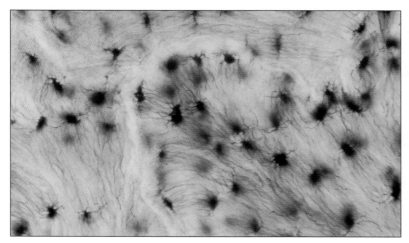

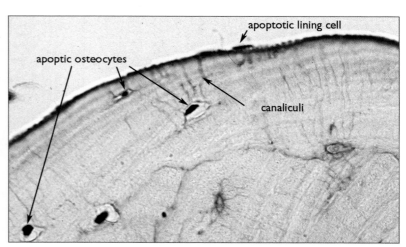

Figure 2-24. After staining with India ink, the osteocyte–canaliculi network of cortical bone can be seen to branch out in a dendritic fashion like a circuit board, reflecting its role as a strain sensor. Magnification ×630 is shown.

Figure 2-25. Long-term glucocorticoid therapy causes the accumulation of apoptotic osteocytes and lining cells. Note that the osteocyte–canaliculi lining cell network now links dead cells. Disruption of this network may interfere with repair of fatigue damage and increase bone fragility [11]. Toluidine blue counterstain with the transferase-mediated biotin-deoxy uridine triphosphate nick-end labeling reaction, magnification ×250, is shown.

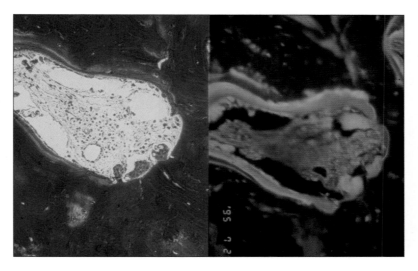

Figure 2-26. This cutting cone is seen eroding through cortical bone traveling from left to right. The *left panel* shows multinucleated osteoclasts at the front and osteoblasts lining new seams of osteoid (*red*) bring up the rear. The central cavity of this basic multicellular unit (BMU) contains vascular structures that are the pipelines conveying the new osteoblasts and osteoclasts to work in the advancing BMU [12]. Modified Masson stain, magnification ×100, is shown. The *right panel* shows the tetracycline labeling of the adjacent section. Note the double labels beneath the osteoblasts at the rear.

References

1. Parfitt AM, Drezner MK, Glorieux FH, *et al.*: Bone histomorphometry: standardization of nomenclature, symbols, and units. *J Bone Miner Res* 1987, 2:595–610.

2. Weinstein RS: Human bone biopsy. In *Handbook of Histology Methods for Bone and Cartilage.* Edited by An YH, Martin KL. Totowa, NJ: Humana; 2003:119–128.

3. Hodgson SF, Johnson KA, Mults JM, *et al.*: Outpatient percutaneous biopsy of the iliac crest: methods, morbidity and patient acceptance. *Mayo Clin Proc* 1986, 61:28–33.

4. Weinstein RS: Needle bone biopsy: how, when, why. *Resid Staff Physician* 1979, 25:48–55.

5. Weinstein RS, Manolagas SC: Apoptosis and osteoporosis. *Am J Med* 2000, 108:153–164.

6. Weinstein RS: The clinical use of bone biopsy. In *Disorders of Bone and Mineral Metabolism.* Edited by Coe FL, Favus MJ. New York: Raven; 1992:455–474.

7. Parfitt AM, Podenphant J, Villanueva AR, Frame B: Metabolic bone disease with and without osteomalacia after intestinal bypass surgery: a bone histomorphometric study. *Bone* 1985, 6:211–220.

8. Weinstein RS, Jilka RL, Parfitt AM, Manolagas SC: Inhibition of osteoblastogenesis and promotion of apoptosis of osteoblasts and osteocytes by glucocorticoids: potential mechanisms of the deleterious effects on bone. *J Clin Invest* 1998, 102:274–282.

9. Weinstein RS: Glucocorticoid-induced osteoporosis. *Rev Endocr Metab Disorders* 2001, 2:65–73.

10. Parfitt AM: Misconceptions V: activation of osteoclasts is the first step in the bone remodeling cycle. *Bone* 2006, 39:1170–1172.

11. Weinstein RS, Nicholas RW, Manolagas SC: Apoptosis of osteocytes in glucocorticoid-induced osteonecrosis of the hip. *J Clin Endocrinol Metab* 2000, 85:2907–2912.

12. Weinstein RS, Manolagas SC: Apoptosis and osteoporosis. *Am J Med* 2000, 108:153–164.

Bone Acquisition and Peak Bone Mass

3

Connie M. Weaver and Laura K. Bachrach

The foundation of bone health is established in the first three decades of life [1]. Peak bone mass, acquired by early adulthood, serves as the bone bank for the remainder of adult life. The more robust the skeletal mass at its peak, the greater the amount of bone loss (from aging, menopause, and other factors) that can be tolerated without clinical signs of osteoporosis. Peak bone mass accounts for at least half of the variability in skeletal mass in the elderly, with the remainder attributable to subsequent bone loss [1]. The pace of bone mineral acquisition is similar to that of linear bone growth, with rapid gains in infancy, slower increases during childhood, and major gains at puberty [2]. Approximately half of peak bone mass is gained during the teenage years, making this a critical period for optimizing conditions for skeletal health. Unlike growth patterns, however, peak bone mineral acquisition lags 8 months behind peak height velocity [3]. This is a period of increased incidence of fracture and the numbers of fractures have been increasing over the last 3 decades [4].

Peak bone mass is largely predetermined by heritable factors. Family and twin studies suggest that 60% to 80% of the differences in peak bone mass between individuals can be attributed to genetics [5,6]. Ethnic and racial differences in bone mass have also been observed [7]. Although some of these differences appear to be artifacts of densitometry technique, healthy blacks have been shown to achieve greater true bone density than nonblacks during adolescence [8,9]. The gene or genes linked to osteoporosis have not yet been identified, although several have been considered, including the vitamin D and estrogen receptors [10]. Genes associated with pubertal timing and bone mass acquisition may be linked [2].

Lifestyle factors also have a substantial influence on bone acquisition, accounting for 20% to 40% of the variability in young adult skeletal mass. Maximal bone mineral gains occur only when nutrition, physical activity, and hormone production are adequate. Body mass, especially the fat-free component, is a consistent correlate of bone mineral density in healthy youth [11–13]. The positive relationship between weight and bone mineral density may reflect common genetic determinants, overall nutritional status, or the effects of mechanical loading on the skeleton [13]. Calcium intake influences rates of bone accrual, as shown in calcium supplementation trials; children given added calcium gained more bone mineral than did those in the control group [14–16]. A recent meta-analysis of calcium supplementation trials in children, which have typically focused on white populations with habitual intakes over 700 mg/d, suggested that while the effect of calcium supplementation on bone is positive, it is small [17]. This report was criticized for using bone mineral density rather than bone mineral content as the outcome measure [18]. Recommended calcium intakes are based on the calcium intake that is needed to achieve maximal calcium retention [19]. Racial and gender differences in calcium retention as a function of intake are not associated with different calcium needs for optimal calcium retention [20,21]. Weight-bearing physical activity can stimulate bone mineral accrual by as much as 5% to 17% and may modify bone geometry [22]. Activity may boost bone acquisition and strength only when calcium intake is sufficient [22,23] and results depend on the stage of maturation when physical activity begins. Normal endocrine function is necessary for optimal bone mineral acquisition. Bone mass in adolescents is more highly correlated with pubertal stage than with chronologic age, reflecting the pivotal role of sex steroids in bone accrual [24]. Peak bone mass is reduced in patients with sex steroid deficiency or resistance [25]. Growth hormone deficiency, hyperthyroidism, and glucocorticoid excess have also been associated with low bone mass in children as well as in adults [26–28].

The costs of osteoporosis exceed $20 billion annually in the United States and $30 billion worldwide [29]. Stemming the rise of these costs will require an effective intervention directed at increasing peak bone mass and reducing subsequent bone loss. A bone health program for all youth includes maintaining adequate body weight, appropriate calcium intake, and regular physical activity. Unfortunately, the gap between the recommended and actual intakes of calcium in the United States continues to widen; more than 90% of girls and 50% of boys consume less than the optimal amount of calcium during their teen years [30]. In addition, American youth have become less active over time; only half of teens (age 12–21 years) exercise vigorously on a regular basis and 25% report no vigorous physical activity [31]. Girls are less active than boys and black girls are less active than are white girls. Skeletal health is an immediate concern in youth, with a variety of chronic disorders that have been associated with early deficits in bone mass [25]. Anorexia nervosa, exercise-associated amenorrhea, cystic fibrosis, immobilization disorders, and therapy with systemic glucocorticoids are among the conditions that can compromise gains in bone mass or size or accelerate the loss of bone mineral. In severe cases of skeletal fragility, bone fractures can occur with minimal or no trauma, a condition termed *osteoporosis*. Whether deficits in bone that develop in childhood can be reversed with prompt recognition and treatment remains uncertain. Continued efforts are needed to define ways of optimizing peak bone mass and to deliver the message that osteoporosis prevention begins in childhood.

Bone Mineral Acquisition

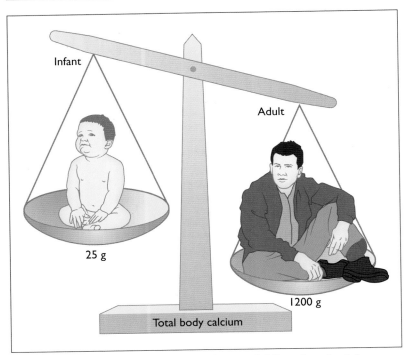

Figure 3-1. Accrual of bone mass during childhood and adolescence. Total skeletal calcium increases dramatically from infancy until adulthood. Half of these gains occur during adolescence, making this period critical in establishing bone health [2,3].

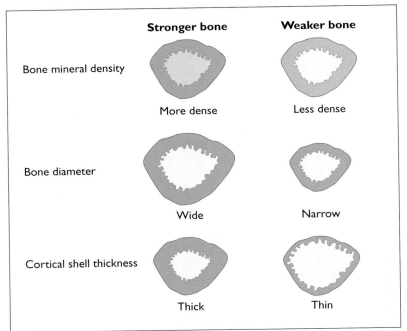

Figure 3-2. Bone characteristics that affect bone strength. Bone material properties include bone mineral content (measured in grams), bone mineral density (the mass of mineral per unit volume of bone, most commonly measured by dual-energy x-ray absorptiometry), and bone geometry. Bone geometry includes bone length and cross-sectional dimensions and can be measured by peripheral quantitative computed tomography. Bones with greater mass or density and greater diameter are stronger and considered more resistant to fracture. (*Adapted from* Kalkwarf [32].)

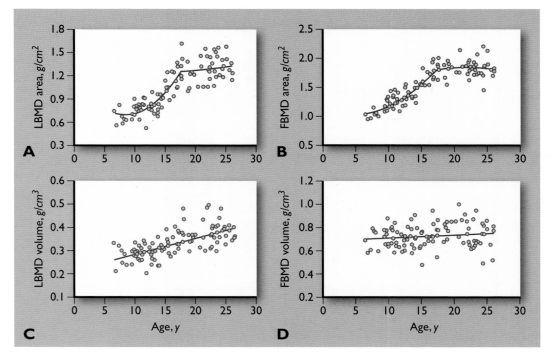

Figure 3-3. Bone mineral acquisition and bone growth. Gains in bone mineral during childhood and adolescence vary by skeletal size and the measurement term used [33–36]. The areal bone mineral density (BMD) area increases with age at all sites, including the lumbar spine and femoral shaft (**A** and **B**). In contrast, volumetric BMD increases at the spine but not at the femoral shaft (**C** and **D**). These findings suggest that gains in bone mass during adolescence are due largely to increases in bone size; volumetric BMD increases as well within the vertebrae [36]. Data from healthy boys are shown; similar differences in areal and volumetric BMD are observed in girls [33]. LBMD—lumbar spine bone mineral density; FBMD—femoral shaft bone mineral density. (*Adapted from* Lu *et al.* [33].)

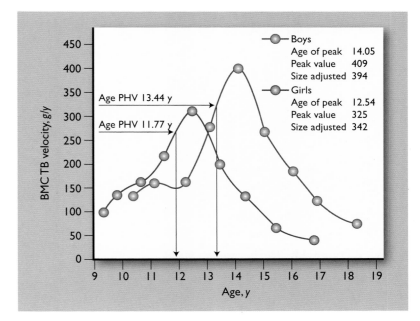

Figure 3-4. Bone mineral content acquisition during puberty. The tempo of bone mineral acquisition during adolescence is more closely linked to pubertal development than to chronological age [2,3]. Peak height velocity (PHV) preceeds peak bone mass accrual by approximately 0.7 years. At the age of PHV (11.6 years for girls and 13.5 for boys), adolescents have reached 90% of adult height but only 60% of adult total body bone mineral content (BMC). The discrepancy between bone size and BMC during the adolescent growth spurt results in a transient period of relative bone weakness, which corresponds to the higher incidence of fracture at this age [4]. Peak bone mineral velocity is higher in boys than girls and occurs about 1.5 years later in boys. BMC TB—bone mineral content total body. (*From* Bailey *et al.* [3]; with permission.)

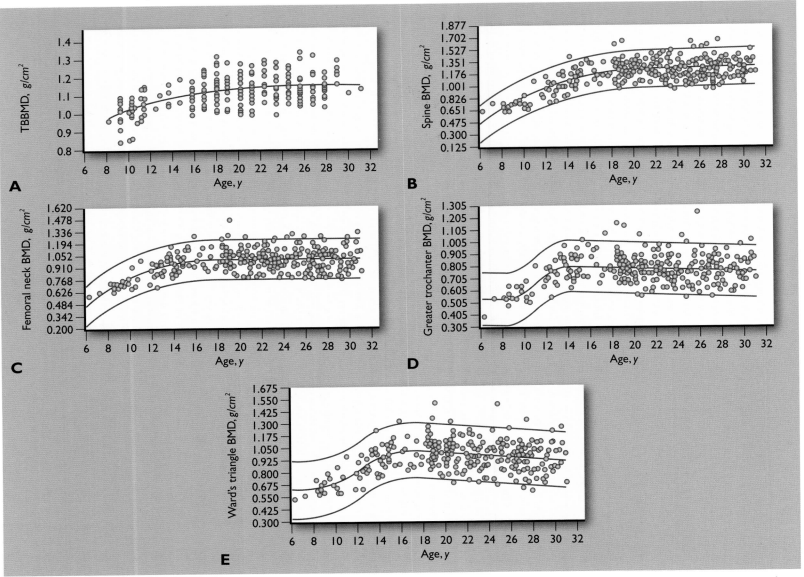

Figure 3-5. Bone mineral density (BMD) accumulation with age in females. Gains in BMD vary with skeletal site. Ninety-five percent of adult peak total body (TB) BMD is achieved by an age of 16.2 years and 99% by an age of 22.1 years (**A**). The highest BMD occurs by an age of 23 years for the spine (**B**), by an age of 18.5 years for the femoral neck (**C**), by an age of 14.2 years for the greater trochanter (**D**), and by an age of 15.8 years for Ward's triangle (**E**). (**A** and **B** from Teegarden *et al.* [37] and **C–E** *from* Lin *et al.* [38]; with permission.)

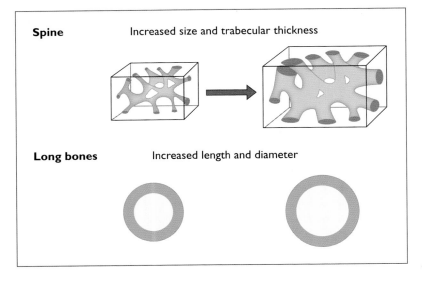

Figure 3-6. Adolescent changes in bone geometry. Changes in bone geometry accompany gains in bone size and mineral throughout childhood as the medullary cavity expands. Spinal vertebrae increase not only in size but also in the thickness of trabeculae with the bone [36]. Long bones increase in length and in cross-sectional area. The increases in cortical thickness are largely proportional to the increase in bone diameter, so volumetric bone density of long bones changes little throughout childhood and adolescence [36]. Hip axis length (HAL) increases during puberty; however, the ratio of HAL to height does not change [39]. These skeletal changes are important clinically because bone size and shape influence bone strength, independently of bone mineral content [40,41]. (*Adapted from* Seeman [36].)

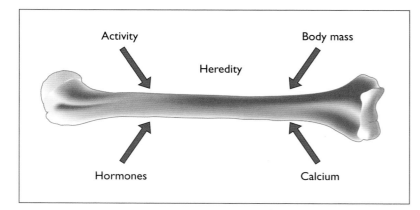

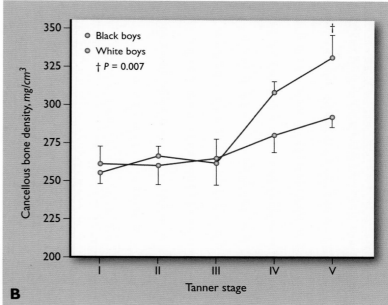

Figure 3-7. Determinants of peak bone mass. Peak bone mass is largely determined by genetic factors, which account for 60% to 80% of the observed variance in adult bone mineral [5,6]. Several lifestyle factors influence the remaining 20% to 40%. Weight-bearing physical activity can stimulate changes in bone geometry and mineral accrual, whereas immobility leads to accelerated bone loss [3]. Body mass is highly correlated with bone mass, perhaps because weight reflects bone size and nutritional status [11,13]. Additionally, body weight may act as a mechanical load to the skeleton [13]. The lean mass component of total body weight is associated more highly with bone mass than is total body fat mass [12]. Calcium intake modifies rates of bone gain and resorption [14,15]. Finally, sex steroids and growth hormone contribute to bone mineral accrual, whereas glucocorticoids in excess can impair bone acquisition or result in bone loss [25–28].

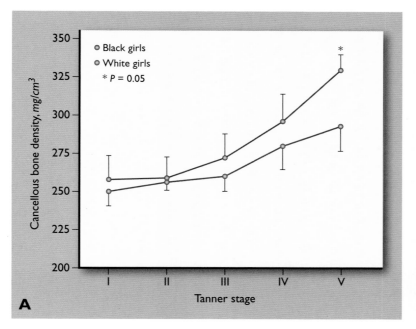

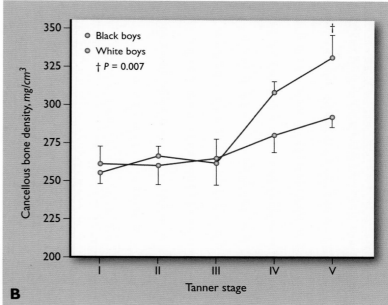

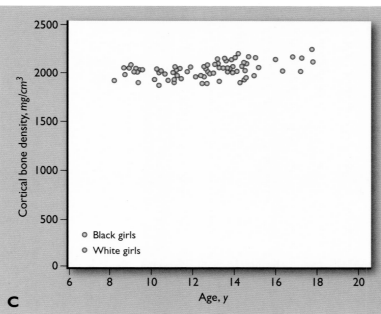

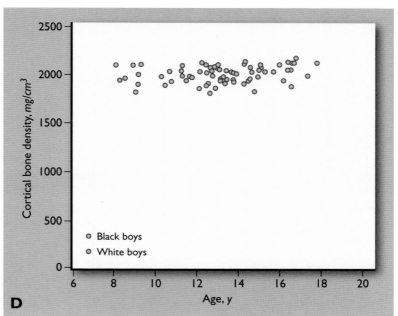

Figure 3-8. Racial differences in bone mass. There are few racial differences in bone mass between Asian, Hispanic, and white youths once adjustments are made for bone size [39–42]. By late adolescence, however, black youths have significantly greater bone mass than do white youths [8]. Using quantitative computed tomography, Gilsanz *et al.* [8] found racial differences in bone density, but not bone size, at the spine (**A** and **B**). In contrast, bone density at the femoral shaft (**C** and **D**) did not differ by race; however, blacks had greater cross-sectional area at that site than did whites. The observed differences in bone density and size probably contribute to the lower incidence of osteoporosis in blacks [7]. (*Adapted from* Gilsanz *et al.* [8].)

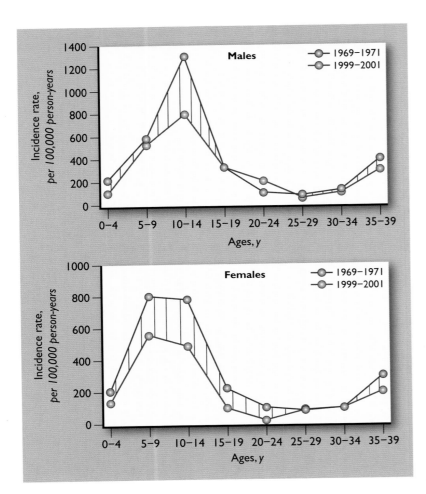

Figure 3-9. Forearm fracture incidence from 1969 to 1971 and from 1999 to 2001. The incidence of childhood fracture has risen 32% among males (*top*) and 56% among females (*bottom*) in the last three decades and has been related to low calcium intakes, increased sedentary behavior, and increased body weight in youth. The greatest incidence and increase over time was in boys 11 to 14 years old and girls 8 to 11 years old when peak total body bone mineral content lags behind peak height velocity. (*Adapted from* Heaney and Weaver [43] and Khosla *et al.* [4].)

Gene Polymorphisms that Influence Bone Mass During Childhood

Gene	Role in bone metabolism	Polymorphisms
VDR	Vitamin D acts through its receptor to influence calcium absorption, bone differentiation, and mineralization	Bsml/Apal/Taq 1. Intronic polymorphisms, function unknown; Fok 1 alters the VDR translational start site and receptor/protein size
Estrogen receptor	Estrogen acts through its receptor to influence skeletal growth, maturation, and bone loss after menopause	Pvu II/Xba I intronic polymorphisms, function unknown
Lipoprotein receptor	Encodes for high bone mass	LRP 5 mediates binding of Wnt growth factor to the receptor to promote osteoblast differentiation
Interleukin-6	Regulates osteoclasts' growth and differentiation; may mediate the effects of sex steroids on bone	Polymorphisms, function unknown
IGF	Mediates action growth hormone	IGF-1 stimulates osteoblast proliferation and differentiation
Collagen 1 α 1	Major protein in bone; mutations occur in type 1 collagen genes in osteogenesis imperfecta	COLIA 1 polymorphism, function unknown

Figure 3-10. Genes that influence bone mass. Heritable factors are major determinants of peak bone mass, explaining an estimated 60%–80% of the variability in peak bone mass between individuals [5,6]. Racial, ethnic, and familial similarities in bone mineral density have been observed, supporting the contribution of genetics in bone acquisition. Many genes have been associated with determining bone mass, but the magnitude of the effects of these polymorphisms in childhood are unknown [10]. COLIA 1—type IA collagen; IGF-1—insulin-like growth factor 1; LRP 5—lipoprotein receptor-related protein 5; VDR—vitamin D receptor.

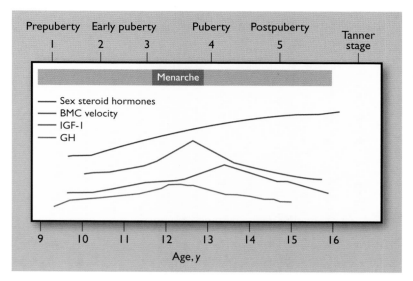

Figure 3-11. Changes in bone mineral content (BMC) velocity and hormonal regulators throughout growth. In prepuberty, bone growth remains gradual due to constant levels of growth hormone (GH) and insulin-like growth factor-1 (IGF-1). Pulses of gonadotropin-releasing hormone receptor released into circulation trigger the production and release of sex steroids that mark the onset of puberty. Increased estrogen triggers GH and IGF-1 production and the growth spurt begins. Patients with rare disorders of estrogen resistance or impaired synthesis (aromatase deficiency) have osteopenia and delayed epiphyseal closure [25]. Estrogen therapy results in skeletal maturation and increases bone mineral acquisition except in cases of estrogen resistance [44]. Androgens may also be essential for normal bone mineral accrual and growth, especially for long bones [45]. Patients with androgen insensitivity syndrome have androgen-receptor abnormalities that confer partial or complete resistance to androgens. Many of these patients have reduced areal and volumetric bone mineral density after gonadectomy despite estrogen-replacement therapy, indicating an essential role for androgens in mineral accrual [45]. (*Adapted from* MacKelvie *et al.* [46].)

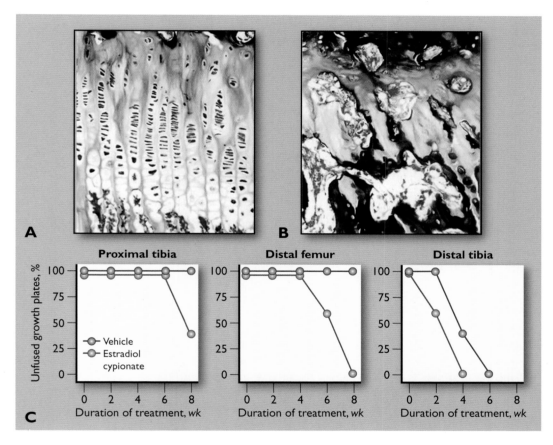

Figure 3-12. Estrogen treatment and epiphyseal fusion. Proximal tibial growth plates are unfused (**A**) in saline-treated ovariectomized rabbits, but fused (**B**) after 8 weeks of estrogen treatment. Chondrocyte columns have been replaced by vascular and bone tissue. **C**, The percentage of animals that have unfused growth plates decreases over time in proximal tibia, distal femur, and distal tibia of rats treated with intramuscular estradiol cypionate (*green circles*) compared to vehicle (*red circles*). Growth plate senescence following the pubertal growth spurt may be triggered by a local mechanism in the growth plate involving the depletion of stem-like cells in the resting zone of epiphyseal chondrocytes [47,48]. (*From* Weise *et al.* [49]; with permission.)

Calcium Economics and Bone Health

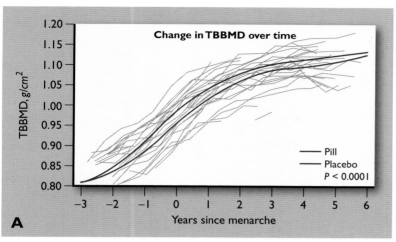

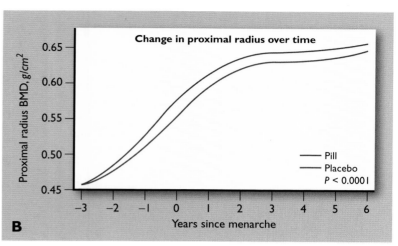

Figure 3-13. Calcium supplementation and bone mineral density (BMD) accrual. More than 10 controlled trials have shown that calcium intake in childhood and adolescence results in gains in BMD [50]. Matkovic *et al.* [16] studied girls, randomized to treatment, from 10 to 18 years old; total body (TB) BMD (**A**) and proximal radius BMD (**B**) were significantly higher in the group assigned to a daily 1-g calcium supplement. There was a significant interaction with body size; significant effects of calcium supplementation at young adulthood remained in the metacarpals and forearm of those above the median for height. (*Adapted from* Matkovic *et al.* [16].)

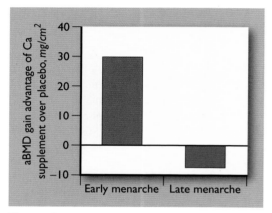

Figure 3-14. Interaction between menarcheal age and calcium intake. Prepubertal girls who had been randomized to supplemented calcium foods of 850 mg/d or a placebo from an age of 7.9 to 8.9 years were followed for bone accrual until a mean age of 16.4 years. Age of menarche was negatively correlated ($r = -0.32$, $P < 0.001$, $n = 122$) with mean areal bone mineral density (aBMD) gains at six skeletal sites. Earlier menarche implies longer exposure to estrogen and calcium intake was negatively correlated with menarcheal age ($r = -0.35$, $P < 0.001$). The mean gain in six skeletal site aBMD from 7.9 to 16.4 years was greater in girls who received calcium-fortified foods relative to the placebo group in girls who had early menarche (*$P = 0.009$) compared to girls who had late menarche (nonsignificant). Thus, the level of calcium intake during prepuberty may influence the timing of menarche, which in turn may influence gain in bone mineral density in response to calcium supplementation. (*Adapted from* Chevalley *et al.* [51].)

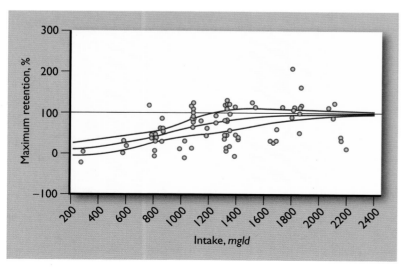

Figure 3-15. Optimal calcium intake for maximal calcium retention in adolescents. Calcium retention (reflective of bone accrual) increases with greater calcium intake until a threshold is reached. Using data from Jackman *et al.* [52], the mean and 95% CI calcium accrual did not rise significantly with a calcium intake above 1300 mg calcium/d so 1300 mg/d was adopted as the recommended calcium intake by the Institute of Medicine [19]. (*From* Weaver and Heaney [50]; with permission.)

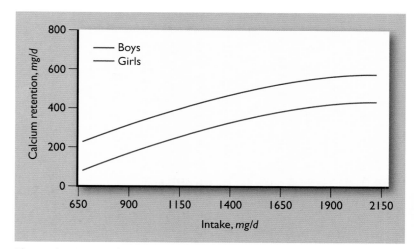

Figure 3-16. Gender comparison of calcium intake for maximal retention. White boys retain 171 mg more calcium per day across all calcium intakes than girls, but the intake that leads to maximal retention is not significantly different for boys than girls. Boys achieve a larger skeleton than girls by utilizing calcium more efficiently, rather than requiring more calcium. (*Adapted from* Braun *et al.* [20].)

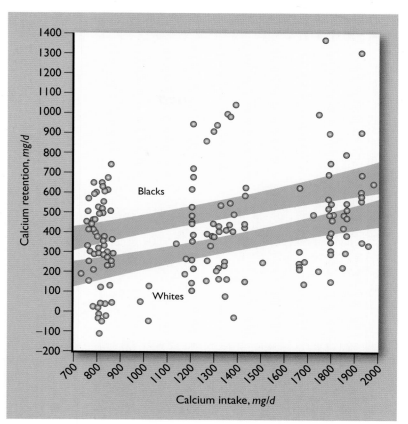

Figure 3-17. Racial comparison of calcium retention as a function of calcium intake in girls. Black girls retained 185 mg more calcium per day than white girls across a wide range of calcium intakes. Calcium intake explained 12.3% of the variance in calcium retention and race explained an additional 13.7% of the variation. (*Adapted from* Braun *et al.* [21].)

Dietary Reference Intake for Calcium

Age, y	Calcium intake, mg/d
1–3	500
4–8	800
9–18	1300
19–50	1000
51+	1200

Figure 3-18. Dietary reference intake for calcium. In 1997, the National Academy of Science issued new dietary guidelines for substances related to bone health, including calcium, phosphorus, magnesium, vitamin D, and fluoride. The recommended intake of calcium for each age group is shown, as well as the upper tolerable level. The calcium recommendations for children and adolescents were raised based on data linking increased calcium with greater bone accrual [19]. Calcium intake of 1300 mg/d is the equivalent of 4.3 cups of milk.

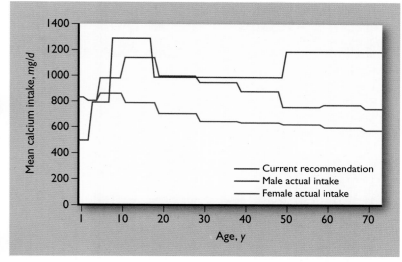

Figure 3-19. The gap in calcium intake. The mean daily calcium intake falls well below the recommended level, especially during adolescence. Data shown here from the 1994 to 1995 Continuing Survey of Food Intakes by Individuals (CSI) indicates that 86% of girls and 65% of boys 12 to 18 years old failed to meet the previous recommended daily calcium allowance of 1200 mg/d [30]. The optimal intake for calcium has now been set at 1300 mg/d; thus, the gap between the recommended and actual intakes of dietary calcium has widened in American youth.

Comparison of Sources for Absorbable Calcium

Source	Serving size, *g*	Estimated calcium content, *mg/serving*	Food amount to absorption efficiency, %	Equals the calcium in 1 c milk
Foods				
Milk	240	300	32.1	1.0 c
Beans (pinto)	86	44.7	26.7	4.1 c
Beans (red)	172	40.5	24.4	4.8 c
Beans (white)	110	113	21.8	2.0 c
Bok choy	85	79	53.8	1.2 c
Broccoli	71	35	61.3	2.3 c
Cheddar cheese	42	303	32.1	1.5 oz
Cheese food	42	241	32.1	1.8 oz
Chinese cabbage flower leaves	85	239	39.6	0.5 c
Chinese mustard greens	85	212	40.2	0.6 c
Chinese spinach	85	347	8.36	1.7 c
Kale	85	61	49.3	1.6 c
Spinach	85	115	5.1	8.1 c
Sugar cookies	15	39	91.9	35 cookies
Sweet potatoes	164	44	22.2	4.9 c
Rhubarb	120	174	8.5	4.7 c
Whole wheat bread	28	20	82.0	5.8 slices
Whole bran cereal	28	20	38.0	12.8 oz
Yogurt	240	300	32.1	1.0 c
Fortified foods with added calcium				
Tofu, calcium set	126	258	31.0	0.6 c
Orange juice with calcium citrate malate	240	300	36.3	0.9 c
Soy milk with calcium phosphate	240	300	24.0	1.3 c
Bread with calcium sulfate	17	300	43.0	1 slice

Foods that have been intrinsically labeled during growth of the plant or animal ingredient or during preparation or processing of fortified foods are represented.

Figure 3-20. Comparing sources for absorbable calcium. Calcium content is substantial in few foods and absorption efficiency varies widely due to the presence of inhibitors in many foods of plant origin. The number of common servings (cup of beverage and yogurt, half cup of vegetables) required to replace a cup of milk show that it would be difficult to achieve recommended calcium intakes without dairy products in the diet. Dairy products provide approximately 75% of calcium in the American diet. Calcium-fortified foods offer a means of boosting calcium consumption through nondairy foods. (*Adapted from* Weaver and Heaney [50].)

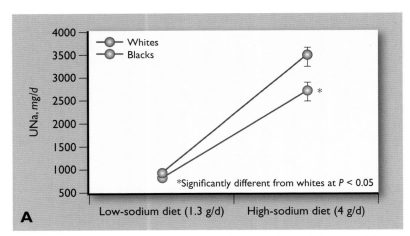

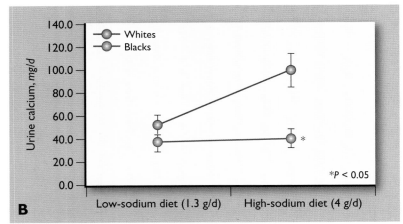

Figure 3-21. Calcium economics and sodium intake in adolescents. The net amount of calcium that is available for bone metabolism reflects the balance of calcium intake and excretion. Calcium intake has declined over recent decades. To compound this problem, increased dietary sodium increases calcium loss through the surine, leaving less available for bone acquisition. This loss is greater for white than black children. As dietary sodium increases, more sodium is excreted in the urine (**A**), especially in white girls. Because calcium and sodium share common transporters in the kidney, increased sodium excretion leads to increased calcium excretion (**B**). The result is that calcium retention is reduced in high-sodium diets.

Continued on the next page

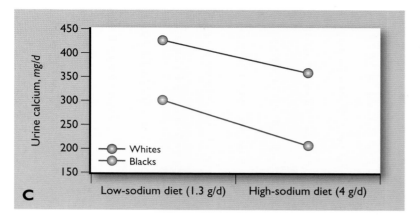

C

Low-sodium diet (1.3 g/d) High-sodium diet (4 g/d)

Figure 3-21. *(Continued)* (**C**) This loss is greater in white than black girls [53]. UNa—urinary sodium excretion.

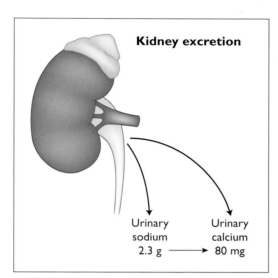

Figure 3-22. Calcium economics and sodium intake in adults. The net amount of calcium that is available for bone metabolism reflects the balance of calcium intake, absorption, and excretion. Calcium consumption has declined in recent years and only 30% to 40% of what is consumed is absorbed [54]. To compound these problems, urinary calcium losses are likely to be on the rise due to increased sodium intake. Calcium and sodium excretion are linked. In studies of white adults, 10 mg of calcium is lost for every 500 mg of urinary sodium [54]. Americans are consuming more sodium, which is contained in prepackaged and fast foods. Decreased calcium intake coupled with increased urinary losses may translate to inadequate calcium for optimal bone maintenance.

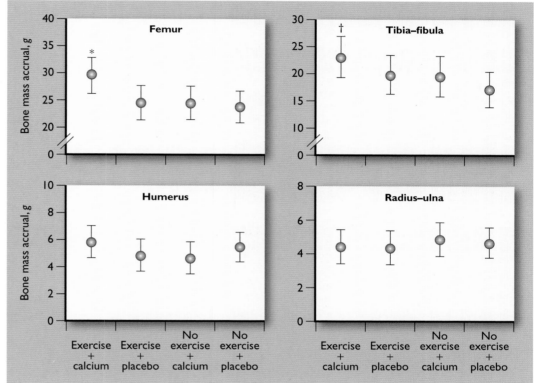

Figure 3-23. Jumping activities, calcium intake, and bone accrual in children. Several controlled trials have shown that brief periods of jumping activity increased bone mass and bone area in prepubertal or peripubertal children. Subjects who jumped for several minutes three times a week gained more bone mass at the hip or spine and more bone strength at the distal tibia than those in the control group [55–58]. Introducing jumping activities into the school physical education curriculum may help offset the trend toward inactivity among American youth [31]. Exercise plus calcium interventions have shown to be the best response in bone accrual. The advantage of an 8.5-month intervention of exercise plus calcium on bone mass accrual was 2% for the femur (*$P < 0.002$) and 3% ($^{\dagger}P < 0.002$) in the tibia–fibula over either intervention alone or control group in pre- and early-pubertal boys, underscoring the important interaction of diet and exercise. There was no advantage at the unloaded skeletal sites to either intervention *(From Bass et al. [23]; with permission.)*

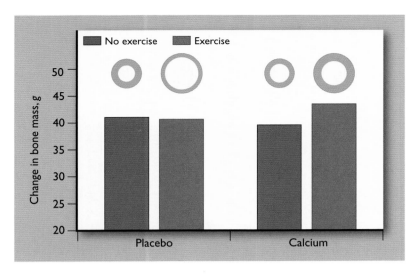

Figure 3-24. Physical activity and calcium interact to influence bone geometry. In a 12-month randomized trial of physical activity and calcium in children age 3 to 5 years, bone mass accrual was higher only in the combined exercise and calcium group, but 20% of the tibia cross-section was greater in both exercise groups regardless of calcium intake. In another study, tennis players who began their sport before menarche had greater results on cross-sectional area of cortical bone, cortical wall thickness, and tortional bone strength than did those who began the sport after menarche [57]. These studies confirm the importance of both loading activity for building bone strength and calcium for building bone mass, particularly during growth. (*Adapted from* Specker *et al.* [22].)

Common Risk Factors for Poor Skeletal Health

Nutritional
  Malabsorption
  Vitamin D deficiency
  Calcium deficiency
  Protein deficiency
  Calorie deficiency

Endocrine
  Sex steroid deficiency
  Glucocorticoid excess
  Immobility

Figure 3-25. Fostering skeletal health. Even the modest gains in bone mass seen in persons with a healthy lifestyle may produce a measurable benefit. Although it may be difficult to convince youths of the relevance of bone health, health care professionals, educators, and the media need to spread the word that osteoporosis prevention, which includes adequate calcium intake, vitamin D status, and weight-bearing exercise, begins in childhood.

Pediatric Disorders Associated with Low Bone Mass

Anorexia nervosa
Endocrinopathies
  Cushing syndrome and iatrogenic glucocorticoid excess
  Diabetes
  Growth hormone deficiency
  Hyperprolactinemia
  Hyperthyroidism
  Hypogonadism
Exercise-associated amenorrhea

Idiopathic juvenile osteoporosis
Systemic diseases
  Asthma
  Celiac disease
  Cystic fibrosis
  Leukemia
  Postorgan transplantation
  Rheumatologic disorders

Figure 3-26. Pediatric disorders associated with bone fragility in childhood. A variety of chronic conditions may threaten bone health during the first two decades of life [26]. In some cases, such as in patients with diabetes or growth hormone deficiency, the deficits may be mild. Osteoporosis and atraumatic fractures have been reported in patients with anorexia nervosa, cystic fibrosis, and glucocorticoid excess, and after organ transplantation. Idiopathic juvenile osteoporosis is a poorly understood syndrome of bone pain, low bone mass, and fractures that improves spontaneously at puberty.

Pediatric Reference Data for Dual-Energy X-Ray Absorptiometry

Study	Equipment	Number	Age, y	Sex	Ethnicity	Sites
59	Hologic QDR 4500	1554	6–16	Male, female	All (US)	Whole body, lumbar spine (L1–4), hip, forearm
60	Hologic QDR	442	6–17	Male, female	White	Whole body, spine, femoral neck
61	Lunar DPXL/PED	444	4–23	Male, female	White (Neth)	Whole body, spine
62	Lunar DPX/DPX-L	1218	6–18	Male, female	All	Whole body
63	Lunar DPX-L	646	5–18	Male, female	Unknown (US)	Whole body, spine

Figure 3-27. Pediatric reference data for dual-energy x-ray absorptiometry. Bone growth and pubertal stage should be considered when interpreting bone mineral density (BMD) results. Normative reference pediatric data are now available. When one uses these data to interpret BMD results, it is important to select reference data collected with the software version and equipment from the same manufacturer used to study patients, because there are systematic differences in results [64]. Standard deviation scores will vary, depending on the normative data employed. In particular, the percentage of boys defined as having low bone mass is greater when gender-specific data are not employed [65]. Patients with chronic disease often have growth retardation as well as delayed sexual and skeletal maturation, which result in lower BMD values. It may be more appropriate to compare the BMD results from these patients based on bone age or pubertal stage, rather than chronologic age. To correct for smaller bone size, volumetric bone density can be estimated and compared with published values [33,39].

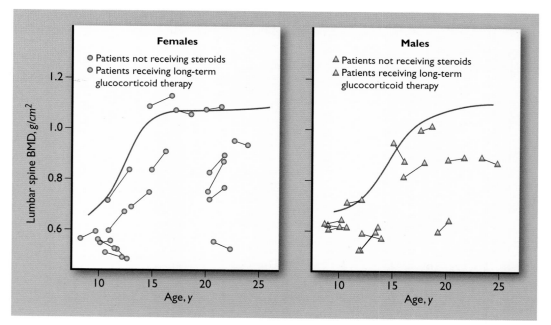

Figure 3-28. The spectrum of bone mineral density (BMD) in cystic fibrosis. Low bone mass is common in several chronic disorders due to reduced bone acquisition or increased bone loss. Bhudhikanok *et al.* [66] found that spinal BMD was below the mean for age (dark line) in many young patients with cystic fibrosis at study entry. At follow-up 1.5 years later, most patients had gained bone mineral but failed to reach expected values. Bone loss was more common in patients on glucocorticoid therapy. Mean bone mineral values remained low even when corrected for small bone size [63]. (*Adapted from* Bhudhikanok *et al.* [66].)

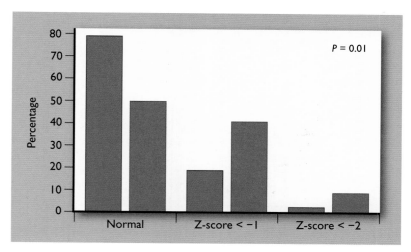

Figure 3-29. Bone mineral density (BMD) in anorexia nervosa. Girls with anorexia nervosa have significantly lower z-scores for BMD of the spine and femoral neck than healthy control subjects. The difference in prevalence by z-score in the spine of healthy (*purple bars*) and disordered subjects (*green bars*) is shown. Dietary fat and calorie intakes are reduced in girls with anorexia nervosa; the lower the fat intake, the lower the circulating insulin-like growth factor-1 level [67]. Even when women are clinically recovered from anorexia nervosa for weight and menstrual function, they may still suffer from low bone mass and an increased lifetime risk of fracture [68,69]. (*Adapted from* Misra *et al.* [70].)

Determinants of Skeletal Status in Athletes

Age at onset of training

Body mass

Menstrual status

Skeletal site

  Trabecular vs cortical bone

  Weight-bearing vs non–weight-bearing

Sport

  Running

  Gymnastics

  Ballet

  Swimming

Figure 3-30. Determinants of skeletal status in the athlete. Exercise-associated amenorrhea is another frequent cause of reduced bone mass. The risk of low bone mass in young women who train intensively is dependent on a number of variables. The most profound deficits have been observed as part of the "athletic triad" of disordered eating, amenorrhea, and osteoporosis. Earlier onset of training, low body mass, and delayed or absent menses have been identified as risk factors for low bone mass. Deficits in bone mineral density have been observed at the spine, hip, femoral shaft, and tibia, indicating that weight-bearing activity may not be sufficient to protect against the deleterious effects of hypogonadism [71]. However, the risks to bone health are not equal for all activities. Female gymnasts have greater spinal and hip bone mass (after correcting for bone size) than do runners and nonathletes, despite a high incidence of menstrual dysfunction [72]. By contrast, elite swimmers have no greater bone mass at these sites than do persons in the nonathletic control group [73]. These observations underscore the importance of high-impact activity as a stimulus for bone formation (*see* Fig. 3-23).

Evaluation of Low Bone Mass in Childhood

History
  Calorie, protein, and calcium intake
  Activity patterns
  Fractures
  Medications
  Family history of osteoporosis
Laboratory tests
  Calcium, phosphorus, creatinine, alkaline phosphatase, blood urea nitrogen
  25-hydroxyvitamin D (to assess stores)
  1,25-dihydroxyvitamin D (to test conversion to active form)
  Intact parathyroid hormone
  Thyroid function
  Estradiol and testosterone (if adolescent)
  Genetic studies (optional)
Bone densitometry

Figure 3-31. Evaluation of low bone mass or fragility fractures in childhood. The cause of poor skeletal health may be apparent from the clinical history, such as chronic glucocorticoid use, anorexia nervosa, and cystic fibrosis. When the cause of low bone mass is unknown, laboratory studies serve to rule out endocrine or renal disorders. The diagnosis of inherited disorders of bone metabolism (such as osteogenesis imperfecta) may be established from DNA analysis of blood or skin biopsies. Bone densitometry is indicated to assess bone mass and to establish a baseline bone mineral density if therapy is initiated. Dual-energy x-ray absorptiometry is currently the preferred method of assessing bone mass in children because of its speed, precision, low radiation exposure, and pediatric reference data.

Therapy for Low Bone Mass in Young Patients

Risk-free therapies
  Address nutritional deficits
    Increase calorie and protein intake
    Supplement calcium intake
    Supplement vitamin D intake
  Treat endocrinopathies
    Hyperthyroidism
    Glucocorticoid excess—endogenous, iatrogenic
    Diabetes
    Growth hormone deficiency
  Avoid immobility
Possible beneficial therapy
  Sex steroids
Experimental therapies
  Antiresorptive agents
    Bisphosphonates
  Anabolic agents

Figure 3-32. Therapy for low bone mass in young patients. Treatment begins by addressing the multiple nutritional and hormonal risk factors. Weight-bearing physical activity should be encouraged, if possible, balancing the risks of slower weight gain or pathologic fracture against the benefits of mechanical loading. For patients requiring glucocorticoid therapy, the minimal effective dose should be used. Sex steroid-replacement therapy should be considered for patients with hypogonadism; however, this therapy has not proved sufficient to correct the osteopenia associated with anorexia nervosa [74]. Furthermore, to date, estrogen replacement has not been shown to increase bone mass or to prevent fractures in athletes with amenorrhea in any controlled trial. Antiresorptive agents have not yet been proved safe or effective in children and remain experimental. In theory, anabolic agents such as insulin-like growth factor I or parathyroid hormone may be more promising because low bone density acquired early in life probably reflects a failure to gain bone without or with increased bone loss [66,74]. These agents have not been approved for this purpose in pediatric patients [75,76].

References

1. Hui SL, Slemenda CW, Johnston CC: The contribution of bone loss to post menopausal osteoporosis. *Osteoporosis Int* 1990, 1:30–34.

2. Bonjour J-P, Chevalley T: Pubertal timing, peak bone mass and fragility fracture risk. *Bonekey Osteovision* 2007, 4:30–48.

3. Bailey DA, McKay HA, Mirwald RL, *et al.*: A six-year longitudinal study of the relationship of physical activity to bone mineral accrual in growing children: the University of Saskatchewan bone mineral accrual study. *J Bone Miner Res* 1999, 14:1672–1679.

4. Khosla S, Melton IJ III, Delatoski MB, *et al.*: Incidence of childhood distal forearm fractures over 30 years. *JAMA* 2003, 290:1479–1485.

5. Kelly PJ, Eisman JA, Sambrook PN: Interaction of genetic and environmental influences on peak bone density. *Osteoporosis Int* 1990, 1:56–60.

6. Krall EA, Dawson-Hughes B: Heritable and lifestyle determinants of bone mineral density. *J Bone Miner Res* 1993, 8:1–9.

7. Villa ML, Nelson L, Nelson D: Race, ethnicity, and osteoporosis. In *Osteoporosis*, vol 1, edn 2. Edited by Marcus R, Kelsey J, Feldman D. San Diego: Academic; 2001, 569–584.

8. Gilsanz V, Skaggs DL, Kovanlikaya A, *et al.*: Differential effect of race on the axial and appendicular skeletons of children. *J Clin Endocrinol Metab* 1998, 83:1420–1427.

9. Seeman E: Growth in bone mass and size: are racial and gender differences in bone mineral density more apparent than real? *J Clin Endocrinol Metab* 1998, 83:1414–1419.

10. Davis JH, Evans BAJ, Gregory JW: Bone mass acquisition in healthy children. *Arch Dis Child* 2005, 90:373–378.

11. Miller JZ, Slemenda CW, Meaney FJ, *et al.*: The relationship of bone mineral density and anthropometric variables in healthy male and female children. *Bone Miner* 1991, 4:137–152.

12. Cadogan J, Blumsohn A, Barker ME, Eastell R: A longitudinal study of bone gain in pubertal girls: anthropometric and biochemical correlates. *J Bone Miner Res* 1998, 13:1602–1612.

13. Moro M, van der Meulen MCH, Kiratli BJ, *et al.*: Body mass is the primary determinant of midfemoral bone acquisition during adolescent growth. *Bone* 1996, 19:519–526.

14. Johnston CC Jr, Miller JZ, Slemenda CW, *et al.*: Calcium supplementation and increases in bone mineral density in children. *N Engl J Med* 1992, 327:82–87.

15. Bonjour J-Ph, Carrie A-L, Ferrari S, *et al.*: Calcium-enriched foods and bone mass growth in prepubertal girls: a randomized, double-blind, placebo-controlled trial. *J Clin Invest* 1997, 99:1287–1294.

16. Matkovic V, Goel PK, Badenkop-Stevens NE, *et al.*: Calcium supplementation and bone mineral density in females from childhood to young adulthood: a randomized controlled trial. *Am J Clin Nutr* 2005, 81:175–188.

17. Winzenberg TM, Shaw K, Fryer J, Jones G: Effects of calcium supplementation on bone density in healthy children: meta analysis of randomized controlled trials. *Br Med J* 2006, 333:775–781.

18. Heaney RP, Weaver CM: Rapid response (letter to the editor). *Br Med J* September 2006. Available at http://www.bmj.com/cgi/eletters/bmj.38950.561400.55v1#142646

19. Institute of Medicine: *Dietary Reference Intakes for Calcium, Phosphorus, Magnesium, Vitamin D, and Fluoride. Standing Committee on the Scientific Evaluation of Dietary Reference Intakes, Food and Nutrition Board.* Washington, DC: National Academy Press; 1997.

20. Braun M, Palacios C, Wigertz K, *et al.*: Racial differences in skeletal calcium retention in adolescent girls on a range of controlled calcium intakes. *Am J Clin Nutr* 2007, 85:1657–1663.

21. Braun MM, Martin BR, Kern M, *et al.*: Calcium retention in adolescent boys on a range of controlled calcium intakes. *Am J Clin Nutr* 2006, 84:414–418.

22. Specker B, Binkley T, Wermers J: Randomized trial of physical activity and calcium supplementation BMC in 3–5 year old healthy children: The South Dakota Children's Health Study. *J Bone Miner Res* 2002, 17:S398.

23. Bass SL, Naughton G, Saxon L, *et al.*: Exercise and calcium combined results in a greater osteogenic effect than either factor alone: a blinded randomized placebo-controlled trial in boys. *J Bone Miner Res* 2007, 22:458–464.

24. Bonjour J-B, Chevalley T: Pubertal timing peak bone mass and fragility fracture risk. *Bonekey Osteovision* 2007, 4:30–48.

25. Bachrach BE, Smith EP: The role of sex steroids in bone growth and development: evolving new concepts. *Endocrinologist* 1996, 6:362–368.

26. Bachrach LK: Osteoporosis in childhood and adolescence. In *Osteoporosis*, vol 2, edn 2. Edited by Marcus R, Kelsey J, Feldman D. San Diego: Academic; 2001:151–167.

27. Saggese G, Baroncelli BI, Bertelloni S, *et al.*: Effects of long-term treatment with growth hormone on bone and mineral metabolism in children with growth hormone deficiency. *J Pediatr* 1993, 122:37–45.

28. Kotaniemi A, Savolainen A, Kautiainen H, Kroger H: Estimation of central osteopenia in children with chronic polyarthritis treated with glucocorticoids. *Pediatrics* 1993, 91:1127–1129.

29. Sambrook P, Coocer C: Osteoporosis. *Lancet* 2006, 367:2010–2018.

30. Agricultural Research Service: *USDA Continuing Survey of Food Intakes by Individuals, 1994–95.* Washington, DC: US Department of Agriculture.

31. Gordon-Larsen P, McMurray RG, Popkin BM: Adolescent physical activity and inactivity vary by ethnicity: The National Longitudinal Study of Adolescent Health. *J Pediatr* 1999, 135:301–306.

32. Kalkwarf HJ: Forearm fractures in children and adolescents. *Nutr Today* 2006, 41:171–177.

33. Lu PW, Cowell CT, Lloyd-Jones SA, *et al.*: Volumetric bone mineral density in normal subjects, aged 5–27 years. *J Clin Endocrinol Metab* 1996, 81:1586–1590.

34. Katzman DK, Bachrach LK, Carter DR, Marcus R: Clinical and anthropometric correlates of bone mineral acquisition in healthy adolescent girls. *J Clin Endocrinol Metab* 1991, 73:1332–1339.

35. Kroger H, Kotaniemi A, Vainio P, Alhava E: Bone densitometry of the spine and femur in children by dual-energy x-ray absorptiometry. *Bone Miner Res* 1992, 17:75–85.

36. Seeman E: From density to structure: growing up and growing old on the surfaces of bone. *J Bone Miner Res* 1997, 12:509–521.

37. Teegarden D, Proulx WR, Martin BR, *et al.*: Peak bone mass in young women. *J Bone Miner Res* 1995, 10:711–715.

38. Lin Y-C, Lyle RM, Weaver CM, *et al.*: Peak spine and femoral neck bone mass in young women. *Bone* 2003, 32:546–553.

39. Wang M-C, Aguirre M, Bhudhikanok GS, *et al.*: Bone mass and hip axis length in healthy Asian, Black, Hispanic and White American youths. *J Bone Miner Res* 1997, 12:1922–1935.

40. Gilsanz V, Loro ML, Roe TF, *et al.*: Vertebral size in elderly women with osteoporosis: mechanical implications and relationship to fractures. *J Clin Invest* 1995, 95:2332–2337.

41. Faulkner KG, Cummings SR, Black D, *et al.*: Simple measurement of femoral geometry predicts hip fracture: the study of osteoporotic fractures. *J Bone Miner Res* 1993, 8:1211–1217.

42. Bachrach LK, Hastie T, Wang M-C, *et al.*: Bone mineral acquisition in healthy Asian, Hispanic, Black and Caucasian youth. A longitudinal study. *J Clin Endocrinol Metab* 1999, 84:4702–4712.

43. Heaney RP, Weaver CM: Newer perspectives on calcium and bone quality. *J Am Coll Nutr* 2005, 24:574S–581S.

44. Bilezikian JP, Morishima A, Bell J, Grumbach MM: Increased bone mass a result of estrogen therapy in a man with aromatase deficiency. *N Engl J Med* 1998, 339:599–603.

45. Wiren KM, Orwell ES: Skeletal biology of androgens. In *Osteoporosis*. Edited by Marcus R, Feldman D, Kelsey J. San Diego: Academic; 2001:339–359.

46. MacKelvie KJ, Khan KM, McKay HA: Is there a critical period for bone response to weight-bearing exercise in children and adolescents? A systematic review. *Br J Sports Med* 2002, 36:250–257.

47. Nilsson O, Baron J: Impact of growth plate senescence on catch-up growth and epiphyseal fusion. *Pediatr Nephrol* 2005, 20:319–322.

48. Schrier L, Ferus SP, Barnes KM, *et al.*: Depletion of resting zone chondrocytes during growth plate senescence. *J Endocrinol* 2006, 189:27–36.

49. Weise M, De-Levi S, Barnes KM, *et al.*: Effects of estrogen on growth plate senescence and epiphyseal fusion. *Proc Natl Acad Sci U S A* 2001, S98:6871–6876.

50. Weaver, CM, Heaney, RP, Eds. *Calcium in Human Health*, Totowa, NJ: Humana; 2006.

51. Chevalley T, Rizzoli R, Hans D, *et al.*: Interaction between calcium intake and menarcheal age on bone mass gain: an eight-year follow-up study from prepuberty to postmenarche. *J Clin Endocrinol Metab* 2005, 90:44–51.

52. Jackman LA, Millane SS, Martin BR, *et al.*: Calcium retention in relation to calcium intake and postmenarcheal age in adolescent females. *Am J Clin Nutr* 1997, 66:327–333.

53. Wigertz K, Palacios C, Jackman LA, *et al.*: Racial differences in calcium retention in response to dietary salt in adolescent girls. *Am J Clin Nutr* 2005, 81:845–850.

54. Nordin BEC, Polley RJ: Metabolic consequences of the menopause. A cross-sectional, longitudinal, and intervention study on 557 normal postmenopause women. *Calcif Tissue Int* 1987, 41:S1–S59.

55. McKay HA, Petit MA, Schutz RW, *et al.*: Augmented trochanteric bone mineral density after modified physical education classes: a randomized school-based exercise intervention study in prepubescent and early pubescent children. *J Pediatr* 2000, 136:156–162.

56. Fuchs RK, Bauer JJ, Snow CM: Jumping improves hip and lumbar spine bone mass in prepubescent children: a randomized controlled trial. *J Bone Miner Res* 2001, 16:148–156.

57. Kontulainen S, Sievanen H, Kannus P, *et al.*: Effect of long-term impact-loading on mass, size, and estimated strength of humerus and radius of female racquet-sports players: a peripheral quantitative computed study between young and old starters and controls. *J Bone Miner Res* 2002, 17:2281–2289.

58. Macdonald HM, Kentulainen SA, Khan KM, McKay HA: Is a school-based physical activity intervention effective for increasing tibial bone strength in boys and girls? *J Bone Miner Res* 2007, 22:434–446.

59. Kalkwarf HJ, Zemel BS, Gilsang V, *et al.*: The bone mineral density childhood study: bone mineral content and density according to age, sex, and race. *J Clin Endocrinol Metab* 2007, 92:2087–2099.

60. Ward KA, Ashby RL, Roberts SA, *et al.*: UK reference data for the Hologic QDR Discovery duel-energy x-ray absorptiometry scanner in healthy children and young adults aged 6-17 years. *Arch Dis Child* 2007, 923:53–59.

61. van der Sluis IM, de Ridder MA, Boot AM, *et al.*: Reference data for bone density and body composition measured with dual energy x-ray absorptiometry in white children and young adults. *Arch Dis Child* 2002, 87:341–347.

62. Horlick M, Wang J, Pierson, RN Jr, Thornton JC: Prediction models for evaluation of total-body bone mass with dual-energy x-ray absorptiometry among children and adolescents. *Pediatrics* 2004, 114:337–345.

63. Crabtree NJ, Kibirige MS, Fordham JN, *et al.*: The relationship between lean body mass and bone mineral content in paediatric health and disease. *Bone* 2004, 35:965–972.

64. Genant HK: Universal standardization for dual x-ray absorptiometry: patient and phantom cross-calibration results. *J Bone Miner Res* 1995, 10:997–998.

65. Leonard MB, Propert KJ, Zemel BS, *et al.*: Discrepancies in pediatric bone mineral density reference data: potential for misdiagnosis of osteopenia. *J Pediatr* 1999, 135:182–188.

66. Bhudhikanok GS, Wang M-C, Marcus R, *et al.*: Bone acquisition and loss in children and adults with cystic fibrosis: a longitudinal study. *J Pediatr* 1998, 133:18–27.

67. Misra M, Tsai P, Anderson EJ, *et al.*: Nutrient intake in community-dwelling adolescent girls with anorexia nervosa in healthy adolescents. *Am J Clin Nutr* 2006, 84:698–706.

68. Herzog W, Minne H, Deter C, *et al.*: Outcome of bone mineral density in anorexia nervosa 11.7 years after first admission. *J Bone Miner Res* 1993, 8:597–605.

69. Bachrach LK, Katzman DK, Litt IF, *et al.*: Recovery from osteopenia in adolescent girls with anorexia nervosa. *J Clin Endocrinol Metab* 1991, 72:602–606.

70. Misra M, Aggarual A, Killer KK, *et al.*: Effects of anorexia nervosa on clinical, hematologic, biochemical, and bone density parameters in community-dwelling adolescent girls. *Pediatrics* 2004, 114:1574–1583.

71. Young N, Formica C, Szmukler G, Seeman E: Bone density at weight-bearing and nonweight-bearing sites in ballet dancers: the effects of exercise, hypogonadism, and body weight. *J Clin Endocrinol Metab* 1994, 78:449–454.

72. Robinson TL, Snow-Harter C, Taaffe DR, *et al.*: Gymnasts exhibit higher bone mass than runners despite similar prevalence of amenorrhea and oligomenorrhea. *J Bone Miner Res* 1995, 10:26–35.

73. Taaffe DR, Snow-Harter C, Connolly DA, *et al.*: Differential effects of swimming versus weight-bearing activity on bone mineral status of eumenorrheic athletes. *J Bone Miner Res* 1995, 10:586–593.

74. Grinspoon S, Thomas L, Miller K, *et al.*: Effects of recombinant human IGF-1 and oral contraceptive administration on bone density in anorexia nervosa. *J Clin Endocrinol Metab* 2002, 87:2883–2891.

75. Rauch F, Glorieux FH: Bisphosphonate treatment in osteogenesis imperfecta: which drug, for whom, for how long? Ann Med 2005, 37:295–302.

76. Ward L, Tricco AC, Phuong P, et al.: Bisphosphonate therapy for children and adolescents with secondary osteoporosis. Cochrane Database Syst Rev 2007, 4:CD005324.

Genetics of Osteoporosis

Robert F. Klein

Osteoporosis is one of the most common bone and mineral disorders in all aging communities. It is characterized by low bone mass (and, thus, low bone strength) resulting in fractures from relatively minor trauma. Although osteoporotic fractures are most commonly observed among the elderly, the pathogenesis of osteoporosis starts early in life and involves the interaction of multiple factors [1,2]. Genetic epidemiological studies provide convincing descriptive data demonstrating population and ethnic differences. In addition, studies of familial aggregation, familial transmission patterns, and comparisons of twin concordance rates consistently identify a significant portion of those with the vulnerability to develop osteoporosis as being inherited. The distributions of quantitative skeletal phenotypes in the general population do not conform to a monogenic mode of inheritance. Rather, susceptibility to osteoporosis appears to involve a complex interplay between both genetic and environmental factors. Initial association studies examined polymorphisms in the vitamin D receptor and the impact of dietary calcium and vitamin D intake. Studies on other candidate genes such as the estrogen receptor or the collagen type I alpha 1 gene also showed associations that could explain at least part of the genetic background of osteoporosis. Genome-wide linkage studies in humans have revealed a number of chromosomal regions that show probable linkage to bone mineral density, but so far the causative genes remain to be identified. It is hoped that new techniques, such as whole genome association analyses, will likely provide important new directions for the genetic analysis of osteoporosis risk.

Although there are multiple genetic determinants of the common forms of osteoporosis, recent family studies indicate that this disease can also occur as the result of mutations in a single gene. Examples are the osteoporosis–pseudoglioma syndrome, caused by inactivating mutations in the lipoprotein receptor-related protein 5 gene and the high bone mass syndrome described in two kindreds thus far, which is caused by activating mutations of the same gene. While recent clinical reports show promise, unraveling the very complex genetic basis of skeletal development will be difficult due to the genetic and cultural heterogeneity of the patient populations. A number of laboratories are now using appropriate animal models to pinpoint candidate genes for more focused human investigation. With the steadily increasing body of information evolving from studies on the genetics of osteoporosis, an improved understanding of skeletal biology and metabolic bone disease is emerging. The identification of genes that predispose people to osteoporosis will provide numerous opportunities to influence the screening, prognosis, and diagnosis, but perhaps the most important application of the discovery of osteoporosis genes will be to identify target molecules for new therapeutic approaches.

Genetic Concepts

Common Genetic Terms

Term	Definition
Allele	An alternative form of the same gene that is present at a given genetic locus
Complex disorder	A disorder resulting from the inheritance of more than one genetic locus, environmental factors, or genotype–environment interactions
Genetic map	The diagram of a particular chromosome in which the relationship of one genetic locus to another, with respect to linear order and distance along the chromosome, is depicted
Genotype	The specific set of alleles inherited by a given individual: it is not uncommon to refer to the genotype of a given individual as the allele present at a particular location along the genome
Haplotype	The specific alleles on a chromosome inherited from one parent (haploid genotype); because physically distant alleles on a chromosome are easily separated during meiosis, a haplotype typically refers to closely grouped loci
Linkage	The inheritance of genetic material at two loci that, because of their physical proximity on the chromosome, do not assort independently
Linkage disequilibrium	The nonrandom distribution (ie, deviation from the distribution expected from the allele frequencies) of alleles at different loci in haplotypes
LOD score	The results of a statistical test to determine if two genetic loci are linked, in which the logarithm (to the base 10) of the odds that the two loci are linked is given
Multigenic trait	A phenotype that is influenced by more than one gene
Mutation	An alteration in the DNA sequence
Phenotype	The biochemical, physiological, or behavioral profile of an individual based on genetic and environmental factors
Pleiotropism	The multiple phenotypic effects of a gene
Polygenic trait	A multigenic trait in which each influential gene exerts a small effect
Polymorphism	The existence of two or more alleles at a frequency of at least 1% in the population
Positional cloning	The cloning of a gene on the basis of its chromosomal location without knowledge of the gene product or function
QTL mapping	A strategy used to identify the chromosomal locations of genes in multigenic or polygenic traits
Synteny	When two or more genetic loci are present on the same chromosome: when genetic loci are present in a similar chromosomal order between different species (such as humans and mice), the loci are in a region of conserved synteny

Figure 4-1. Glossary of common genetic terms. Genetics is the study of inheritance, of its patterns and consequences. Over the past three decades, the study of genetic influences has impacted every medical discipline. However, the language of genetics remains quite specialized and certain terms may be unfamiliar. Therefore, a number of very brief definitions to assist the reader in understanding the information in this chapter is provided in this figure. LOD—logarithm of odds; QTL—quantitative trait locus.

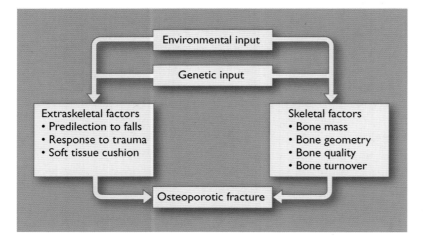

Figure 4-2. Osteoporosis is a multifactorial disorder. It is a disease characterized by an inadequate amount or faulty structure of bone, resulting in fractures from relatively minor trauma. A fragility fracture is a highly complex event with extraskeletal risk factors controlling predilection and response to trauma as well as other factors determining skeletal integrity. Both sets of risk factors have environmental and genetic inputs. Considerable past research has centered on the influence of environmental (nutritional or lifestyle) factors on the occurrence of osteoporotic fracture. With the advent of new molecular genetic approaches, the focus of research has shifted toward genetic factors.

Figure 4-3. Characteristics of multifactorial disorders. Osteoporosis, like many other common chronic diseases, best fits into the category of multifactorial genetic disease. This category should be suspected when the pedigree of the disease does not support inheritance in a simple dominant or recessive manner. Multifactorial genetic diseases have both polygenic and environmental components of causative factors. In the population at large, risk genes are present in low frequency. If any one individual has a particularly large number of risk genes, the latent disorder becomes overt. For another family member to develop the same disease, that individual would have to inherit the same or a very similar combination of genes. The likelihood of such an occurrence is clearly greater in first-degree than in more distant relatives. The chance of another relative inheriting the right combination of risk genes also decreases as the number of genes required to express a given trait increases. Elegant and complex mathematical models have been advanced for polygenic multifactorial disease, but these models should not obscure the fact that each of the risk genes must, like any other gene, express itself by a specific biochemical product.

Characteristics of Multifactorial Disorders

Characteristics	Description
Multifactorial influence	Contribution of genetic as well as environmental factors for disease development
Phenotypic heterogeneity	Large variety in clinical phenotypes within a syndrome
Polygenicity	The effect of many genes that contribute to a disease
Genetic heterogeneity	Different genes, or even different alleles of the same gene, may contribute to the development of the same phenotype
Variable disease onset	The onset of the disease may vary between individuals; onset is often late in life

Contribution of Genetics to Skeletal Characteristics

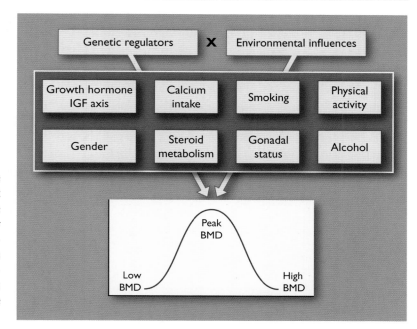

Figure 4-4. Interaction of genetic and nongenetic factors on peak bone mass. The risk of osteoporosis depends, in large degree, on the achievement of peak bone mass, which is mostly determined by changes in bone size and volumetric density. These developmental processes are controlled by complex and selective genetic, hormonal, nutritional, and other environmental factors, which tightly interact. Because of the multiple influences on bone homeostasis and the heterogeneity of the mechanisms governing skeletal growth, the genetic control of bone mass implicates numerous genes of variable importance during an individual's lifespan. BMD—bone mineral density; IGF—insulin-like growth factor.

Figure 4-5. Mendelian versus polygenic determination of bone mineral density (BMD). Mendelian inheritance explains phenotypes that depend on the transmission of alleles at one genetic locus. Polygenic inheritance explains phenotypes that depend on alleles at multiple genetic loci, aggregates in a sense of Mendelian effects. Within biologic populations, continuous traits often fall along a bell-shaped curve that depends on two factors: a mean value and the extent of variation about the mean. Continuous variation in the phenotype is partly attributable to the joint segregation of alleles at multiple genetic loci and by truly continuous environmental variation. By contrast, variation for a Mendelian disorder is discrete and has a single genetic basis. **A,** The discrete BMD produced by an inactivating mutation at the low-density lipoprotein receptor-related protein 5 (LRP5) locus is contrasted with a hypothetical curve generated by alternative genotypes at two loci. Note that the mutant LRP5 allele, which is responsible for the osteoporosis–pseudoglioma syndrome, truncates the continuous distribution of BMD, while **B** illustrates the continuous range of BMD that is standard in human populations. For the purpose of this illustration, the normal BMD distribution is produced by five combinations of alleles at two susceptibility loci. In fact, the number of loci that determine BMD is unknown but undoubtedly large.

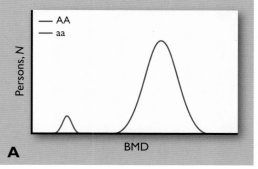

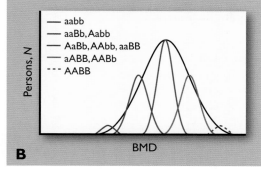

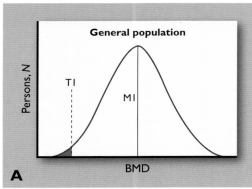

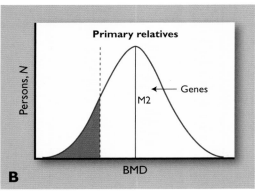

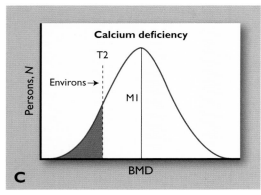

A **B** **C**

Figure 4-6. Threshold of liability for osteoporosis. Although most bone-strength traits follow a bell-shaped distribution, osteoporotic fractures are either present or absent in individuals. A commonly used explanation for such a relationship is that there is an underlying liability distribution for osteoporosis and fractures in the general population. Using bone mineral density (BMD) as an example, those individuals who are on the high end of the BMD distribution have little chance of developing osteoporosis (*ie*, they have few alleles or environmental factors that contribute to skeletal fragility), while those who are closer to the low end of the BMD distribution have more of the disease-causing genes and environmental factors and, therefore, are more likely to experience an osteoporotic fracture. Thus, it is thought that a threshold of liability must be crossed before the disease is expressed. Above the BMD threshold, the individual appears normal; below it he or she is osteoporotic and at high risk for subsequent fracture. As shown in this figure, both genetics and the environment can increase the likelihood for osteoporosis. **A,** Distribution of BMD in the general population is shown. **B,** Distribution of BMD in primary relatives of osteoporosis patients shows genetic factors. **C,** Distribution of BMD in calcium-deficient offspring of osteoporotic mothers illustrates an environmental factor. M1—general population; M2—primary relatives; T1—threshold 1; T2—threshold 2.

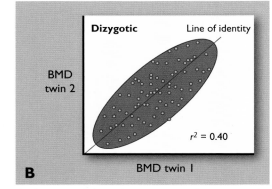

A **B**

Figure 4-7. Similarity of bone density in monozygotic (**A**) and dizygotic (**B**) twins. Twin studies have consistently demonstrated a significant genetic contribution to bone mass. Bone density is more similar between monozygotic twins, who are genetically identical, than between dizygotic twins, who share on average half of their genes. Analysis of these data suggests that 75% to 80% of the variance in bone density in individuals matched for age, sex, and general health is genetically determined. However, the consistent evidence across several studies [3–7] of extremely high heritability values may indicate confounding interactions among a relatively small number of genes. BMD—bone mineral density.

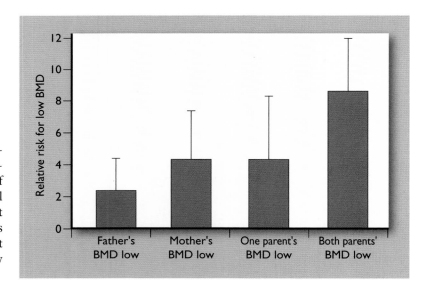

Figure 4-8. Similarity of bone density among members of healthy families. Numerous family studies have demonstrated significant familial correlation for bone mineral density (BMD). An early study in a series of mother–daughter pairs estimated the heritability of radial bone mineral content to be 72% [8]. More recently, Jouanny *et al.* [9] found a significant correlation between the BMD of children over age 15 and their parents ($r = 0.27$; $P < 0.0001$). As depicted here, logistic regression revealed that offspring had a 4.3-fold higher risk of low BMD if one parent had low BMD and an 8.6-fold higher risk when both parents had low BMD.

Figure 4-9. Heritability estimates for various skeletal traits. Inheritance studies over the past three decades have consistently demonstrated a large genetic contribution to many bone phenotypes. Shown are heritability estimates derived from a large set of sib pairs [10,11]. Thus far, however, most studies have only sampled women and not enough studies have examined men to determine if there are significant gender differences in the heritability of certain skeletal traits [12]. This is an important issue given the well-described sex differences in the clinical prevalence of osteoporosis and fragility fracture. In this regard, it is significant that studies of laboratory mice have provided evidence of gender-specific genetic influences on both bone density [13] and bone geometry [14]. BMD—bone mineral density.

Heritability Estimates for Various Skeletal Traits	
Phenotype	Heritability
Lumbar spine BMD	0.89
Femoral neck BMD	0.77
Femoral neck axis length	0.81
Femoral neck width	0.61
Femoral shaft width	0.58

Methods in Genetic Investigation

Figure 4-10. Methods for determining the heritability of common diseases. Although it is not possible to assess an individual's liability for a particular disorder, it is possible to estimate what proportion results from genetic factors as opposed to environmental factors. This assessment is referred to as heritability, which can be defined as the proportion of the total phenotypic variance of a condition that is caused by additive genetic variance. Heritability is expressed either as a proportion of 1 or as a percentage. Estimates of the heritability of a condition or trait indicate the relative importance of genetic factors in its causation, so that the greater the value for the heritability the greater the role for genetic factors. The best studies of heritability ascertain all patients and their relatives who have a disease, then evaluate concordance as a function of relationship. Twin studies are the most powerful method for estimating heritability. Concordance in identical (monozygotic) twins is weighed against the concordance in fraternal (dizygotic) twins to produce an estimate of heritability. Although very powerful, twin studies are susceptible to bias. Other methods for evaluating heritability include ethnic differences and familial aggregation of disease, but these methods are weaker than twin studies, because environmental factors may differ among ethnic groups and increasingly mobile families.

Methods for Determining the Heritability of Common Diseases	
Method	Example
Twin studies	Higher incidence in monozygotic versus dizygotic twins
Familial aggregation	Higher incidence in relatives of affected patients
Ethnic differences	Higher incidence in certain ethnic groups
Adoption studies	Higher incidence in biological versus adoptive parents
Presence in Mendelian disorders	Mendelian disorders with osteoporosis as one component

Figure 4-13. Common marker genotyping assays. To identify an osteoporosis gene, its influence on a skeletal trait must be detected amid considerable "noise" from other quantitative trait loci and nongenetic sources of variation. To accomplish this, laboratory techniques have been developed to detect polymorphisms of loci distributed throughout the genome. Such genetic variation provides a means to distinguish the maternal and paternal chromosomes in an individual, as well as provide markers of different regions along the chromosomes. This approach

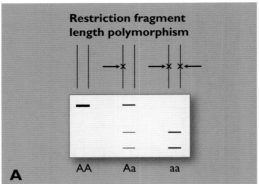
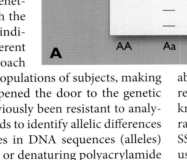
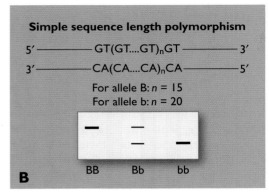

has greatly facilitated the analysis of large populations of subjects, making it possible to trace inheritance, and has opened the door to the genetic analysis of quantitative traits that have previously been resistant to analysis. Two of the more commonly used methods to identify allelic differences are illustrated and each exploits differences in DNA sequences (alleles) that are easily detected on standard agarose or denaturing polyacrylamide gels. **A,** Schematic electrophoretic pattern for restriction fragment length polymorphisms. Each pair of parallel lines represents a DNA segment. The three possible genotypes are inferred from the electrophoretic pattern; A,

absence of the restriction site and a, presence of the restriction site. More recent mapping efforts have primarily utilized microsatellite markers, also known as simple sequence length polymorphisms (SSLPs), which are naturally occurring variations in the number of repetitive base pair sequences. SSLPs are readily genotyped by polymerase chain reaction amplification using oligodeoxynucleotide primer pairs that are specific to each marker. **B,** Schematic electrophoretic pattern for SSLPs. Unique DNA sequences, depicted as lines, flank a tract of (GT/AC)n repeats. The number of repeat units *n* varies with genotype, as indicated.

Figure 4-14. Sib-pair allele-sharing methods. Nonparametric techniques have become popular for localizing genes that confer increased susceptibility for complex diseases because they do not rely on a precise specification of an inheritance model. The objective of allele-sharing methods is to determine whether related individuals who are affected by a given disease or phenotype inherit copies of particular genomic regions that are identical by descent (IBD) more often than would be expected by chance under independent segregation. These experiments are based on the premise that siblings exhibiting similar

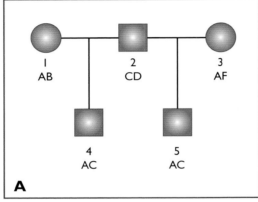
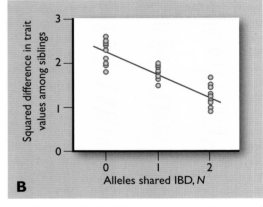

values for a quantitative trait would be more likely to share a common chromosomal region near a quantitative trait locus (QTL) influencing that trait. Studies examining affected sibling pairs often do not include parents; therefore, only identity by state (IBS) information is available. It cannot be determined with certainty whether siblings share alleles that are descended from the same allele in an ancestral generation (IBD) or whether the alleles are coincidentally the same size and, hence, inferred to be identical (IBS). If many siblings are available, however, it may be possible to infer the IBD status without parental genotype. IBD allele sharing provides information about linkage, while IBS allele sharing provides information about the population-level association between the marker and the trait of interest. **A,** Restriction fragment-length polymorphism. Individuals 4 and 5, who are half-siblings, share the C allele IBD because both inherited it from a common ancestor, their father. Alternatively, while they both have an A allele, these alleles are not IBD but rather IBS, since they were inherited

from the unrelated mothers of the two half-siblings and cannot be traced back to a common ancestor. In addition, while individuals 1 and 3 cannot share any alleles IBD, as they are unrelated, they share the A allele IBS. Sib-pair linkage analysis for quantitative traits involves the linear regression of the (squared) difference in trait values within sibling pairs (the dependent variable) on the number or proportion of alleles shared IBD (the independent variable). If a particular trait is influenced by genetic factors, individuals who are more similar with respect to a given trait—those exhibiting a smaller squared difference—are expected to share a greater number of alleles IBD at marker loci close to a gene influencing the trait of interest. **B,** Simple sequence length polymorphism. A regression coefficient greater than or equal to zero suggests that the genetic marker does not occur close to a gene influencing the trait, but a significant negative regression coefficient indicates linkage between the marker and a trait-influencing gene.

Genes and Metabolic Bone Disease

Figure 4-15. Monogenic bone disease genes. Using linkage analysis in extended families, considerable progress has been made in initially identifying chromosomal loci and then eventually the causative genes for a number of rare monogenic bone diseases. Some of these monogenic disease genes may contribute to regulation of bone mineral density in the normal population. For example, polymorphisms in the TGFβ1 gene have been associated with osteoporosis in population studies [15,16].

Monogenic Bone Disease Genes

Disease	OMIM No.	Gene	Genomic locus
Pycnodysostosis	601105	CTSK	1q21
Camurati Engelmann disease	131300	TGFβ1	9q13
Osteopetrosis, autosomal recessive	604592	TCIRG1	11q12
Osteoporosis–pseudoglioma/high bone mass	259770	LRP5	11q12
Osteopetrosis, autosomal dominant	602727	CLCN7	16p13
Sclerosteosis/van Buchem's disease	605740	SOST	17q12
Osteogenesis imperfecta	120150	COL1A1	17q12
Paget's disease/familial expansile osteolysis	603499	TNFRSF11A	18q21

Figure 4-16. Low-density lipoprotein (LDL) receptor-related protein (LRP5) and peak bone mass. One approach to identify genes for bone density is through families segregating apparently Mendelian forms of abnormal bone density. In human pedigrees, significant linkage to the centromeric portion of chromosome 11 (11q12-13) has been observed in two different clinical settings. The first is the autosomal recessive, osteoporosis–pseudoglioma (OPPG) syndrome [17,18] and the second is an autosomal dominant trait characterized by high bone mass [19,20]. Recent studies have succeeded in identifying the genetic origin of these two syndromes; they are allelic disorders resulting from different mutations of the same gene, LDL LRP5. OPPG patients harbor inactivating mutations in LRP5 while an activating mutation (Gly171Val) in LRP5 is responsible for the high bone mass syndrome. LRP5 is involved in the Wnt canonical signaling pathway. Secreted Wnts are thought to interact with serpentine transmembrane receptors of the Frizzled gene family and co-receptors such as LRP5. Members of the Wnt family of secreted signaling molecules have been implicated in regulating chondrocyte differentiation and skeletal morphogenesis. The further role of LRP5 in the determination of bone mass is unclear. However, these results highlight a new pathway that is likely to play a role in attaining peak bone mass and, therefore, could be an important pathway for understanding more common forms of osteoporosis. Unraveling the exact mechanisms of the LRP5–Wnt signaling cascade has become an important area in the field of bone research [21,22].

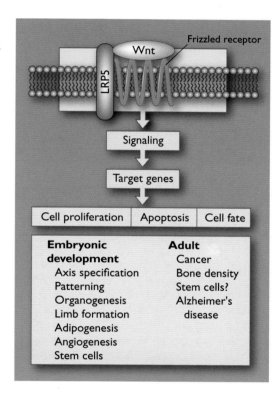

Candidate Gene Polymorphisms Implicated in the Pathogenesis of Osteoporosis

Category	Candidate Gene	Location
Bone matrix proteins	Collagen type I alpha 1	17q22
	Collagen type II alpha 2	7q22
	Osteocalcin	1q25
	Matrix Gla protein	12p12
	Collagenase	11q22.2
	Alpha HS2 glycoprotein	3q27
Cytokines and growth factors	Interleukin-1	2q13
	Interleukin-6	7p21
	Insulin-like growth factor I	12q23.2
	Transforming growth factor beta	19q13
Calciotropic hormones and receptors	Vitamin D receptor	12q13
	Estrogen receptor	6q25.1
	Androgen receptor	Xq12
	Parathyroid hormone	11p15
	Parathyroid hormone receptor, type 1	3p22
	Calcitonin receptor	7q21.3
	Calcium-sensing receptor	3q21-24
Miscellaneous	Aromatase	15q21.1
	Apolipoprotein E	19q13
	Methylenetetrahydrofolate reductase	1p36.3
	Peroxisome proliferator-activated receptor gamma	3p25.2
	Lipoprotein receptor-related protein 5	11q13.2
	Core-binding factor A1	6p12.3
	Chloride channel 7	16p13.3
	Tumor necrosis factor receptor superfamily 1B	1p36.22

Figure 4-17. Candidate gene polymorphisms implicated in the pathogenesis of osteoporosis. There are numerous experimental approaches that can be employed to identify genetic loci that contribute to the risk of osteoporosis. One of the most commonly employed experimental designs is that of candidate gene analysis, which seeks to test the association between a particular genetic variant (*ie*, allele) and a specific trait. Many of these candidate gene studies use population-based association methods. As applied to the study of osteoporosis, two samples are collected: a group of osteoporotic patients and a control group of nonosteoporotic subjects. The allele frequencies at a polymorphism within or near the candidate gene are then compared in the two groups. Evidence of differences in allele frequencies within the two populations (association) may be the result of linkage disequilibrium with the candidate gene or possibly with another gene in close proximity; however, in practice, the candidate gene is thought to be likely causative for disease. Unfortunately, it is well recognized that admixture, heterogeneity, or stratification of a population may result in significant association, even when there is no susceptibility locus in the chromosomal region [23]. Therefore, the results of population-based association tests are often suspect and difficult to interpret. Despite the known limitations of population-based association study, it is a commonly used experimental design. Polymorphisms of many skeletally relevant candidate genes have been examined in relation to bone mineral density and other osteoporosis-related phenotypes. (A subset is presented here; for a more complete review, *see* Liu *et al.* [24].)

To date, candidate gene studies of osteoporosis have been met with limited achievement, most likely reflecting the current imperfect understanding of disease etiology. However, the recent development of array-based platforms for simultaneously testing hundreds of thousands of single-nucleotide polymorphisms (SNPs) in a single DNA sample offers the prospect of identifying genes (or at least genomic regions harboring as yet undiscovered genes) that contribute to complex disorders such as osteoporosis. The rationale for these studies is that these SNPs will be in linkage disequilibrium with causal variants in genes that predispose to the disease under study. Coupled with the availability of well-characterized cohorts of patients and controls, this approach now allows for so-called genome-wide association (GWA) studies. Spectacular success with GWA in identifying genetic risk factors for various complex disorders, including type 2 diabetes mellitus, myocardial infarction, prostate cancer, Crohn's disease, and obesity [25–30], have raised hopes for identifying risk variants for osteoporosis. The only limiting factor for the wide-spread application of GWA is the very high costs of such studies, but recently described pooling strategies may serve to drastically reduce the cost of such investigations [31].

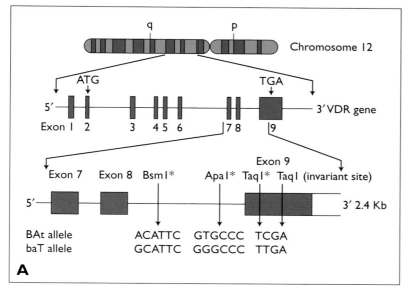

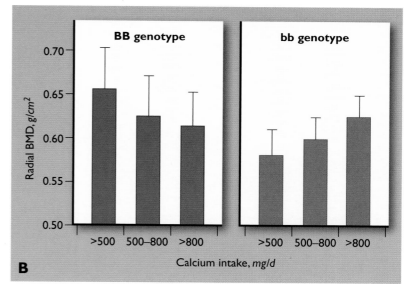

Figure 4-18. Association between vitamin D receptor (VDR) gene alleles and bone mineral density (BMD). Among the several candidate osteoporosis genes, the gene encoding the VDR was the first to be proposed as a major locus for the genetic effect on bone mass. Morrison *et al.* [32] identified three common polymorphisms in the 3-foot region of the VDR gene, which were recognized by the restriction enzymes BsmI, ApaI, and TaqI (**A**). These polymorphisms were found to be associated with BMD in the Australian population [32]. However, results of subsequent association studies in other populations have been conflicting and a meta-analysis incorporating the results from 16 studies concluded that the VDR genotype was associated with only modest effects on BMD [33]. Of some interest: calcium balance experiments in patients with different VDR–BsmI genotypes indicate an influence on intestinal calcium absorption [34]. Furthermore, in the setting of calcium deficiency, the bb genotype is associated with low BMD [35] as compared to

the other genotypes (**B**). In calcium deficiency, patients with the bb genotype may, therefore, be especially sensitive toward calcium deprivation. Failure to take into account dietary calcium (or, for that matter, other yet-to-be-discovered confounding factors) in prior population studies may have limited their ability to detect significant associations. More recently, a new polymorphism detectable by the restriction enzyme FokI in exon 2 of the VDR gene has been identified. This polymorphism results in a 3-amino acid difference in VDR length between FF and ff individuals and in vitro studies found that transcriptional activation was higher with the short form (FF) of the VDR gene [36]. A number of association studies in populations from around the world have shown that postmenopausal women with the ff genotype have lower BMD than those women with the FF genotype [37–39]. In contrast to these association studies, two large sib-pair studies failed to find evidence of linkage with the VDR locus at 12q13 [10,40].

Figure 4-19. Association between type I collagen gene alleles and bone mineral density (BMD). Type I collagen is the major structural protein of bone. Abnormalities in type I collagen have been shown to result in osteogenesis imperfecta and mutations in the COL1A1 and COL1A2 genes, which encode the type I collagen proteins and have been well documented in patients with osteogenesis imperfecta. As a result, more subtle polymorphisms in COL1A1 and COL1A2 were hypothesized to account, in part, for the genetic determination of BMD [41]. Some studies of the regulatory region of COL1A1 have supported an association with bone mass [42,43]. In the results of a study of postmenopausal British women shown here, a common polymorphism was identified that results in a G to T substitution at the first base of a consensus site for the transcription factor Sp1 in the first intron of COL1A1 [42]. Lumbar spine BMD values were significantly higher in women homozygous for the wild-type allele (a genotype termed SS) as compared to women who were heterozygous (the Ss genotype). Moreover, the unfavorable Ss and ss genotypes were over-represented in patients with severe osteoporosis and vertebral fractures (54%), as compared

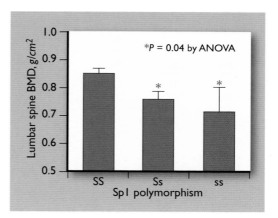

with controls (27%), equivalent to a relative risk of 3 (95% confidence interval 1.6–9.6). The mechanism by which the Sp1 polymorphism predisposes to osteoporosis is not yet fully defined, but preliminary data have shown evidence of differences in allele-specific transcription and collagen protein production [44]. ANOVA—analysis of variance.

QTL Associated with Bone Density or Size

Genetic Analysis	Phenotype	QTL	Study
Linkage	Low BMD	1p36	[45]
		2p23-24	
		4qter	
Sib pairs	Forearm BMD	2q	[46]
		13q	
Sib pairs	Lumbar or femoral BMD	1q21-33	[10]
		5q33-35	
		6p11-12	
Linkage	Lumbar or femoral BMD	4q32.1	[47]
		10q26.3	
		12q24.3	
Linkage	Lumbar or femoral BMD	7q31	[48]
		21q22	
Sib pairs	Femoral neck axis length	5q11-12	[11]
		4q11-12	
Linkage	Femoral neck cross-sectional geometry	20q12	[49]
		Xq25	
Linkage	Proximal hip geometry	2p21	[50]
		21q11	
		Xq25-26	

Figure 4-20. Quantitative trait loci (QTL) associated with bone density or size. To date, traditional linkage analysis has been successfully employed to discover major contributory genes in monogenic disorders (see Figure 4-15), but this mapping approach has a limited ability to detect genes with more modest effects. In the latter case, different approaches, such as nonparametric allele-sharing methods (ie, affected sib-pair analyses, transmission/disequilibrium testing) are considerably more powerful. In this respect, recent studies have revealed a number of chromosomal regions (quantitative trait loci, QTL) containing genes that appear to regulate bone density or femoral bone geometry. A major goal of current research is the identification of the particular osteoporosis gene(s) residing within each of these QTL.

Figure 4-21. Quantitative trait loci (QTL) for bone mineral density (BMD) in inbred strains of mice. In searching for osteoporosis-susceptibility genes, animal studies are essential. For a number of reasons, the laboratory mouse has proven to be an especially powerful tool for the identification and mapping of skeletal QTLs. First, there is a wide range of bone phenotypic variation in genetically characterized animals, which is a prerequisite for QTL analysis. Second, factors such as short generation interval, the ability to make designed matings and raise very large populations relatively inexpensively, and the capacity to control or experimentally alter environmental factors enable QTL experiments in mice to have increased power, precision, and flexibility. Third, the mouse is an anchor species in comparative genome maps representing homology among mammalian species. It has been estimated that 80% of the mouse genome shows linkage homology with portions of the human genome [56]. This factor makes it likely that a QTL mapping result in the mouse will immediately suggest a map location in the human genome, and vice versa. Since QTL mapping is much easier in the mouse, this genetically well-studied laboratory species has become an important tool in mapping human QTLs. It is encouraging to note that a number of these QTLs are

QTL for BMD in Inbred Strains of Mice

Chromosome	Map Position Mb	Human Syntenic Region	Studies
1	170	1q23*	[51–53]
2	19	10p15-13/9q33-34	[54]
2	81	2qter	[51]
4	122	1p36*	[51,53]
5	76	4p12-4q21	[52]
6	117	3p26-25/12p12-13	[53]
7	19	19q13	[51,54]
7	115	10q25-26*	[53]
9	87	6q14-15	[53]
11	64	17p13	[51,53,55]
11	90	17q22	[54]
13	21	5q31-35*	[52,55]
13	56	1q41-43/7p14-13	[53]
14	64	13q14-21*	[53]
15	75	8q24/22q13	[52]
18	47	5q23-31	[53]

replicable (ie, identified in more than one laboratory) and that five of these murine loci homologous regions in the human genome (indicated by the asterisks) have also been identified.

Figure 4-22. Utility of mouse models in complex traits. Workers investigating the determinants of bone mass in humans have a limited ability to intervene in the genetics, personal environment, or skeletal biology of their subjects. While association studies can, to some extent, implicate a particular genetic locus, they can never be proof of a causal relation. For this, a functional assay is needed, a way to alter the genetic sequence and see whether this modification results in a different phenotype. Such experiments are possible only in animals and may be the sole way to understand how genetic differences result in individual variations in bone mass [57]. New methods, such as targeted and random mutagenesis, quantitative trait loci (QTL) mapping, and gene-expression arrays as well as classical genetic methods such as artificial selection and the study of inbred strains,

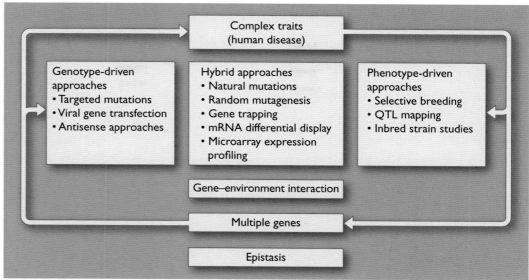

are currently being applied to unravel the complex genetics of osteoporosis and other complex human diseases [58]. Beyond the identification of individually important genes, the power of mouse genetics can be exploited to investigate gene–gene interactions (epistasis), composite effects of a single gene (pleiotropism), and the dependence of gene effects upon environmental conditions.

Figure 4-23. 12/15-lipoxygenase (Alox15) and biology. Recently, investigators employing a combination of quantitative trait loci analysis and global mRNA expression profiling in mice identified the gene encoding Alox15 as a negative determinant of peak bone mineral density (BMD) [59]. Experiments showed that Alox15 knockout mice had higher BMD than normal mice and pharmacological inhibitors of Alox15 activity improved BMD and bone strength in two rodent models of osteoporosis. Armed with this new information, clinical investigators have subsequently confirmed that polymorphisms in the human homologs of Alox15 (ALOX12 and ALOX15) are associated with BMD in four separate association studies [60–63]. The enzyme Alox15 converts arachidonic and linoleic acids into endogenous ligands (15-HETE and 13-HODE) for the peroxisome proliferator-activated receptor-γ (PPARγ) [64]. Activation of this pathway in marrow-derived mesenchymal progenitors stimulates adipogenesis and inhibits osteoblastogenesis [65,66]. Prior to the mouse work, the Alox15 had not been

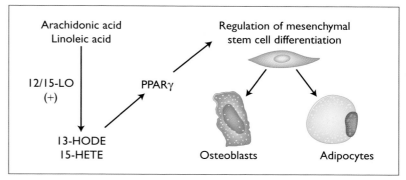

explored as a determinant of bone mass and previous work had focused on the contribution of lipoxygenases and their products on atherosclerosis. This recent example clearly demonstrates the power of animal models to pinpoint candidate genes for more focused investigation.

Figure 4-24. Transcriptional profiling with microarrays. Advances in technology are providing tools that allow for new and abundant levels of information on genome-wide patterns of transcription. A microarray comprises a set of thousands of nucleic acid spots on a solid support. Each spot represents an expressed sequence and consists of an oligonucleotide or cDNA probe. When a labeled cRNA is hybridized to the array, the amount of hybridization to each spot is quantified as an intensity reading that represents individual gene activity, which provides a global picture of gene transcription. The chromosomal region encompassing a quantitative trait loci (QTL) is generally large, containing thousands of genes, and extensive additional work is required to identify the specific gene or genes involved. Recent studies suggest that regulatory variation is important in a variety of complex traits [67]. Quantitative microarray expression studies can reveal regulatory variation in genes for complex traits, including traits for which

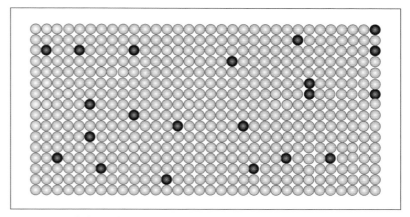

a priori candidates do not exist. By combining QTL mapping with global expression profiling, it is possible to nominate positional candidate genes for a phenotype of interest [68,69].

References

1. Peacock M, Turner CH, Econs MJ, Foroud T: Genetics of osteoporosis. *Endocr Rev* 2002, 23:303–326.

2. Ralston SH: Genetic control of susceptibility to osteoporosis. *J Clin Endocrinol Metab* 2002, 87:2460–2466.

3. Smith DM, Nance WE, Kang KW, *et al.*: Genetic factors in determining bone mass. *J Clin Invest* 1973, 52:2800–2808.

4. Pocock NA, Eisman JA, Hopper JL, *et al.*: Genetic determinants of bone mass in adults: a twin study. *J Clin Invest* 1987, 80:706–710.

5. Christian JC, Yu PL, Slemenda CW, Johnston CC: Heritability of bone mass: a longitudinal study in aging male twins. *Am J Hum Genet* 1989, 44:429–433.

6. Slemenda CW, Christian JC, Williams CJ, *et al.*: Genetic determinants of bone mass in adult women: a reevaluation of the twin model and the potential importance of gene interaction on heritability estimates. *J Bone Miner Res* 1001, 6:561–567.

7. Flicker L, Hopper JL, Rodgers L, *et al.*: Bone density determinants in elderly women: a twin study. *J Bone Miner Res* 1995, 10:1607–1613.

8. Lutz J: Bone mineral, serum calcium, and dietary intakes of mother/daughter pairs. *Am J Clin Nutr* 1986, 44:99–106.

9. Jouanny P, Guillemin F, Kuntz C, *et al.*: Environmental and genetic factors affecting bone mass: similarity of bone density among members of healthy families. *Arthritis Rheum* 1995, 38:61–67.

10. Koller DL, Econs MJ, Morin PA, *et al.*: Genome screen for QTLs contributing to normal variation in bone mineral density and osteoporosis. *J Clin Endocrinol Metab* 2000, 85:3116–3120.

11. Koller DL, Liu G, Econs MJ, *et al.*: Genome screen for quantitative trait loci underlying normal variation in femoral structure. *J Bone Miner Res* 2001, 16:985–991.

12. Gennari L, Brandi ML: Genetics of male osteoporosis. *Calcif Tissue Int* 2001, 69:200–204.

13. Orwoll ES, Belknap JK, Klein RF: Gender specificity in the genetic determinants of peak bone mass. *J Bone Miner Res* 2001, 16:1962–1971.

14. Klein RF, Turner RJ, Skinner LD, *et al.*: Mapping quantitative trait loci that influence femoral cross-sectional area in mice. *J Bone Miner Res* 2002, 17:1752–1760.

15. Yamada Y, Hosoi T, Makimoto F, *et al.*: Transforming growth factor beta-1 gene polymorphism and bone mineral density in Japanese adolescents. *Am J Med* 1999, 106:477–479.

16. Langdahl BL, Knudsen JY, Jensen HK, *et al.*: A sequence variation: 713-8delC in the transforming growth factor-beta 1 gene has higher prevalence in osteoporotic women than in normal women and is associated with very low bone mass in osteoporotic women and increased bone turnover in both osteoporotic and normal women. *Bone* 1997, 20:289–294.

17. Gong Y, Vikkula M, Boon L, *et al.*: Osteoporosis-pseudoglioma syndrome, a disorder affecting skeletal strength and vision, is assigned to chromosome region 11q12-13. *Am J Hum Genet* 1996, 59:146–151.

18. Gong Y, Slee RB, Fukai N, *et al.*: LDL receptor-related protein 5 (LRP5) affects bone accrual and eye development. *Cell* 2001, 107:513–523.

19. Little RD, Carulli JP, Del Mastro RG, *et al.*: A mutation in the LDL receptor-related protein 5 gene results in the autosomal dominant high-bone-mass trait. *Am J Hum Genet* 2002, 70:11–19.

20. Boyden LM, Mao J, Belsky J, *et al.*: High bone density due to a mutation in LDL-receptor-related protein 5. *N Engl J Med* 2002, 346:1513–1521.

21. Ferrari SL, Deutsch S, Antonarakis SE: Pathogenic mutations and polymorphisms in the lipoprotein receptor-related protein 5 reveal a new biological pathway for the control of bone mass. *Curr Opin Lipidol* 2005, 16:207–214.

22. Balemans W, Van Hul W: The genetics of low-density lipoprotein receptor-related protein 5 in bone: a story of extremes. *Endocrinology* 2007, 148:2622–2629.

23. Econs MJ, Speer MC: Genetic studies of complex diseases: let the reader beware. *J Bone Miner Res* 1996, 11:1835–1840.

24. Liu YJ, Shen H, Xiao P, *et al.*: Molecular genetic studies of gene identification for osteoporosis: a 2004 update. *J Bone Miner Res* 2006, 21:1511–1535.

25. Sladek R, Rocheleau G, Rung J, *et al.*: A genome-wide association study identifies novel risk loci for type 2 diabetes. *Nature* 2007, 445:881–885.

26. Rioux JD, Xavier RJ, Taylor KD, *et al.*: Genome-wide association study identifies new susceptibility loci for Crohn disease and implicates autophagy in disease pathogenesis. *Nat Genet* 2007, 39:596–604.

27. McPherson R, Pertsemlidis A, Kavaslar N, *et al.*: A common allele on chromosome 9 associated with coronary heart disease. *Science* 2007, 316:1488–1491.

28. Helgadottir A, Thorleifsson G, Manolescu A, *et al.*: A common variant on chromosome 9p21 affects the risk of myocardial infarction. *Science* 2007, 316:1491–1493.

29. Haiman CA, Patterson N, Freedman ML, *et al.*: Multiple regions within 8q24 independently affect risk for prostate cancer. *Nat Genet* 2007, 39:638–644.

30. Frayling TM, Timpson NJ, Weedon MN, *et al.*: A common variant in the FTO gene is associated with body mass index and predisposes to childhood and adult obesity. *Science* 2007, 316:889–894.

31. Chanock SJ, Manolio T, Boehnke M, *et al.*: Replicating genotype-phenotype associations. *Nature* 2007, 447:655–660.

32. Morrison NA, Qi JC, Tokita A, *et al.*: Prediction of bone density from vitamin D receptor alleles. *Nature* 1994, 367:284–287.

33. Cooper GS, Umbach DM: Are vitamin D receptor polymorphisms associated with bone mineral density? A meta-analysis. *J Bone Miner Res* 1996, 11:1841–1849.

34. Krall EA, Parry P, Lichter JB, Dawson-Hughes B: Vitamin D receptor alleles and rates of bone loss: influence of years since menopause and calcium intake. *J Bone Miner Res* 1995, 10:978–984.

35. Kiel DP, Myers RH, Cupples LA, *et al.*: The BsmI vitamin D receptor restriction fragment length polymorphism (bb) influences the effect of calcium intake on bone mineral density. *J Bone Miner Res* 1997, 12:1049–1057.

36. Arai H, Miyamoto K, Taketani Y, *et al.*: A vitamin D receptor gene polymorphism in the translation initiation codon: effect on protein activity and relation to bone mineral density in Japanese women. *J Bone Miner Res* 1997, 12:915–921.

37. Gross C, Eccleshall TR, Malloy PJ, *et al.*: The presence of a polymorphism at the translation initiation site of the vitamin D receptor gene is associated with low bone mineral density in postmenopausal Mexican-American women. *J Bone Miner Res* 1996, 11:1850–1855.

38. Harris SS, Eccleshall TR, Gross C, *et al.*: The vitamin D receptor start codon polymorphism (FokI) and bone mineral density in premenopausal American black and white women. *J Bone Miner Res* 1997, 12:1043–1048.

39. Gennari L, Becherini L, Mansani R, *et al.*: FokI polymorphism at translation initiation site of the vitamin D receptor gene predicts bone mineral density and vertebral fractures in postmenopausal Italian women. *J Bone Miner Res* 1999, 14:1379–1386.

40. Zee RY, Myers RH, Hannan MT, *et al.*: Absence of linkage for bone mineral density to chromosome 12q12-14 in the region of the vitamin D receptor gene. *Calcif Tissue Int* 2000, 67:434–439.

41. Prockop DJ, Constantinou CD, Dombrowski KE, *et al.*: Type I procollagen: the gene-protein system that harbors most of the mutations causing osteogenesis imperfecta and probably more common heritable disorders of connective tissue. *Am J Med Genet* 1989, 34:60–67.

42. Grant SF, Reid DM, Blake G, *et al.*: Reduced bone density and osteoporosis associated with a polymorphic Sp1 binding site in the collagen type I alpha 1 gene. *Nat Genet* 1996, 14:203–205.

43. Uitterlinden AG, Burger H, Huang Q, *et al.*: Relation of alleles of the collagen type I alpha1 gene to bone density and the risk of osteoporotic fractures in postmenopausal women. *N Engl J Med* 1998, 338:1016–1021.

44. Mann V, Hobson EE, Li B, *et al.*: A COL1A1 Sp1 binding site polymorphism predisposes to osteoporotic fracture by affecting bone density and quality. *J Clin Invest* 2001, 107:899–907.

45. Devoto M, Shimoya K, Caminis J, *et al.*: First-stage autosomal genome screen in extended pedigrees suggests genes predisposing to low bone mineral density on chromosomes 1p, 2p and 4q. *Eur J Hum Genet* 1998, 6:151–157.

46. Niu T, Chen C, Cordell H, *et al.*: A genome-wide scan for loci linked to forearm bone mineral density. *Hum Genet* 1999, 104:226–233.

47. Deng HW, Xu FH, Huang QY, *et al.*: A whole-genome linkage scan suggests several genomic regions potentially containing quantitative trait loci for osteoporosis. *J Clin Endocrinol Metab* 2002, 87:5151–5159.

48. Streeten EA, McBride DJ, Pollin TI, *et al.*: Quantitative trait loci for BMD identified by autosome-wide linkage scan to chromosomes 7q and 21q in men from the Amish Family Osteoporosis Study. *J Bone Miner Res* 2006, 21:1433–1442.

49. Xiong DH, Shen H, Xiao P, *et al.*: Genome-wide scan identified QTLs underlying femoral neck cross-sectional geometry that are novel studied risk factors of osteoporosis. *J Bone Miner Res* 2006, 21:424–437.

50. Demissie S, Dupuis J, Cupples LA, *et al.*: Proximal hip geometry is linked to several chromosomal regions: genome-wide linkage results from the Framingham Osteoporosis Study. *Bone* 2007, 40:743–750.

51. Klein RF, Carlos AS, Vartanian KA, *et al.*: Confirmation and fine mapping of chromosomal regions influencing peak bone mass in mice. *J Bone Miner Res* 2001, 16:1953–1961.

52. Beamer WG, Shultz KL, Churchill GA, *et al.*: Quantitative trait loci for bone density in C57BL/6J and CAST/EiJ inbred mice. *Mamm Genome* 1999, 10:1043–1049.

53. Beamer WG, Shultz KL, Donahue LR, *et al.*: Quantitative trait loci for femoral and lumbar vertebral bone mineral density in C57BL/6J and C3H/HeJ inbred strains of mice. *J Bone Miner Res* 2001, 16:1195–1206.

54. Benes H, Weinstein RS, Zheng W, *et al.*: Chromosomal mapping of osteopenia-associated quantitative trait loci using closely related mouse strains. *J Bone Miner Res* 2000, 15:626–633.

55. Shimizu M, Higuchi K, Bennett B, *et al.*: Identification of peak bone mass QTL in a spontaneously osteoporotic mouse strain. *Mamm Genome* 1999, 10:81–87.

56. Copeland NG, Jenkins NA, Gilbert DJ, *et al.*: A genetic linkage map of the mouse: current applications and future prospects. *Science* 1993, 262:57–66.

57. Flint J, Corley R: Do animal models have a place in the genetic analysis of quantitative human behavioural traits? *J Mol Med* 1996, 74:515–521.

58. Phillips TJ, Belknap JK, Hitzemann RJ, *et al.*: Harnessing the mouse to unravel the genetics of human disease. *Genes Brain Behav* 2002, 1:14–26.

59. Klein RF, Allard J, Avnur Z, *et al.*: Regulation of bone mass in mice by the lipoxygenase gene Alox15. *Science* 2004, 303:229–232.

60. Mullin BH, Spector TD, Curtis CC, *et al.*: Polymorphisms in ALOX12, but not ALOX15, are significantly associated with BMD in postmenopausal women. *Calcif Tissue Int* 2007, 81:10–17.

61. Cheung CL, Chan V, Kung AW: A differential association of ALOX15 polymorphisms with bone mineral density in pre- and post-menopausal women. *Hum Hered* 2007, 65:1–8.

62. Ichikawa S, Koller DL, Johnson ML, *et al.*: Human ALOX12, but not ALOX15, is associated with BMD in white men and women. *J Bone Miner Res* 2006, 21:556–564.

63. Urano T, Shiraki M, Fujita M, *et al.*: Association of a single nucleotide polymorphism in the lipoxygenase ALOX15 5'-flanking region (-5229G/A) with bone mineral density. *J Bone Miner Metab* 2005, 23:226–230.

64. Kuhn H, Walther M, Kuban RJ: Mammalian arachidonate 15-lipoxygenases structure, function, and biological implications. *Prostaglandins Other Lipid Mediat* 2002, 68-69:263–290.

65. Khan E, Abu-Amer Y: Activation of peroxisome proliferator-activated receptor-γ inhibits differentiation of preosteoblasts. *J Lab Clin Med* 2003, 142:29–34.

66. Lecka-Czernik B, Moerman EJ, Grant DF, *et al.*: Divergent effects of selective peroxisome proliferator-activated receptor-gamma 2 ligands on adipocyte versus osteoblast differentiation. *Endocrinology* 2002, 143:2376–2384.

67. Mackay TFL: The genetic architecture of quantitative traits. *Annu Rev Genet* 2001, 35:303–339.

68. Aitman TJ, Glazier AM, Wallace CA, *et al.*: Identification of CD36 (Fat) as an insulin-resistance gene causing defective fatty acid and glucose metabolism in hypertensive rats. *Nat Genet* 1999, 21:76–83.

69. Wayne ML, McIntyre LM: Combining mapping and arraying: an approach to candidate gene identification. *Proc Natl Acad Sci U S A* 2002, 99:14903–14906.

Biomechanics of Bone

5

Karl J. Jepsen

Biomechanics is the study of how variable biological processes affect bone strength and the risk of fracture. Biomechanics provides functional meaning to biological processes, which is critical for advancing our understanding of how the skeleton grows into a mechanically functional structure, how each bone adapts to changes in its loading environment, and how cellular processes during aging compromise or promote the maintenance of strength [1]. The goal of this chapter is to review basic biomechanical principles and to step through some of the analyses that are available at each hierarchical level of structure.

Measures of mass and size are important predictors of strength and fragility [2], and bone mineral density (BMD) is a useful clinical tool for identifying individuals at higher risk of fracturing [3]. BMD decreases with age [4], and low BMD has been associated with an increased risk of fracturing [5]. Aging is associated with complex changes in both, and BMD shows a decline with age despite structural changes that are thought to maintain bone strength [6]. These age-related structural changes may be telling us that there is more going on with the aging skeleton than simple bone loss [7]. Khosla *et al.* [7] showed that aging is associated with specific structural modifications, suggesting that increased fragility of the aging skeleton is not a simple bone-loss problem, but that the relative amount and location of bone loss and gain need to be investigated to provide new insight into the biological basis of bone fragility. Engineering principles have been used to improve our understanding of how age-related changes in bone structure affect bone strength [8–10], and in so doing have identified critical biological targets for treatment.

Whole Bone Mechanical Properties

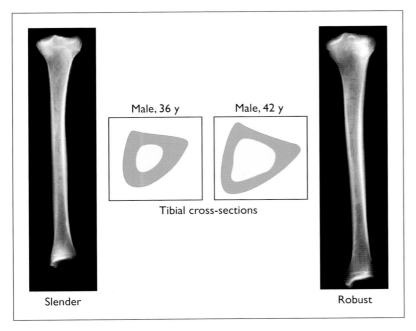

Male, 36 y   Male, 42 y

Tibial cross-sections

Slender   Robust

Figure 5-1. Understanding biomechanical principles is important for many reasons. Bones come in various sizes and shapes, which arise among individuals from variable genetic and environmental factors affecting skeletal growth and aging. Traits of individuals can vary from being slender (narrow relative to length) to robust (wide relative to length). Individuals with slender bones, often associated with lower bone mineral density [11], tend to be at higher risk of fracturing throughout life [12–18]. For the aging skeleton, biomechanical principles provide a systematic way to understand how the cellular processes that affect bone size, shape, mass, and tissue quality contribute to fracture risk.

Quantification and Interpretation of Morphological Traits

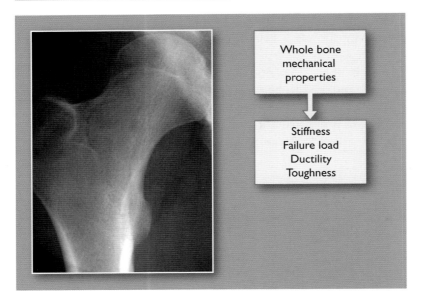

Whole bone mechanical properties

Stiffness
Failure load
Ductility
Toughness

Figure 5-2. There are many important whole bone mechanical properties, each of which has a specific meaning. Properties such as stiffness, failure load, ductility, and toughness are particularly important because they play unique roles in health and disease. Stiffness, which is a measure of the amount of deflection the bone undergoes when loaded, is important for loads engendered during daily activities. Extreme loading conditions (*eg*, those that occur such as during a fall) require that bones are strong and tough to resist fracturing [19]. Failure load, which is often called *whole bone strength*, is a measure of the amount of force required to break the bone. Ductility refers to the amount of deflection at the point of failure and is generally used to measure the degree of brittleness. Toughness, or work-to-failure, is a measure of the amount of energy required to break a bone. This property is particularly important during a fall due to the large amount of energy associated with this event.

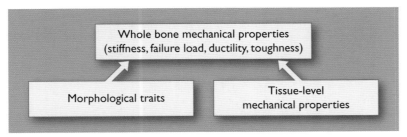

Whole bone mechanical properties
(stiffness, failure load, ductility, toughness)

Morphological traits   Tissue-level mechanical properties

Figure 5-3. Whether studying buildings, bridges, or bones, the mechanical properties of all structures are defined by physical traits that can be broadly classified into two categories. First, the size and shape of a structure define its morphological traits. For bone, this also includes the spatial distribution of cortical and trabecular tissue. Second, the composition and organization of the extracellular matrix define the tissue-level mechanical properties. Many different combinations of traits arise due to genetic and environmental factors that affect growth and aging. The particular set of traits determines, for instance, whether a bone will be stiff, strong, and tough or whether it will be stiff, strong, and brittle [20].

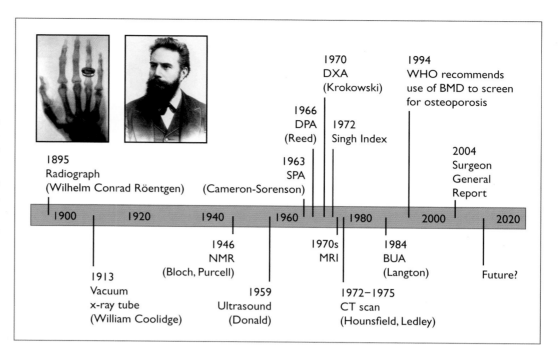

Figure 5-4. Bone size and shape can be assessed noninvasively by using the large number of imaging techniques that are currently available. Bone mineral density (BMD) is currently used to identify individuals that may be at risk of fracture. Ongoing research studies hold tremendous promise for using dual-energy x-ray absorptiometry (DXA) [8], computed tomography [21], and engineering analyses [22] to predict bone strength and identify individuals at risk of fracturing. BUA—broadband ultrasound attenuation; DPA—dual-photon absorptiometry; NMR—nuclear magnetic resonance; SPA—single-photon absorptiometry; WHO—World Health Organization.

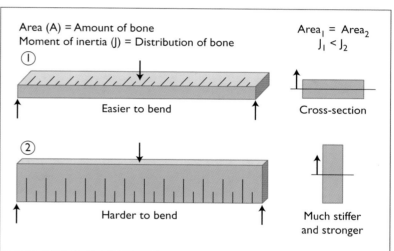

Figure 5-5. Skeletal structures have complex shapes and it is necessary to quantify multiple traits to determine how a structure will respond to loads applied during daily activities and to loads engendered during extreme events such as a fall. For most long bones, these loads are complex and involve tension (or compression), bending, and torsion. Consequently, measures of both the amount and distribution of the material in bone are needed to relate the morphological traits to whole bone stiffness and strength. Moment of inertia is an assessment of the way bone is distributed around its central axis, and it is particularly important because this trait is proportional to the stiffness of bone when it is subjected to bending and torsional loads. Stiffness during bending and torsion depends on how the material of the structure is distributed in space. As such, the moment of inertia is calculated about a specified axis. The general rule of thumb is that stiffness increases as the material is positioned further from the geometric center. For example, bending a ruler about its flat axis is much easier than if the ruler was rotated 90 degrees and bending was attempted along its long axis.

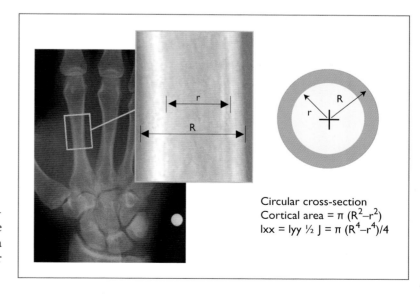

Figure 5-6. Most morphological traits in bone can be estimated with reasonable accuracy from 2-D radiographs using assumptions that the bone is circular or elliptical. For circular cross-sections, the moment of inertia is the same in all directions and is related to the fourth power of the inner and outer radii.

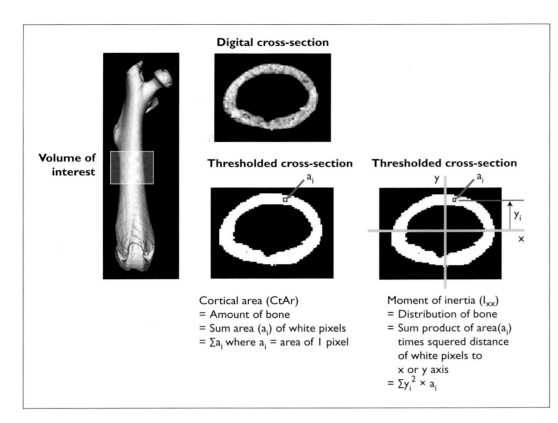

Digital cross-section

Volume of interest

Thresholded cross-section

a_i

Cortical area (CtAr)
= Amount of bone
= Sum area (a_i) of white pixels
= Σa_i where a_i = area of 1 pixel

Thresholded cross-section

y a_i

y_i

x

Moment of inertia (I_{xx})
= Distribution of bone
= Sum product of area(a_i)
   times squered distance
   of white pixels to
   x or y axis
= $\Sigma y_i^2 \times a_i$

Figure 5-7. If digital 3-D tomographic data are available, there are straightforward methods available to calculate morphological traits more accurately, which involves thresholding the image to delineate bone (*white*) from nonbone (*black*) pixels. In this figure, cortical area can be defined as the sum of all bone pixels (*white*) in a cross-section. The moment of inertia of this slice is the sum of all bone pixels multiplied by the square of the distance of each pixel from the geometric centroid of the cross-section.

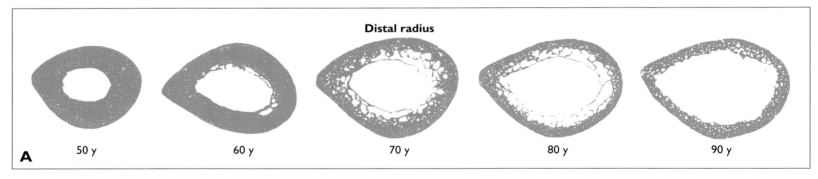

Distal radius

A   50 y   60 y   70 y   80 y   90 y

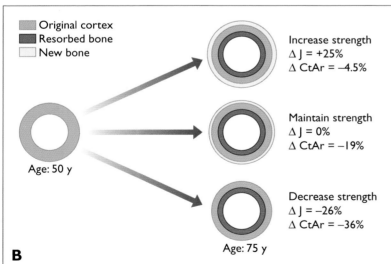

Original cortex
Resorbed bone
New bone

Age: 50 y

Increase strength
Δ J = +25%
Δ CtAr = −4.5%

Maintain strength
Δ J = 0%
Δ CtAr = −19%

Decrease strength
Δ J = −26%
Δ CtAr = −36%

Age: 75 y

B

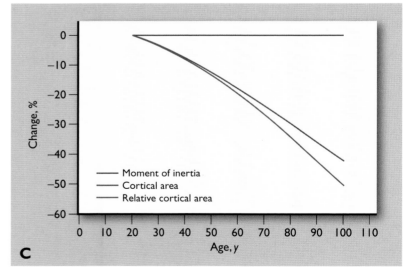

Moment of inertia
Cortical area
Relative cortical area

Change, %

Age, y

C

Figure 5-8. Correlating age-related changes in bone to changes in whole bone stiffness and strength can be challenging, because this relationship is not simply related to the amount of bone loss. **A,** Subendosteal intracortical resorption results in a progressive expansion of the marrow space, which can contribute to an age-related decline in bone strength. However, many individuals show an age-related periosteal expansion [23]. **B,** Because the moment of inertia is calculated based on the fourth power of the radius, small additions of bone to the periosteal surface will result in large improvements in the moment of inertia, which may help to compensate for the endosteal loss and help to maintain whole bone stiffness and strength with aging [24]. **C,** Thus, engineering principles show that the pattern (*ie*, location) of bone loss and gain during aging, not simply the amount of loss (as measured by bone mass or cortical area) is a critical factor needed to relate biological processes to whole bone strength and fracture risk.

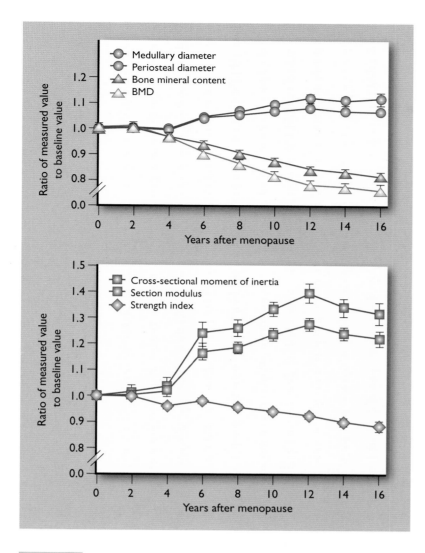

Figure 5-9. Ahlborg *et al.* [10] followed more than 200 white women 48 years of age for 19 years. They reported changes in bone morphology and bone mass of the distal radius as a function of years after menopause. The age-related increase in medullary diameter is consistent with subendosteal resorption and marrow-space expansion. Importantly, they reported an age-related increase in periosteal diameter, providing evidence that women are capable of showing continued periosteal apposition in a nonweight-bearing bone. The net effect of the periosteal and endosteal surface movements resulted in an age-related decline in bone mineral density (BMD), but an age-related increase in moment of inertia. An estimate of strength was based on the product of section modulus multiplied by the apparent BMD; this property showed only small changes with age, despite the sharp decline in measures of bone mass. Thus, measuring changes in bone structure over time may provide a valuable clinical tool to supplement BMD data. (*From* Ahlborg *et al.* [10]; with permission.)

Tissue-Level Mechanical Properties

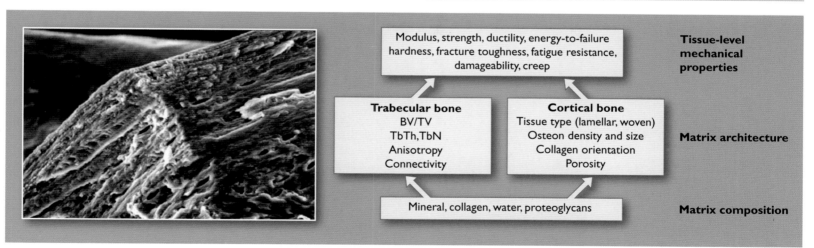

Figure 5-10. Variable cellular processes that affect the construction of bone such as matrix mineralization, collagen organization, water content, porosity, and lamellar organization also directly impact the mechanical properties of the tissue. Tissue-level mechanical properties define how the material responds to mechanical loads. Just as multiple morphological traits are needed to understand bone, multiple tissue-level mechanical properties are also needed to fully understand how variable material properties contribute to whole bone mechanical properties. At minimum, measures of tissue stiffness (also known as the elastic modulus), tissue strength, postyield strain (for ductility), and energy-to-failure (for toughness) provide an accurate description of the quality of the tissue. BV/TV—bone volume fraction = bone volume/total volume; TbTh—trabecular thickness; TbN—trabecular number.

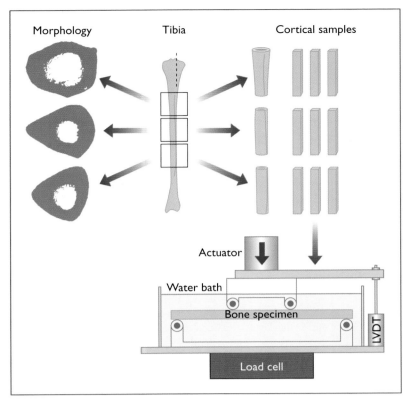

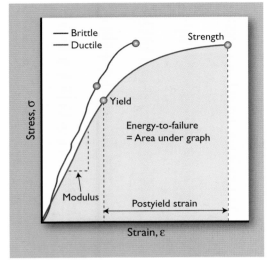

Figure 5-11. The process of measuring tissue-level mechanical properties involves cutting trabecular or cortical bone regions into segments and then further machining these segments into precise shapes. For four-point bending tests, samples are simple beams with a large length-to-height ratio. For tensile, compressive, or torsion tests, the samples can be machined into cylinders with a wasted (thinned) center region. Samples are subjected to destructive tests and the amount of load and deflection are recorded. In this figure, force is applied to bone segments (*via* an actuator) until they fail (*ie*, break) and the movement induced in the bone during this process is recorded.

Figure 5-12. In a destructive test, the load applied to the bone and the deflection or deformation caused can be converted to stress (load normalized for sample size) and strain (deflection normalized for initial bone length). A plot of stress versus strain provides a large amount of information about the material. From these graphs, tissue modulus is calculated as the slope of the initial (linear) portion of the curve, yield is defined as when the initial linear stress–strain curve starts to become nonlinear, strength is calculated as the maximum stress prior to failure, energy-to-failure is calculated as the area under the stress–strain graph, and postyield strain is calculated as the amount of strain from yield to failure. Brittle and ductile materials can have similar moduli and strength, but they differ primarily in terms of postyield strain and energy-to-failure.

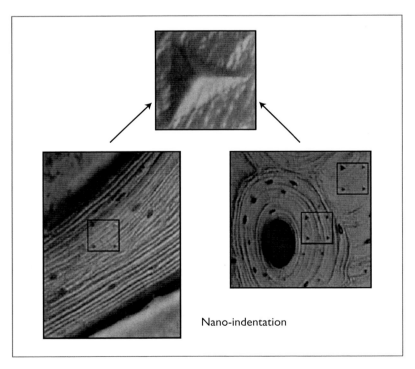

Figure 5-13. Bone mechanical properties can also be assessed at the ultrastructural level. Imaging techniques such as FTIR provide a measure of matrix composition at micron-level resolution [25]. Nano-indentation and atomic force microscopy have been used successfully to quantify the tissue modulus of bone at the lamellar level [26]. (*From* Zysset *et al.* [26]; with permission.)

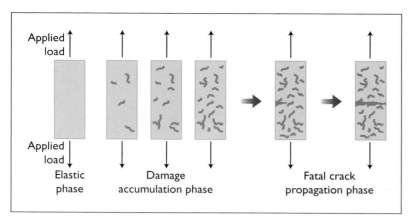

Applied load ↑

Applied load ↓

Elastic phase | Damage accumulation phase | Fatal crack propagation phase

Figure 5-14. The failure process of bone is complex, involving the progressive accumulation of damage and the eventual formation and propagation of a fatal crack [27]. Brittle materials, which fail quickly after reaching the yield point, accumulate very little damage prior to failing. Ductile materials are able to accumulate damage and sustain loads prior to the the fatal crack formation. Healthy bones normally accumulate microscopic cracks, but lamellar and osteonal structures are thought to inhibit excessive crack propagation and accumulations [28], allowing time for biological processes to remove the damaged region [29]. Cellular activities that alter matrix composition, ultrastructural organization, and microstructural organization and lead to a brittle matrix may compromise this crack-blunting trait and reduce fracture toughness.

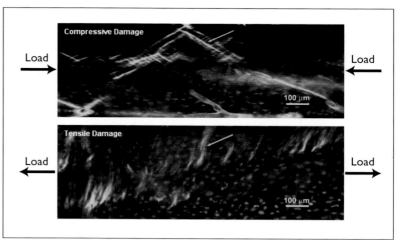

Compressive Damage

Load → | ← Load

100 μm

Tensile Damage

← Load | Load →

100 μm

Figure 5-15. Bone is damaged when it is loaded; this can happen under a large-load magnitude or under smaller loads that are sustained for a long time or are repeated over many cycles [30]. The physical nature of damage differs with the loading mode. Cross-hatched microcracks are typically observed under compressive loading (*upper panel*). These microcracks cross many lamellae and are frequently observed to emanate from vascular canals and lacuna. Compressive microcracks are oriented at approximately 45 degrees to the loading direction, which is consistent with the concept that bone tends to fail along shear (slip) planes. Damage under tensile loading is oriented perpendicular to the loading direction. Tensile damage (*lower panel*) looks less like a crack but tends to be more diffuse and finely structured in appearance, suggesting a more intimate association with the extracellular matrix.

Figure 5-16. Variation in matrix composition has critically important effects on whole bone mechanical behavior. The age-corrected data shown were measured for cortical bone from the diaphyses of male and female tibiae [20]. The amount of mineral incorporated into the matrix plays a particularly crucial role for bone biomechanics [31]. Tissue modulus increases with mineral content, which means that a greater amount of mineral packed into the matrix results in a stiffer material. However, postyield strain, which is a measure of ductility, decreases with mineral content. This means that bone tissue with more mineral packed into the matrix is more brittle. Thus, small variations in mineralization can have reciprocal effects on the properties that are important for daily loads (*ie*, tissue stiffness) and for extreme loading conditions (*ie*, cyclic loading, overloading).

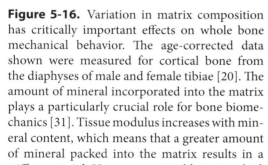
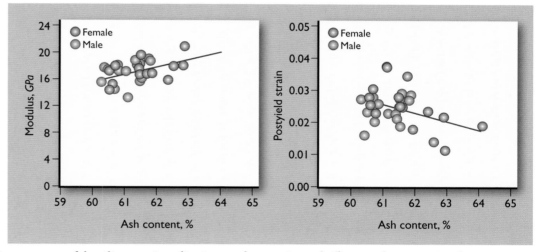

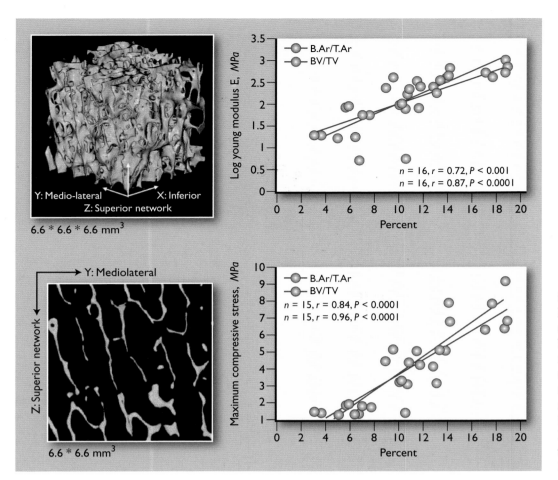

Figure 5-17. The mechanical properties of cancellous bone, like cortical bone, are highly dependent on the underlying physical bone traits. However, because cancellous bone is a porous material, the amount of trabecular bone (*eg*, BV/TV) becomes an important trait, contributing to tissue modulus and strength and emphasizing the importance of maintaining bone mass to sustain the load-carrying capacity of cortico-cancellous structures. (*From* Follet *et al.* [32]; with permission.) BV/TV—bone volume fraction = bone volume/total volume; B.Ar/T.Ar—bone area/total area.

Age-Related Degradation of Mechanical Properties

Mechanical Property	Age-Related Decline, % per decade
Modulus	1.5–4
Strength	2.1–5
Ultimate tensile strain	5.1–9
Energy absorption (work)	6.8–12
Fracture toughness	4.1
Impact energy	300

Figure 5-18. Tissue-level mechanical properties degrade with age; this degradation is evident as early as age 20 [20]. Stiffness and strength degrade 1% to 5% per decade [33,34], whereas ductility and toughness show a more severe degradation of 8% to 12% per decade [34–36]. Age-related changes in collagen cross-linking, formation of advanced glycation endproducts, and increases in mineralization and porosity all affect tissue stiffness and strength, but more importantly these factors have an inordinate effect on tissue ductility and fragility. Knowing how cellular activity affects tissue quality is important because the decline in toughness is thought to contribute to the age-related increase in bone fragility [37].

Summary

Figure 5-19. Most of the discussion thus far has treated morphological traits and tissue-level mechanical properties as having separate contributions to whole bone mechanical function. However, recent data suggests there are functional interactions among morphological traits and tissue-level mechanical properties. This was observed for the bat [38], mouse femora [39] and vertebral bodies [40], and human tibiae [20,41]. Slender tibiae (lower moment of inertia per unit length) tend to have cortical tissue that is stiffer but less ductile compared to robust tibiae, which has tissue that tends to be less stiff and more ductile. The higher tissue modulus of slender bones may help compensate for the small cross-sectional size to increase whole bone stiffness. However, because of their increased stiffness, more slender bones may be at higher risk of fracturing during a fall or at higher risk of developing a stress fracture during intense exercise. (*Adapted from* Tommasini *et al.* [20].) These biomechanical studies reveal that there are important biological controls operating in bone that co-adapt traits to achieve mechanical functionality [42].

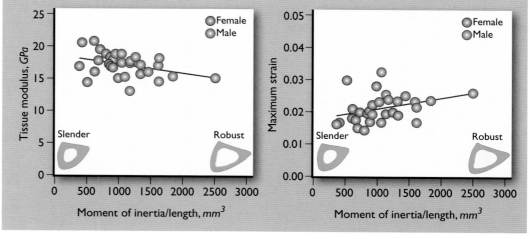

References

1. Seeman E, Delmas PD: Bone quality—the material and structural basis of bone strength and fragility. *N Engl J Med* 2006, 354:2250–2261.

2. van der Meulen MC, Jepsen KJ, Mikic B: Understanding bone strength: size isn't everything. *Bone* 2001, 29:101–104.

3. NIH Consensus Development Panel on Osteoporosis Prevention, Diagnosis, and Therapy. Highlights of the conference. *South Med J* 2001, 94:569–573.

4. Melton LJ III, Khosla S, Atkinson EJ, *et al.*: Cross-sectional versus longitudinal evaluation of bone loss in men and women. *Osteoporos Int* 2000, 11:592–599.

5. Cummings SR, Nevitt MC, Browner WS, *et al.*: Risk factors for hip fracture in white women. Study of Osteoporotic Fractures Research Group. *N Engl J Med* 1995, 332:767–773.

6. Bouxsein ML, Myburgh KH, van der Meulen MC, *et al.*: Age-related differences in cross-sectional geometry of the forearm bones in healthy women. *Calcif Tissue Int* 1994, 54:113–118.

7. Khosla S, Riggs BL, Atkinson EJ, *et al.*: Effects of sex and age on bone microstructure at the ultradistal radius: a population-based noninvasive in vivo assessment. *J Bone Miner Res* 2006, 21:124–131.

8. Beck TJ, Ruff CB, Scott WW, *et al.*: Sex differences in geometry of the femoral neck with aging: a structural analysis of bone mineral data. *Calcif Tissue Int* 1992, 50:24–29.

9. Duan Y, Seeman E, Turner CH: The biomechanical basis of vertebral body fragility in men and women. *J Bone Miner Res* 2001, 16:2276–2283.

10. Ahlborg HG, Johnell O, Turner CH, *et al.*: Bone loss and bone size after menopause. *N Engl J Med* 2003, 349:327–334.

11. Duan Y, Parfitt A, Seeman E: Vertebral bone mass, size, and volumetric density in women with spinal fractures. *J Bone Miner Res* 1999, 14:1796–1802.

12. Albright F, Smith PH, Richardson AM: Post-menopausal osteoporosis. Its clinical features. *JAMA* 1941, 116:2465–2474.

13. Gilsanz V, Loro ML, Roe TF, *et al.*: Vertebral size in elderly women with osteoporosis. Mechanical implications and relationship to fractures. *J Clin Invest* 1995, 95:2332–2337.

14. Vega E, Ghiringhelli G, Mautalen C, *et al.*: Bone mineral density and bone size in men with primary osteoporosis and vertebral fractures. *Calcif Tissue Int* 1998, 62:465–469.

15. Huang Z, Himes JH: Bone mass and subsequent risk of hip fracture. *Epidemiology* 1997, 8:192–195.

16. Schneider P, Reiners C, Cointry GR, *et al.*: Bone quality parameters of the distal radius as assessed by pQCT in normal and fractured women. *Osteoporos Int* 2001, 12:639–646.

17. Ahlborg HG, Nguyen ND, Nguyen TV, *et al.*: Contribution of hip strength indices to hip fracture risk in elderly men and women. *J Bone Miner Res* 2005, 20:1820–1827.

18. Seeman E, Duan Y, Fong C, Edmonds J: Fracture site-specific deficits in bone size and volumetric density in men with spine or hip fractures. *J Bone Miner Res* 2001, 16:120–127.

19. Hayes WC, Myers ER, Robinovitch SN, *et al.*: Etiology and prevention of age-related hip fractures. *Bone* 1996, 18:77S–86S.

20. Tommasini SM, Nasser P, Jepsen KJ: Sexual dimorphism affects tibia size and shape but not tissue-level mechanical properties. *Bone* 2007, 40:498–505.

21. Li W, Sode M, Saeed I, Lang T: Automated registration of hip and spine for longitudinal QCT studies: integration with 3D densitometric and structural analysis. *Bone* 2006, 38:273–279.

22. Crawford RP, Cann CE, Keaveny TM: Finite element models predict in vitro vertebral body compressive strength better than quantitative computed tomography. *Bone* 2003, 33:744–750.

23. Smith RW, Walker RR: Femoral expansion in aging women: implications for osteoporosis and fractures. *Science* 1964, 145:156–157.

24. Szulc P, Seeman E, Duboeuf F, *et al.*: Bone fragility: failure of periosteal apposition to compensate for increased endocortical resorption in postmenopausal women. *J Bone Miner Res* 2006, 21:1856–1863.

25. Boskey AL: Assessment of bone mineral and matrix using backscatter electron imaging and FTIR imaging. *Curr Osteoporos Rep* 2006, 4:71–75.

26. Zysset PK, Guo XE, Hoffler CE, *et al.*: Elastic modulus and hardness of cortical and trabecular bone lamellae measured by nanoindentation in the human femur. *J Biomech* 1999, 32:1005–1012.

27. Akkus O, Yeni YN, Wasserman N: Fracture mechanics of cortical bone tissue: a hierarchical perspective. *Crit Rev Biomed Eng* 2004, 32:379–426.

28. Burr DB, Schaffler MB, Frederickson RG: Composition of the cement line and its possible mechanical role as a local interface in human compact bone. *J Biomech* 1988, 21:939–945.

29. Martin RB, Burr DB: A hypothetical mechanism for the stimulation of osteonal remodelling by fatigue damage. *J Biomech* 1982, 15:137–139.

30. Schaffler M, Radin, EL, Burr, DB: Long-term fatigue behavior of compact bone at low strain magnitude and rate. *Bone* 1990, 11:321–326.

31. Currey JD: Effects of differences in mineralization on the mechanical properties of bone. *Philos Trans R Soc Lond B Biol Sci* 1984, 304:509–518.

32. Follet H, Bruyere-Garnier K, Peyrin F, *et al.*: Relationship between compressive properties of human os calcis cancellous bone and microarchitecture assessed from 2D and 3D synchrotron microtomography. *Bone* 2005, 36:340–351.

33. Burstein AH, Reilly DT, Martens M: Aging of bone tissue: mechanical properties. *J Bone Joint Surg Am* 1976, 58:82–86.

34. McCalden RW, McGeough JA, Barker MB, Court-Brown CM: Age-related changes in the tensile properties of cortical bone. The relative importance of changes in porosity, mineralization, and microstructure. *J Bone Joint Surg Am* 1993, 75:1193–1205.

35. Currey JD: Changes in the impact energy absorption of bone with age. *J Biomech* 1979, 12:459–469.

36. Zioupos P, Currey JD: Changes in the stiffness, strength, and toughness of human cortical bone with age. *Bone* 1998, 22:57–66.

37. Kanis JA, Johnell O, Oden A, *et al.*: Ten year probabilities of osteoporotic fractures according to BMD and diagnostic thresholds. *Osteoporos Int* 2001, 12:989–995.

38. Papadimitriou HM, Swartz SM, Kunz TH: Ontogenetic and anatomic variation in mineralization of the wing skeleton of the Mexican free-tailed bat, Tadarida brasiliensis. *J Zool (Lond)* 1996, 240:411–426.

39. Jepsen KJ, Hu B, Tommasini SM, *et al.*: Genetic randomization reveals functional relationships among morphologic and tissue-quality traits that contribute to bone strength and fragility. *Mamm Genome* 2007, 18:492–507.

40. Tommasini SM, Morgan TG, van der Meulen M, Jepsen KJ: Genetic variation in structure-function relationships for the inbred mouse lumbar vertebral body. *J Bone Miner Res* 2005, 20:817–827.

41. Tommasini SM, Nasser P, Schaffler MB, Jepsen KJ: Relationship between bone morphology and bone quality in male tibias: implications for stress fracture risk. *J Bone Miner Res* 2005, 20:1372–1380.

42. Olson EC, Miller RL: *Morphological Integration*. Chicago: University of Chicago Press; 1958.

Epidemiology of Osteoporosis and Fractures

6

Elsa S. Strotmeyer and Jane A. Cauley

Osteoporosis is a skeletal disorder characterized by compromised bone strength, a combination of bone density and bone quality, which predisposes an individual to an increased risk of fracture [1]. Osteoporotic fractures occur particularly at the hip, spine, and wrist [2], but most fractures appear to be related to low bone density [3]. Osteoporosis and its related fractures are a significant public health issue, particularly in older adults. Osteoporosis affects approximately 8 million women and 2 million men in the United States, and an additional 22 million women and 12 million men have low bone mass [4]. In the United States, 18% of women and 6% of men 50 years of age and older had osteoporosis in 1995, and an additional 50% of women and 47% of men had low bone mass at the femoral neck [5]. For white women 50 years of age with osteoporosis, approximately 40% to 50% are expected to suffer a hip fracture in their lifetime [6,7]. These fractures, particularly at the hip, and their resulting disability are associated with significant health care services usage and costs [2,8].

This chapter provides an overview of the current epidemiologic data on osteoporosis and its related fractures. The magnitude and scope of the public health problem is summarized, including the prevalence and incidence of both low bone density and fractures, risk factors for osteoporosis and its related fractures, the role of falls and trauma in fractures, and the economic impact of fractures. Prevalence is defined as the number of individuals in a population that have had a disease or event (*eg*, osteoporosis, fracture) at any time. Incidence is defined as the number of individuals in a population developing a new disease or event (*eg*, fracture) within a specific period of time. A description by key demographic characteristics of age, sex, and race/ethnic group is given whenever available.

The risk factors for osteoporosis and its related fractures are numerous [9–15] though clearly those most impacted are older adults [11,12,16–18]. Osteoporosis and fractures are more common in women, especially after menopause, with men experiencing an approximately 50% lower fracture incidence due to low bone mineral density (BMD) than women [5,17,19–21]. However, fractures still represent a significant burden for men, particularly at the oldest ages [14,17,21]. Differences also occur by race/ethnic group [5,13,18,22,23]. The genetics of osteoporosis has had many exciting developments recently, with the release of several genome-wide association studies [24,25].

The risk for osteoporosis and fractures has typically been quantified by BMD assessments with dual x-ray absorptiometry (DXA). A BMD that is at least 2.5 SDs below the average for young normal adults is classified as osteoporosis and a BMD between 1.0 and 2.5 SD below the average for young normal adults is classified as low bone mass or osteopenia [5]. BMD is a key technique to assess differences in fracture risk among individuals [14,15,19,20,26,27] and also monitor change in risk over time. In general, 1 SD in BMD is associated with a two- to threefold increase in hip fracture risk [28,29]. However, DXA is a two-dimensional technique that has limitations in its ability to account for bone size. BMD by DXA is known to vary by sex and race groups based on this limitation [30]. Peripheral bone density measurements have become more common. Although these are associated with varied osteoporosis prevalence across devices, overall each SD decrease in peripheral BMD is related to an approximate 50% increase in fracture risk in women [22]. Recently, the World Health Organization and the National Osteoporosis Foundation have implemented a fracture risk-assessment tool, FRAX™ (WHO, Geneva, Switzerland), which calculates the risk of fracture based on BMD and clinical risk factors [10,31–33]. This tool is shown to be more accurate in predicting future fracture risk than BMD alone and is available across international populations for men and women [31–33]. The goal is to move away from defining osteoporosis by BMD measurement alone and to focus instead on the absolute fracture risk when making clinical treatment decisions.

With the well-recognized aging of the population structure across the world, the prevalence of osteoporosis and its related fractures is projected to increase dramatically. This represents an expected increase in the prevalence of osteoporosis of 35% (11 million) in women and of 43% (3 million) in men in the United States by 2020 [4]. Worldwide, an estimated 6.26 million individuals will have suffered a hip fracture in 2050 [34]. In order to prevent disability and mortality related to fractures [21], and to extend disability-free years of life, osteoporotic fractures will need to be effectively prevented and managed.

Epidemiology of Osteoporosis

Diagnostic Criteria for Osteoporosis Established by the World Health Organization and Modified by the International Osteoporosis Foundation* Based on a Comparison to Young Adult Mean Bone Density†

Normal
Bone density is within 1 SD of the young adult mean

Low bone mass (osteopenia)
Bone density is within 1–2.5 SD below the young adult mean

Osteoporosis
Bone density is 2.5 SD or more below the young adult mean

Severe (established) osteoporosis
Bone density is more than 2.5 SD below the young adult mean and there has been one or more osteoporotic fractures

*Specify use of the hip site.
†One SD represents about a 10%–15% decline in bone density.

Figure 6-1. Diagnostic categories for low bone mass (osteopenia), osteoporosis, and severe osteoporosis, established by the World Health Organization and modified by the International Osteoporosis Foundation, are shown. These findings are based on a SD from a young adult reference population and not on biologic criteria. (*Adapted from* Kanis and Glüer [6].)

Risk Factors for Osteoporosis

Older age

Genetic
  Ethnicity
  Female sex
  Family history
  Genes

Anthropometry
  Low body weight or low body mass index
  Weight loss
  Greater height

Environmental
  Nutrition (*eg*, calcium deficiency, vitamin D deficiency)
  Physical inactivity, immobility, and decreased mechanical loading
  Medications (*eg*, glucocorticoids, thiazides–positive)
  Smoking
  Excessive alcohol intake
  Falls or other trauma

Endogenous hormones and chronic diseases
  Estrogen deficiency
  Androgen deficiency
  Chronic conditions (*eg*, endocrine disorders, gastrointestinal disorders, liver diseases, neurological disorders, renal disease, cancer, diabetes mellitus)

Physical characteristics of bone
  Density (mass)
  Size and geometry
  Microarchitecture
  Strength

Figure 6-2. Established risk factors for osteoporosis are given. (*Adapted from* Samelson and Hannan [9] and the National Osteoporosis Foundation [10].)

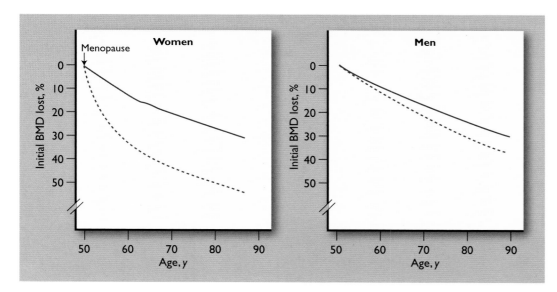

Figure 6-3. Patterns of age-related bone loss in women and men based on multiple cross-sectional and longitudinal studies using dual x-ray absorptiometry are shown. *Dashed lines* represent trabecular bone and *solid lines* represent cortical bone. BMD—bone mineral density. (*Adapted from* Khosla and Riggs [16].)

Prevalence of Osteoporosis* Among an Age-Stratified Sample of Rochester, Minnesota, Residents

Age group, y	Total hip alone, %	Lumbar spine alone, %	Total wrist alone, %	Hip, spine, or wrist, %
Postmenopausal women				
50–59 (n = 50)	4.0	2.0	6.0	8.0
60–69 (n = 50)	10.0	8.0	28.0	30.0
70–79 (n = 51)	19.6	17.6	56.9	56.9
≥ 80 (n = 50)	40.0	4.0	78.0	82.0
Total (n = 201)	13.6†	7.7	32.9	34.7†
Men ≥ 50 y				
50–59 (n = 49)	12.2	2.0	4.1	12.2
60–69 (n = 50)	16.0	0.0	4.0	18.0
70–79 (n = 51)	15.7	2.0	11.8	21.6
≥ 80 (n = 50)	26.0	2.0	30.0	40.0
Total (n = 200)	15.8†	1.4	8.8	19.4†

*By World Health Organization criteria (2.5 SD or more below sex-specific young normal mean).
†Total prevalence per 100 age-adjusted to 1990 US white population ≥ 50 years old.

Figure 6-4. Osteoporosis prevalence by age and skeletal site for an age-stratified sample of women and men from Rochester, Minnesota, is shown. The total is age adjusted to the United States white population 50 years of age and older in 1990. (*Adapted from* Melton *et al.* [17].)

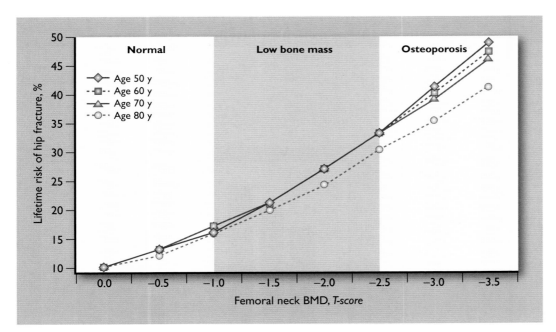

Figure 6-8. Lifetime risk of hip fracture by femoral neck bone mineral density (BMD) by T-score and age group for white women is shown. Overall mortality rates are based on United States vital statistics. (*Adapted from* Cummings *et al.* [7].)

Epidemiology of Fracture

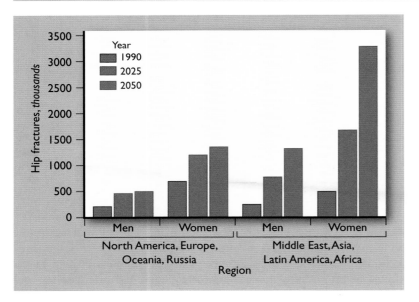

Figure 6-9. The estimated numbers of hip fractures by sex and region of the world in 1990 and projections for 2025 and 2050 are given. The number of hip fractures worldwide is projected to increase from 1.66 million in 1990 to 6.26 million by 2050. Currently, about half of all hip fractures occur in Europe and North America; however, by 2050 these regions will account for only one-fourth of the total and the majority are expected to occur in Asia and Latin America. (*Adapted from* Cooper *et al.* [34].)

Incidence of Hip Fracture (Rates Per 100,000) in 1990 by Age, Sex, and Region of the World

Region	Men by age group, y						
Europe	50–54	55–59	60–64	65–69	70–74	75–79	80+
Western Europe	28	33	67	103	203	331	880
Southern Europe	10	16	34	55	81	190	534
Eastern Europe	38	38	88	88	194	194	475
Northern Europe	58	66	97	198	382	682	1864
North America	33	33	81	123	119	338	1230
Oceania	20	34	63	92	180	445	1157
Asia	20	20	37	47	102	150	364
Africa	6	10	14	27	8	0	116
Latin America	25	40	40	106	106	327	327
World	23	25	47	69	119	219	630
	Women by age group, y						
Europe	50–54	55–59	60–64	65–69	70–74	75–79	80+
Western Europe	33	54	115	184	362	657	1808
Southern Europe	11	21	47	100	170	380	1075
Eastern Europe	58	58	155	155	426	426	1251
Northern Europe	74	78	190	327	612	1294	2997
North America	60	60	117	252	437	850	2296
Oceania	31	63	112	204	358	899	2476
Asia	14	14	38	75	156	252	563
Africa	4	12	17	12	16	50	80
Latin America	20	50	50	163	163	622	622
World	24	28	69	122	240	458	1289

Figure 6-10. The incidence of hip fracture by sex, age, and region of the world is provided. (*Adapted from* Gullberg *et al.* [23].)

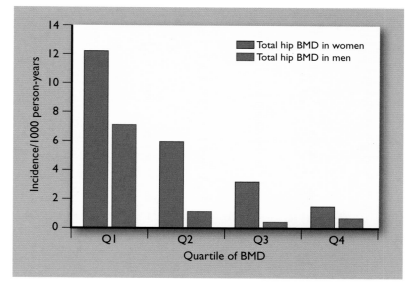

Figure 6-11. Age-adjusted annual hip fracture incidence by the sex-specific quartile of total hip bone mineral density (BMD) for women and men is given. Women are from the Study of Osteoporotic Fractures and men are from the Study of Osteoporotic Fractures in Men. (*Adapted from* Cummings *et al.* [19].)

High- and Low-Trauma Fractures According to T-Score for SOF Women and MrOS Men

BMD T-score	High-trauma fracture Rate per 1000 person-years (95% CI)	Low-trauma fracture Rate per 1000 person-years (95% CI)
Women		
> –1.0*	2.1 (1.3–2.9)	21.4 (18.9–24.0)
≤ –1.0 and > –2.5*	3.4 (2.8–4.0)	40.7 (38.6–42.7)
≤ –2.5*	5.8 (4.6–7.0)	69.0 (64.8–73.3)
Men		
> –1.0*	2.2 (1.4–3.1)	7.0 (5.5–8.5)
≤ –1.0 and > –2.5*	3.3 (2.4–4.1)	12.4 (10.7–14.1)
≤ –2.5*	8.2 (3.5–12.8)	34.7 (25.2–44.2)

*At either the total hip or femoral neck.

Figure 6-12. High- and low-trauma fracture incidence (per 1000 person-years) by T-score for women and men. Women are from the Study of Osteoporotic Fractures (SOF) and men are from the Study of Osteoporotic Fractures in Men (MrOS). BMD—bone mineral density. (*Adapted from* Mackey *et al.* [20].)

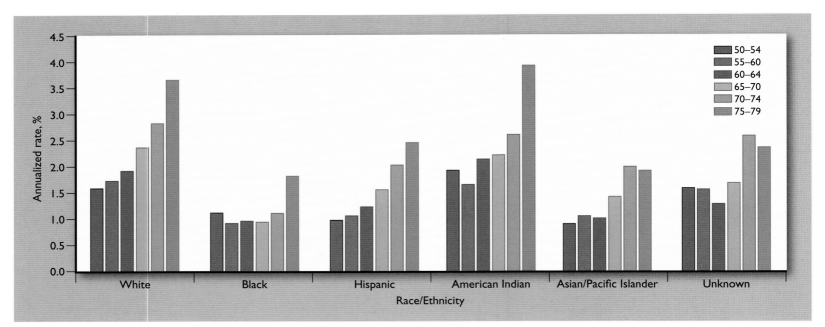

Figure 6-13. Annualized incidence of nonvertebral fractures by ethnicity and age groups for postmenopausal women in the Women's Health Initiative [18] are shown. (*Adapted from* Cauley *et al.* [18].)

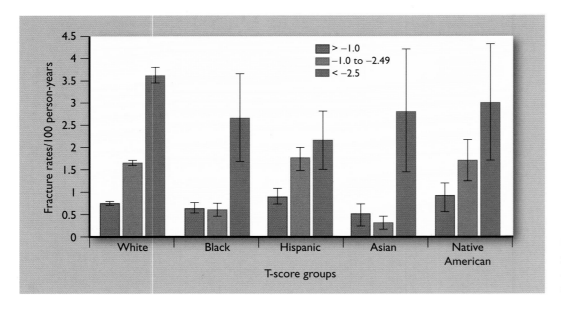

Figure 6-14. Fracture rates (±SE) by ethnicity and T-score group in women over the age of 50 years are given. (*Adapted from* Barrett-Connor *et al.* [22].)

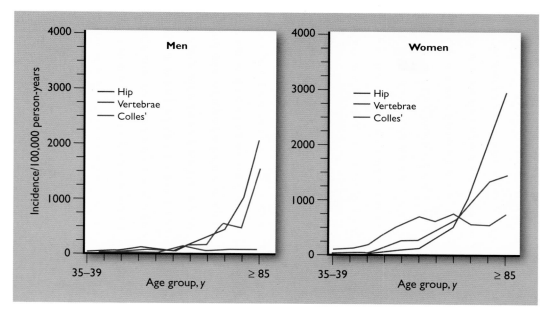

Figure 6-15. Age-specific incidence rates for hip, vertebral, and distal forearm (Colles') fractures in men and women from Rochester, Minnesota, are shown. (*Adapted from* Cooper and Melton [11].)

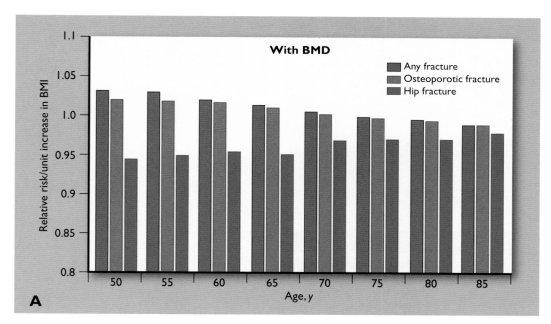

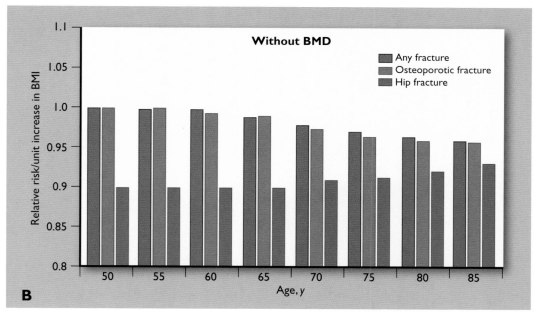

Figure 6-16. Relative fracture risk for any fracture, osteoporotic fracture, and hip fracture per unit increases in body mass index (BMI) by age group with (**A**) and without (**B**) adjustment for bone mineral density (BMD). Men and women were combined for the analyses, as the relative risk/unit changes in BMI were not significantly different for each sex. (*Adapted from* De Laet *et al.* [35].)

Prevalence and Incidence of Vertebral Fracture According to Age Group, the Framingham Study

Age, y	Women		Men	
	Prevalence	Incidence	Prevalence	Incidence
47–50	0.14	0.17	0.09	0.07
51–55	0.14	0.27	0.17	0.11
56–60	0.16	0.26	0.1	0.06
> 60	0.14	0.28	0.1	0.2
Total	0.14	0.24	0.13	0.1

Figure 6-17. The prevalence and incidence of vertebral fractures by age and sex over 25 years are given. (*Adapted from* Samelson *et al.* [36].)

Risk Factors for Osteoporotic Fractures

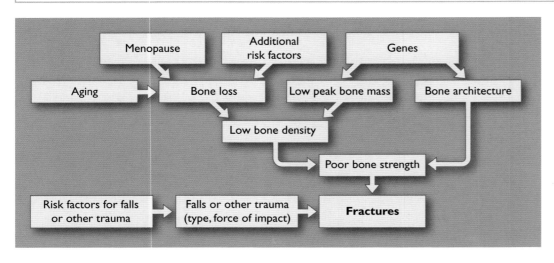

Figure 6-18. Multifactorial determinants of fracture risk are given. (*Adapted from* Cooper and Melton [11].)

Risk Factors for Hip Fracture in Older White Women

Measurement	Approximate increase in hip fracture risk, %
Age (per 5 y)	40
History of maternal hip fracture (vs none)	80
Increase in weight since age 25 (per 20%)	−20
Height at age 25 (per 6 cm)	30
Self-rated health (per 1-point decrease)	60
Previous hyperthyroidism (vs none)	70
Current use of long-acting benzodiazepines (vs no current use)	60
Current use of anticonvulsant (vs no current use)	100
Current caffeine intake (per 190 mg/d)	20
Walking for exercise (vs not walking for exercise)	−30
On feet < 4 h/d (vs > 4 h/d)	70
Inability to rise from a chair (vs no inability)	70
Lowest quartile for distant depth perception (vs other three)	40
Low-frequency contrast sensitivity (per 1-SD decrease)	20
Resting pulse rate > 80 bpm (vs ≤ 80 bpm)	70
Any fracture since age 50 (vs none)	50
Calcaneal BMD (per 1-SD decrease)	60

Figure 6-19. Risk factors for hip fracture in white women and their approximate percentage increase in hip fracture risk are given. BMD—bone mineral density; bpm—beats per minute. (*Adapted from* Cummings *et al.* [12].)

Multivariate Logistic Regression Model: Risk Factors for Hip Fracture in the Women's Health Initiative Observational Study

Risk factors	Odds ratio (95% CI)	P value
Age per each year	1.13 (1.11–1.15)	< 0.001
Self-reported health		
Fair or poor vs excellent	2.38 (1.66–3.40)	< 0.001
Good vs excellent	1.22 (0.90–1.66)	< 0.001
Very good vs excellent	1.11 (0.83–1.49)	< 0.001
Height per each inch	1.11 (1.07–1.16)	< 0.001
Weight per each pound	0.99 (0.98–0.99)	< 0.001
Fracture on or after age 55 y		
Not applicable vs no	1.01 (0.51–2.02)	< 0.001
Yes vs no	1.72 (1.41–2.10)	< 0.001
Race/ethnicity		
Unknown vs white	1.00 (0.47–2.14)	< 0.001
Asian/Pacific Islander vs white	0.26 (0.10–0.70)	< 0.001
American Indian vs white	1.60 (0.50–5.10)	< 0.001
Hispanic vs white	0.32 (0.12–0.86)	< 0.001
Black vs white	0.41 (0.24–0.70)	< 0.001
Physical activity, METs		
5–12 vs ≤ 12	1.32 (1.04–1.67)	0.004
< 5 vs ≤ 12	1.26 (0.97–1.64)	0.004
Inactive 0 vs ≤ 12	1.64 (1.24–2.17)	0.004
Smoking status		
Current vs never	2.33 (1.71–3.18)	< 0.001
Past vs never	0.96 (0.79–1.17)	< 0.001
History		
Parent broke hip, yes vs no	1.50 (1.20–1.87)	< 0.001
Corticosteroid use, yes vs no	1.94 (1.16–3.25)	0.01
Use of hypoglycemic agent, yes vs no	1.74 (1.17–2.60)	0.006

Figure 6-20. Risk factors for the 5-year risk of hip fracture in multiethnic postmenopausal women from the Women's Health Initiative Observational Study is shown. METs—metabolic equivalents. (*Adapted from* Robbins *et al.* [13].)

Multivariable Models of Risk Factors for Nonspine Fracture Including and Excluding BMD in Variable Selection (HR [95% CI])*

Characteristics, *unit*	Model 1: excluding BMD from variable selection	Model 2: model 1 controlling for BMD
Total hip BMD, *g/cm²†*	—	1.53 (1.34–1.74)
Fracture at or after age 50 years	2.35 (1.85–2.99)	2.07 (1.62–2.65)
Age ≥ 80 years	1.51 (1.14–1.99)	1.33 (1.01–1.76)
Any fall in past year	1.56 (1.21–2.02)	1.59 (1.23–2.05)
Use of tricyclic antidepressant	2.39 (1.27–4.51)	2.36 (1.25–4.46)
Unable to complete any narrow walk trial‡	1.80 (1.31–2.47)	1.70 (1.23–2.34)
Depressed mood	1.98 (1.17–3.35)	1.72 (1.00–2.95)

*Models are also controlled for clinical site and race/ethnicity.
†BMD per 1-SD (0.139 g/cm²) decrease.
‡Narrow walk trial reference: able to complete one or more trials.

Figure 6-21. Risk factors for nonvertebral fracture with and without bone mineral density (BMD) adjustment in men are given. HR—hazard ratio. (*Adapted from* Lewis *et al.* [14].)

Measurement (comparison or unit)	Odds ratios and 95% CIs	
	Base MV model	Add radius BMD
Age (+5 y)	1.34 (1.15–1.55)	1.28 (1.11–1.49)
Maternal history of wrist fracture (vs none)	0.10 (0.01–0.69)	0.09 (0.01–0.66)
Paternal history of hip fracture (vs none)	2.27 (1.02–5.07)	2.22 (1.00–4.96)
Milk when pregnant or teen (<1 glass/d)	1.43 (1.05–1.96)	1.42 (1.04–1.94)
Current estrogen user (vs never user)*	0.53 (0.30–0.93)	0.60 (0.33–1.08)
Current smoker (vs never smoked)*	1.70 (1.05–2.76)	1.61 (0.98–2.63)
Walks ≤ 1 block/d and does household chores < 1 h/d	1.59 (1.16–2.18)	1.60 (1.16–2.20)
High to moderate intensity recreational activity (any vs none)	0.54 (0.37–0.80)	0.67 (0.37–0.82)
Use of antacids with aluminum weekly (vs < weekly)	1.54 (1.02–2.36)	1.48 (0.95–2.28)
BMI with knee height quintile 1–2 (vs > 2)†	1.70 (1.25–2.33)	1.53 (1.11–2.08)
One or more falls in first 12 months followup (vs none)	1.71 (1.24–2.35)	1.75 (1.27–2.42)
Nonspine fracture since age 50 (vs none)	1.40 (1.03–1.91)	1.32 (0.96–1.81)
Distal radius BMD (per –1 SD)	—	1.40 (1.17–1.67)

*Models include variables for past estrogen user and past smoking.
†< 258.1 vs ≥ 258.1 kg/m².

Figure 6-22. Risk factors for first vertebral fractures with and without adjustment for bone mineral density (BMD) in women are given. BMI—body mass index; MV—multivariate. (*Adapted from* Nevitt *et al.* [15].)

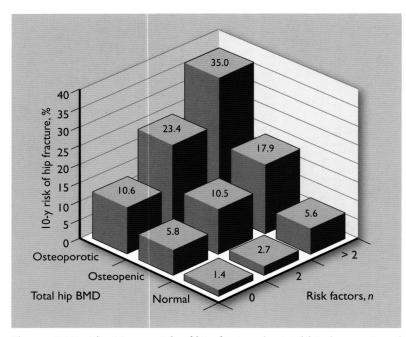

Figure 6-23. The 10-year risk of hip fracture by total hip bone mineral density (BMD) tertile and number of risk factors in women are given. (*Adapted from* Taylor *et al.* [27].)

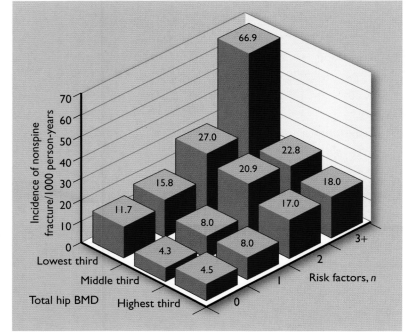

Figure 6-24. Incidence per 1000 person-years of nonvertebral fracture by total hip bone mineral density (BMD) tertile and number of risk factors in men is shown. (*Adapted from* Lewis *et al.* [14].)

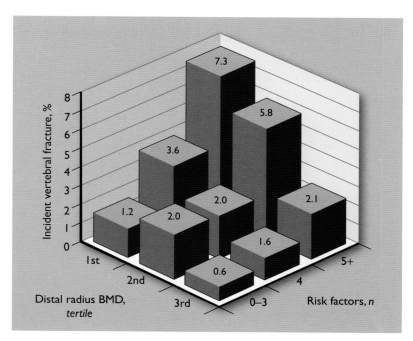

Figure 6-25. Incidence of first radiographic vertebral fracture during 3.7 years of followup by distal radius bone mineral density (BMD) tertile and the number of risk factors in women 65 years of age or older is given. (*Adapted from* Nevitt *et al.* [15].)

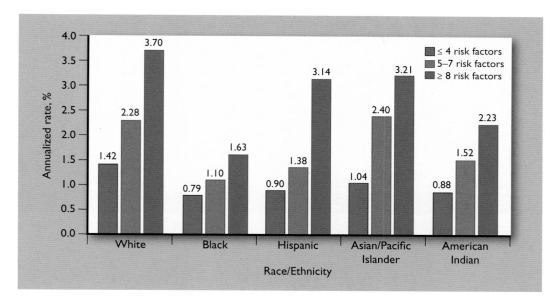

Figure 6-26. The annualized incidence rate of fracture was determined by using the total number of risk factors and ethnicity for postmenopausal women in the Women's Health Initiative. The risk factors included were age greater than 65 years, height greater than 161.9 cm, weight less than 70.5 kg, daily caffeine consumption greater than 188 mg, more than 20 years since menopause, never having used hormone therapy, more than high school education, living without a partner, current smoking, fair or poor health status, fracture at an age of 55 or greater years, arthritis, corticosteroid use for more than 2 years, depression, use of sedatives/anxiolytic, parity 2 or greater, parental history of fracture, and more than 2 falls per year in the last 12 months or the year before the fracture. (*Adapted from* Cauley *et al.* [18].)

RR of Nonspinal Fracture in Black and White Women Per 1-SD Decrease in BMD, BMC, or BMAD

	Black		White	
	RR (95% CI)	AUROC	RR (95% CI)	AUROC
Total hip				
BMD decrease of 1 SD (0.134 g/cm²)				
Age adjusted	1.44 (1.12–1.86)	0.63	1.47 (1.39–1.56)	0.63
Age and body weight adjusted	1.34 (1.01–1.78)	—	1.53 (1.44–1.63)	—
Multivariable adjusted*	1.23 (0.92–1.65)	—	1.42 (1.33–1.52)	—
BMC decrease of 1 SD (6.171 g)				
Age adjusted	1.34 (1.01–1.79)	0.59	1.29 (1.22–1.36)	0.60
Age and body weight adjusted	1.18 (0.85–1.64)	—	1.33 (1.25–1.42)	—
Multivariable adjusted*	1.10 (0.80–1.51)	—	1.25 (1.17–1.35)	—
Femoral neck				
BMD decrease of 1 SD (0.177 g/cm²)				
Age adjusted	1.37 (1.08–1.74)	0.63	1.49 (1.40–1.58)	0.63
Age and body weight adjusted	1.29 (1.00–1.65)	—	1.52 (1.42–1.63)	—
Multivariable adjusted*	1.20 (0.93–1.55)	—	1.42 (1.32–1.52)	—
BMC decrease of 1 SD (0.736 g)				
Age adjusted	1.28 (0.98–1.66)	0.60	1.29 (1.22–1.36)	0.60
Age and body weight adjusted	1.16 (0.88–1.53)	—	1.28 (1.21–1.37)	—
Multivariable adjusted*	1.10 (0.83–1.44)	—	1.20 (1.13–1.29)	—
BMAD decrease of 1 SD (0.034 g/cm²)				
Age adjusted	1.59 (1.16–2.18)	0.64	1.34 (1.26–1.43)	0.61
Age and body weight adjusted	1.50 (1.09–2.07)	—	1.32 (1.24–1.40)	—
Multivariable adjusted*	1.38 (0.99–1.92)	—	1.28 (1.20–1.37)	—

*Multivariable-adjusted model includes age, body weight, height, fracture since age 50 years, walking as form of exercise, current calcium supplement use, current hormone therapy use, alcohol consumption in the past 30 days, diagnosis of osteoarthritis, diagnosis of chronic obstructive pulmonary disease, fallen two or more times in the past year, use arms to stand up from chair, and current smoking.

Figure 6-27. Relative risk (RR) for nonvertebral fractures in black and white women per 1-SD decrease in bone mineral density (BMD), bone mineral content (BMC), or bone mineral apparent density (BMAD) is shown. AUROC—area under the receiver operating characteristic curve. (*Adapted from* Cauley *et al.* [26].)

Risk for Hip and Other Osteoporotic Fractures per SD Change in Risk Score

Age, y	BMD only	Clinical risk factors alone	Clinical risk factors + BMD
Hip fracture			
50	3.68 (2.61–5.19)	2.05 (1.58–2.65)	4.23 (3.12–5.73)
60	3.07 (2.42–3.89)	1.95 (1.63–2.33)	3.51 (2.85–4.33)
70	2.78 (2.39–3.23)	1.84 (1.65–2.05)	2.91 (2.56–3.31)
80	2.28 (2.09–2.50)	1.75 (1.62–1.90)	2.42 (2.18–2.69)
90	1.70 (1.50–1.93)	1.66 (1.47–1.87)	2.02 (1.71–2.38)
Other osteoporotic fractures			
50	1.19 (1.05–1.34)	1.41 (1.28–1.56)	1.44 (1.30–1.59)
60	1.28 (1.18–1.39)	1.48 (1.39–1.58)	1.52 (1.42–1.62)
70	1.39 (1.30–1.48)	1.55 (1.48–1.62)	1.61 (1.54–1.68)
80	1.54 (1.44–1.65)	1.63 (1.54–1.72)	1.71 (1.62–1.80)
90	1.56 (1.40–1.75)	1.72 (1.58–1.88)	1.81 (1.67–1.97)

Figure 6-28. Risk for hip fracture and other osteoporotic fracture per SD change in risk score (with 95% CI) for bone mineral density (BMD), clinical risk factors, or the combination of BMD and clinical risk factors is given. The clinical risk factors included were age, sex, prior fragility fracture after age 50, history of corticosteroid use, parental history of hip fracture, rheumatoid arthritis, secondary osteoporosis, current smoking, alcohol use of more than 2 units daily (a unit is one medium glass of wine or a glass of beer), and body mass index. (*Adapted from* Kanis *et al.* [31].)

Role of Falls and Trauma in Osteoporotic Fracture

Orientation of the Fall, Point of Impact, and Risk of Hip Fracture and Wrist Fracture (vs No Fracture) Among Those Who Fell

Variable, *units*	Odds ratio (95% CIs) for risk of fracture in those who fell*	
	No fracture	Fracture
Hip		
Age (+ 5 y)	1.3 (1.1–1.7)	1.4 (1.1–1.8)
Walking speed (–0.23 m/s)†	1.1	1.0
Fall during stand/turn/transfer (0, 1 = yes)	1.8 (1.1–3.0)	1.4
Fall while descending steps (0, 1 = yes)	1.1	0.9
Fall sideways, straight down (0, 1 = yes)	—	3.3 (2.0–5.6)
Fall on hip/side of leg/buttocks (0, 1 = yes)	—	32.5 (9.9–10)
Wrist‡		
Age (+ 5 y)	1.0	1.1
Walking speed (–0.23 m/s)†	1.0	1.0
Fall while walking/running (0, 1 = yes)	1.3	1.4
Fall backward vs sideways (0, 1 = yes)	—	2.2 (1.3–3.8)
Fall forward vs sideways (0, 1 = yes)	—	0.5 (0.3–0.8)
Fall on hand, wrist (0, 1 = yes)	—	20.4 (11.5–36.0)

*Odds ratios are adjusted for all the other variables in each column plus calcaneus bone density. Confidence limits are shown only for significant odds ratios.
†Odds ratios are for 1-SD decrease.
‡Comparison of subjects who fell and fractured a wrist and those who fell without a fracture. Odds ratios are adjusted for all the other variables in each column plus distal radius bone density.

Figure 6-29. Orientation of the fall, point of impact, and risk of hip and wrist fracture (vs no fracture) in those who fell. White women aged 65 years and older living in the community who suffered hip fractures (*N* = 130) as the result of a fall and a consecutive sample of women who fell without a fracture (*N* = 467) were interviewed about their falls in a case-control study nested in a prospective cohort study, the Study of Osteoporotic Fractures. (*Adapted from* Nevitt *et al.* [37].)

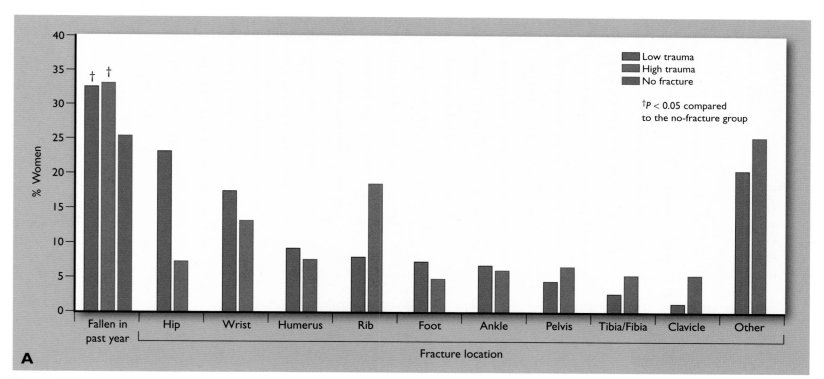

A

Figure 6-30. Prevalence of low- and high-trauma fractures by fall category and fracture location for women (**A**) and men (**B**) is given. Low trauma fractures were defined as those due to: 1) falls from a standing height or less; 2) falls on stairs, steps, or curbs; 3) moderate trauma other than a fall; and 4) minimal trauma other than a fall. High-trauma fractures were defined as those due to severe trauma or falls from greater than a standing height.

Continued on the next page

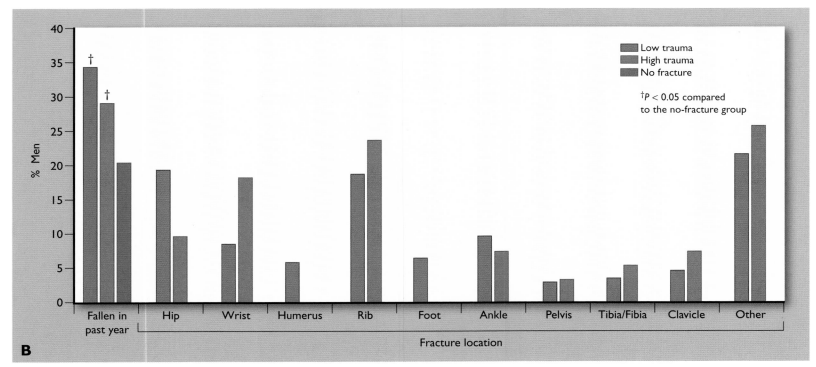

B

Figure 6-30. *(Continued)* Women subjects were from the Study of Osteoporotic Fractures and men subjects were from the Study of Osteoporotic Fractures in Men. The "other" category includes fractures of the skull, face, neck, scapula, shoulder, chest/sternum, elbow, forearm, hand, fingers, tailbone/coccyx/sacrum, femur, patella, toes, heel, hip near prosthesis, knee near prosthesis, and other locations near prosthesis. Each occurred with frequency 8.5% or less in both fracture groups for men and women. *(Adapted from* Mackey *et al.* [20].)

Mortality, Morbidity, and Cost of Osteoporotic Fractures

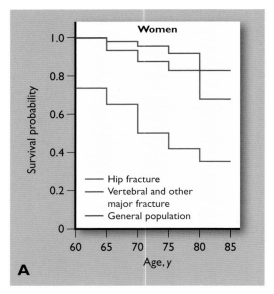

A

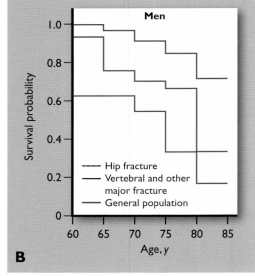

B

Figure 6-31. The cumulative survival probability after fracture by fracture type, age, and sex is listed for women (**A**) and men (**B**). (*Adapted from* Center *et al.* [21].)

Fracture Costs by Fracture Type, Sex, Age, and Race for 2005

Stratus	Costs per fracture type					Total	% of Total
	Hip	Vertebral	Wrist	Pelvic	Other		
Women							
Age, y							
50–64	614	91	130	34	564	1433	8.5
65–74	1045	126	76	67	318	1633	9.7
75–84	3521	253	113	253	461	4601	27.2
≥ 85	4138	193	58	331	410	5129	30.3
Race							
White	8537	573	324	534	1519	11,487	67.9
Black	257	34	19	68	91	469	2.8
Hispanic	291	34	23	55	98	502	3.0
Other	234	21	11	29	44	339	2.0
Total	9319	663	377	686	1752	12,797	75.7
Men							
Age, y							
50–64	263	109	115	34	269	790	4.7
65–74	360	133	22	27	125	667	3.9
75–84	991	101	10	61	129	1292	7.6
≥ 85	1127	71	10	66	95	1370	8.1
Race							
White	2315	355	138	152	503	3464	20.5
Black	151	22	6	10	50	240	1.4
Hispanic	163	21	8	16	45	253	1.5
Other	112	15	5	9	21	162	1.0
Total	2741	414	158	188	619	4119	24.3
Overall Total	**12,060**	**1077**	**535**	**873**	**2372**	**16,916**	**100.0**

Figure 6-32. Health care expenditures (United States dollars in millions) attributable to osteoporotic fracture in the United States by age, race, and type of fracture for women and men are shown. (*Adapted from Burge et al.* [2].)

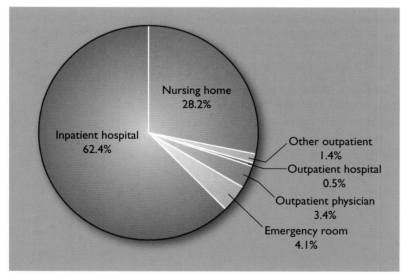

Figure 6-33. Health care expenditures attributable to osteoporotic fracture in the United States by type of health care service are shown. (*Adapted from Ray et al.* [8].)

Aging and Gender

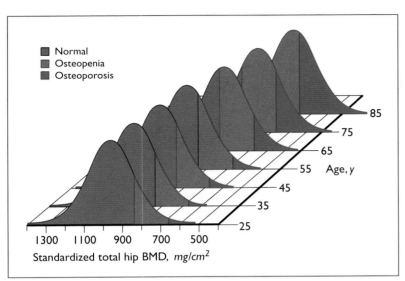

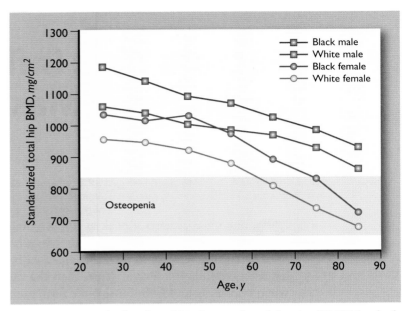

Figure 7-1. Inexorable loss of bone with aging. The normal distribution at age 25 years is the basis for the current World Health Organization definitions of osteoporosis and osteopenia. Whereas less than 1% of young white women have osteoporosis, about 40% of elderly women have bone density in the osteoporotic range. Standardized bone density of the total hip measured by dual-energy x-ray absorptiometry is shown. Although bone mineral density (BMD) is normally distributed at all ages, it gradually declines as age increases. The *green area* shows the proportion of subjects with osteopenia and the *blue area* shows the proportion of women with osteoporosis. (*Data from* Looker *et al.* [1].)

Figure 7-2. Standardized total hip bone mineral density (BMD) by dual-energy x-ray absorptiometry showing the average values for black and white men and women. Both genders and races show bone loss with aging. (*Data from* Looker *et al* [1].)

Clinical Factors that Affect Bone Mass

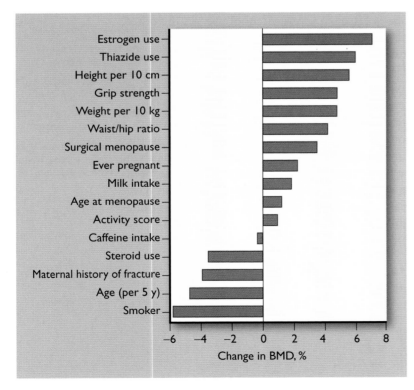

Figure 7-3. Baseline data from the 9704 women in the Study of Osteoporotic Fractures. The subjects were ambulatory women older than 65 years; most were white. The percentage difference in the bone mineral density (BMD) is shown, comparing women who had a risk factor to the group's mean BMD (in the case of categorical variables). For continuous variables, the graph shows the difference in bone density for approximately 1 standard deviation change in the variable. For example, on average, a woman who uses thiazide diuretics has bone density 6% higher than one who does not use thiazides. Similarly, the average BMD decreased about 5% for every 5-year increase in age. (*Data from* Bauer *et al.* [2].)

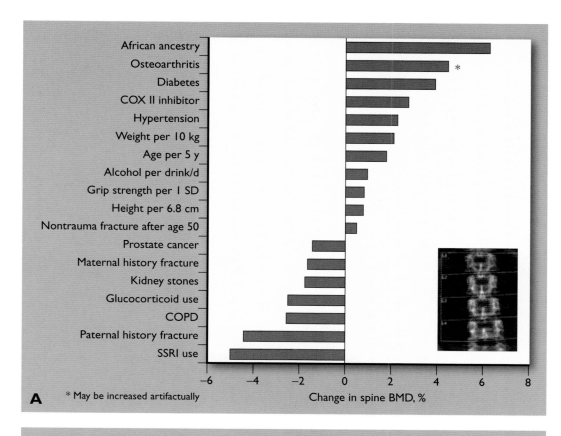

A * May be increased artifactually

Change in spine BMD, %

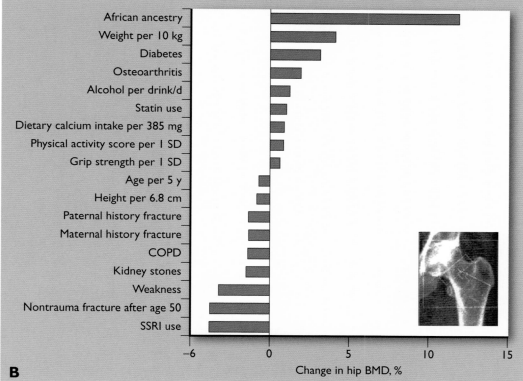

B

Change in hip BMD, %

Figure 7-4. Cross-sectional analyses from the Mr Os study of 5995 men who were older than 65 years is shown. The study was similar to the Study of Osteoporotic Fractures, shown in Figure 7-3. The independent risk factors for bone density are shown for the spine (**A**) and hip (**B**). Only 4% of the men were current cigarette smokers, so it was difficult to evaluate smoking as a risk factor for low bone mineral density (BMD). Osteoarthritis was positively associated with spine and hip bone density; some of this might reflect artifactual errors in measuring with dual energy absorptiometry. COPD—chronic obstructive pulmonary disease; COX—cyclooxygenase; SSRI—selective serotonin reuptake inhibitor. (*Data from* Cauley *et al.* [3].)

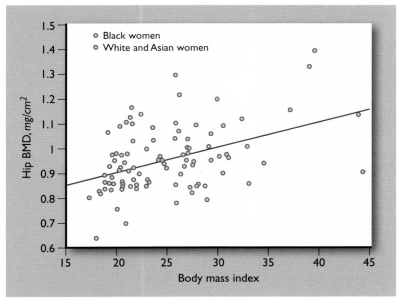

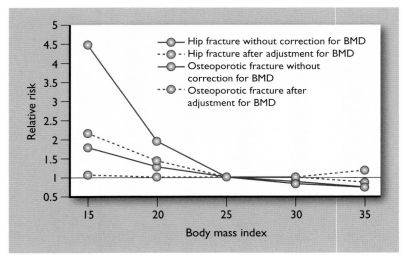

Figure 7-5. Weight is one of the most important factors related to bone mass. The relationship between body mass index (BMI) and total hip bone mineral density (BMD) is shown, measured by dual-energy x-ray absorptiometry (DEXA), in normal women aged 18 to 40 years. Weight itself is even more strongly correlated to the bone density, but weight is related to both fatness and body size. The DEXA measures the amount of mineral within a projected area; thus, bones that are larger will have greater BMD, even when the actual bone density (in three dimensions) is the same. In part, the BMI reflects the contribution of body fat, which may be related to leptin levels. (*Data from* Scholes *et al.* [4].)

Figure 7-6. Relative risk of hip fracture or an osteoporotic fracture, according to the body mass index (BMI). The reference group had a BMI of 25. At low BMI, the risk of fracture went up steeply. The dashed lines show relative risks after adjusting for the bone density and solid lines are without adjustment. These results indicate that some of the risk is independent of bone density, especially at very low BMI. The data are from an international meta-analysis of 58,000 men and women from 12 cohorts. (*Data from* De Laet *et al.* [5].)

Nutritional Factors

Figure 7-7. Protein intake and bone loss in elderly men and women. Evidence suggests that protein undernutrition may be associated with osteoporotic fractures. In contrast, evidence also exists that diets rich in animal protein may actually result in negative calcium balance, which would result in accelerated bone loss. These considerations notwithstanding, there have been few longitudinal studies of protein intake and bone loss among older persons, who may be consuming less protein than the high amounts previously linked to negative calcium balance. Such an evaluation was recently completed as part of the Framingham Osteoporosis Study. Four-year longitudinal data on dietary intake and bone mineral density (BMD) were collected on 391 women and 274 men who were members of the original Framingham Heart Study. Both men and women in the lowest quartile (Q) of protein intake had greater losses of bone mass at the femoral neck than did those in the highest quartile of protein intake. This was true after adjustment for multiple covariates including age, weight, cigarette

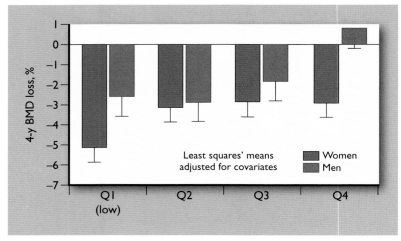

smoking, caffeine intake, calcium intake, physical activity, alcohol consumption, and estrogen-replacement therapy in women. (*Adapted from* Hannan *et al.* [6].)

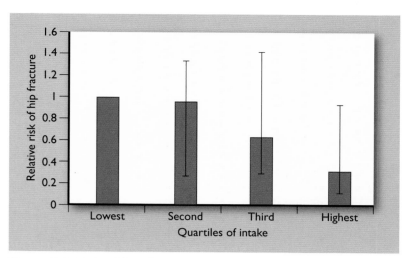

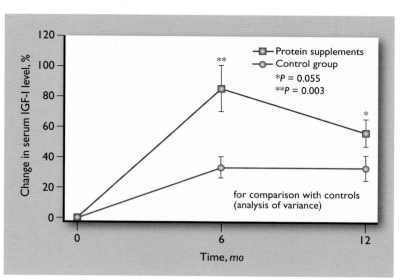

Figure 7-8. Risk of hip fracture according to animal protein intake in postmenopausal women. Data are from a study of 104,338 person-years, showing the 95% confidence intervals using a multivariate model that included body size. (*Data from* Munger et al. [7].)

Figure 7-9. Protein supplementation in patients with hip fracture improves bone mass. Protein restriction has been shown to reduce plasma levels of insulin-like growth factor-I (IGF-I) by inducing resistance to the action of growth hormone in the liver and increasing the metabolic clearance rate of the growth factor. Thus, low protein intake in elderly persons, such as those recovering from hip fracture, may be detrimental to skeletal health. In a recent randomized controlled trial of a protein supplement given to patients recuperating from hip fracture (*n* = 41 treated; 41 in the control group), supplements increased IGF-I levels significantly and slowed the loss of bone mineral density compared with placebo. The *circles* represent patients who received protein supplements and the *squares* represent patients in the control group. (*Adapted from* Schurch et al. [8].)

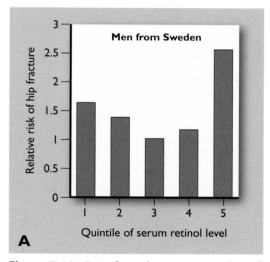

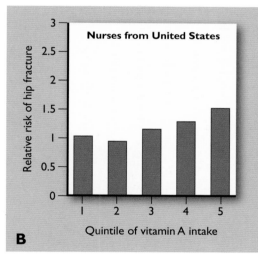

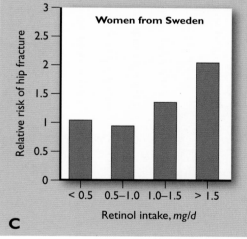

Figure 7-10. Data from three recent studies of vitamin A intake. **A**, Data from 2322 Swedish men. There was a significant increase in the relative risk of hip fracture in those with the highest quintile of serum retinol. **B**, Results from a study of 72,337 American nurses, who had a higher risk of hip fracture with greater vitamin A intake. **C**, Data from 175 Swedish women, in whom the highest quartile of retinol intake was associated with a higher risk of hip fracture. A fourth recent study (*not shown*) from Rancho Bernardo [9] showed that bone mineral density in elderly men and women was related to vitamin A intake in a U-shaped curve; both deficiency and excess were associated with lower bone mass. The best bone mineral density was seen at the recommended intake of vitamin A. (*Data from* Michaelsson et al. [10], Feskanich et al. [11], and Melhus et al. [12].)

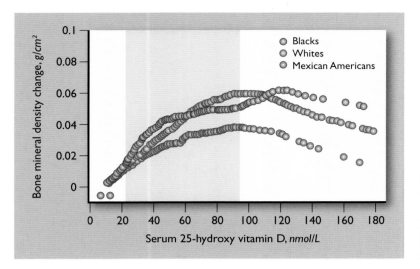

Figure 7-11. Regression plot of bone mineral density by 25-hydroxy vitamin D level in older adults (> 50 y). *Green circles* represent whites, *red circles* represent Mexican Americans, and *blue circles* represent blacks. 100 nmol/L = 40 ng/mL. The shaded area represents the reference range for the Diasorin assay (9–38 ng/mL). The intercept was set to 0 for all racial–ethnic groups. (*Data from* Bischoff-Ferrari *et al.* [13].)

Smoking, Alcohol, and Bone

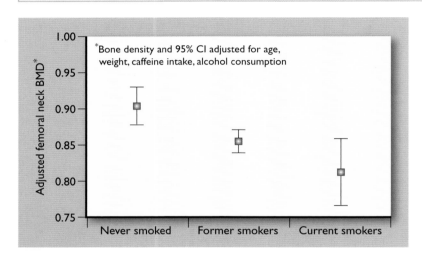

Figure 7-12. Deleterious effects of smoking cigarettes on the skeleton in men. In men, cigarette smoking clearly results in lower bone mineral density (BMD). In this study of 348 elderly men, current smokers had lower BMD at the femoral neck than those who did not smoke. (*Adapted from* Kiel *et al.* [14].)

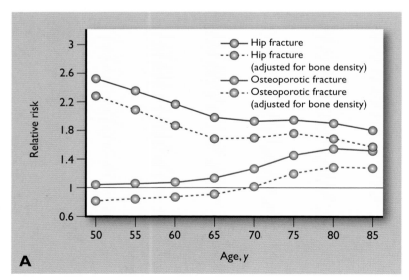

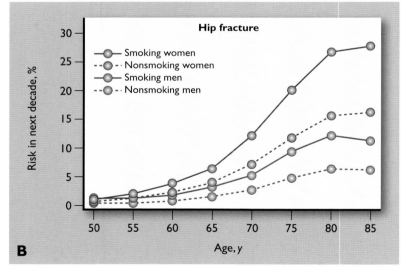

Figure 7-13. A, Relative risk of an osteoporotic or hip fracture in men and women who smoke cigarettes, compared to those who do not smoke. The solid lines are the risk without adjustment for bone density and the dashed lines show the attenuation when bone density is taken into account. **B,** The absolute risk of a fracture in men and women who smoke versus nonsmokers, using the same data as in **A** and calculating the risks based on the fracture prevalence in Sweden [15] and the proportion of smokers in each age range. These results are from an international meta-analysis of 59,232 men and women from 10 prospective cohorts. (*Data from* Kanis *et al.* [16].)

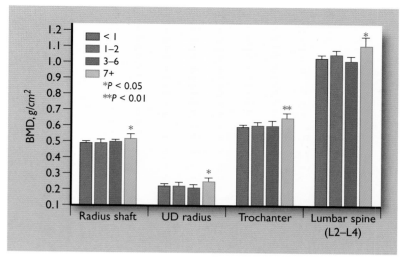

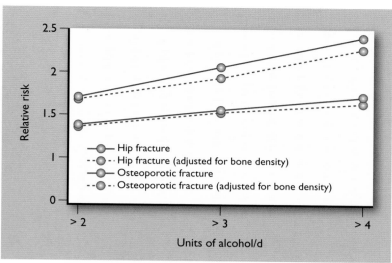

Figure 7-14. Moderate alcohol intake is associated with increased bone mineral density (BMD). Although alcoholics suffer from osteoporosis and increased risk of fracture, consuming less alcohol may favorably impact the skeletal status of women. One mechanism for this may be the recognized effects of alcohol on increasing endogenous estrogen levels or even adrenal androgen levels. In this study of 384 women, BMD was higher in those who drank at least 7 oz/wk of alcohol than in those who drank less than 1 oz/wk. This difference was not explained by differences in age, weight, height, age at menopause, smoking cigarettes, and years of estrogen replacement therapy, which were adjusted for in this analysis. UD—ultradistal. (*Adapted from* Felson *et al.* [17].)

Figure 7-15. International meta-analysis of the effect of alcohol on fractures. Three cohorts including 16,971 men and women were prospectively studied; the risk for osteoporotic fractures (*green circles*) and hip fractures (*red circles*) are shown. Solid lines are not adjusted and the dashed lines are adjusted for bone density. Unlike smoking and BMI, the relative risk was greater when adjusting for the bone density, because alcohol increases bone density as well as fracture risk. Risks are shown, comparing those who drink more than two, three, or four units of alcohol with those drinking less than that amount. One unit of alcohol is 8 grams. A "standard drink" is 14 grams, corresponding to one glass of wine, one can of beer, or about 1 ounce of spirits. (*Data from* Kanis *et al.* [18].)

Pregnancy and Contraception

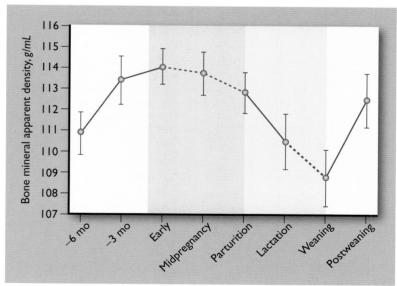

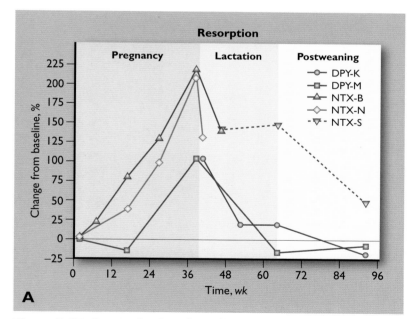

Figure 7-16. Longitudinal study of bone mineral density (BMD) in a primate model. BMD in the spine, measured by dual-energy x-ray absorptiometry and adjusted for three dimensions to avoid size artifact, is shown. The young animals in the study were still growing (analogous to adolescent humans). During pregnancy (*dark shading*), BMD stopped increasing and began to show a loss. Lactation (*light shading*) was associated with a significant decrease in bone density, which promptly recovered after weaning. Bone biopsies were done at the middle of pregnancy and at weaning, which demonstrated a reduced bone-formation rate at midpregnancy and an increased bone formation at weaning. (*Adapted from* Ott *et al.* [19].)

Figure 7-17. Longitudinal studies of human pregnancy and lactation. All the data have been converted to percent change from baseline. In the studies that began after delivery, the baseline from one of the studies of pregnancy was used. **A,** Markers of bone resorption. During the first trimester of pregnancy, bone resorption increased a small amount; it increased to very high levels during the last trimester. Resorption remained high during early lactation and then started to decline. After weaning, resorption returns to baseline levels.

Continued on the next page

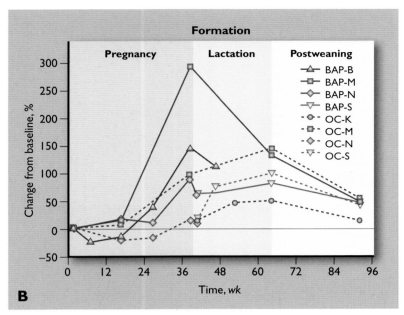

B

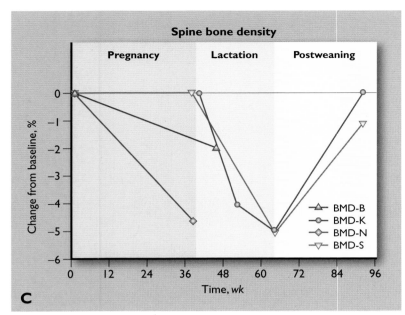

C

Figure 7-17. *(Continued)* **B,** Markers of bone formation. These values are unchanged or depressed during the first half of pregnancy and then start to increase. The data on bone alkaline phosphatase during lactation are variable, but all studies show a return toward baseline following weaning. **C,** Bone mineral density (BMD) of the spine by dual-energy x-ray absorptiometry.

Studies during pregnancy are variable, but losses during lactation approach 1% per month. As in the primate study, rapid recovery is seen after weaning. BAP—bone alkaline phosphatase; DPY—deoxypyridinoline; OC—osteocalcin; NTX—N-telopeptide. (*Data from* studies by Black *et al.* [20], Sowers *et al.* [21–23], Kalkwarf *et al.* [24,25], More *et al.* [26], and Naylor *et al.* [27].)

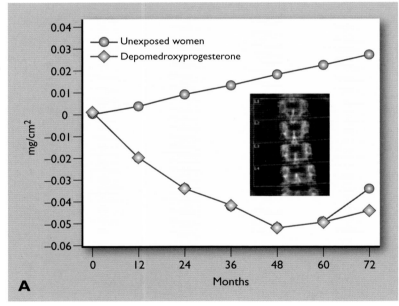

A

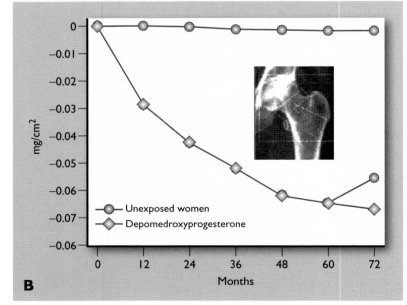

B

Figure 7-18. Loss of bone density at the spine (**A**) and hip (**B**) in young women using depomedroxyprogesterone acetate (*diamonds*) for contraception. Unexposed women (*circles*) had stable bone density at the hip and increasing bone density at the spine. These are calculated from a longitudinal study giving rates of loss every 6 months for women using this

contraception, adjusted for age, race, baseline bone density, and several risk factors. Bone loss was most rapid in those who were just beginning the medication. After discontinuation, the bone density increased (shown between 60 and 72 months). (*Data from* Scholes *et al.* [4].)

References

1. Looker AC, Wahner HW, Dunn WL, *et al.*: Updated data on proximal femur bone mineral levels of US adults. *Osteoporos Int* 1998, 8:468–489.

2. Bauer DC, Browner WS, Cauley JA, *et al.*: Factors associated with appendicular bone mass in older women. The Study of Osteoporotic Fractures Research Group. *Ann Intern Med* 1993, 118:657–665.

3. Cauley JA, Fullman RL, Stone KL, *et al.*: Factors associated with the lumbar spine and proximal femur bone mineral density in older men. *Osteoporos Int* 2005, 16:1525–1537.

4. Scholes D, LaCroix AZ, Ichikawa LE, *et al.*: Injectable hormone contraception and bone density: results from a prospective study. *Epidemiology* 2002, 13:581–587.

5. De Laet C, Kanis JA, Oden A, *et al.*: Body mass index as a predictor of fracture risk: a meta-analysis. *Osteoporos Int* 2005, 16:1330–1338.

6. Hannan M, Dawson-Hughes B, Felson D, Kiel D: Effect of dietary protein on bone loss in elderly men and women: the Framingham Osteoporosis Study. *J Bone Miner Res* 1997, 12:S151.

7. Munger RG, Cerhan JR, Chiu BC: Prospective study of dietary protein intake and risk of hip fracture in postmenopausal women. *Am J Clin Nutr* 1999, 69:147–152.

8. Schurch MA, Rissoli R, Slosman D, *et al.*: Protein supplements increase serum insulin-like growth factor-I levels and attenuate proximal femur bone loss in patients with recent hip fracture: a randomized, double-blind, placebo-controlled trial. *Ann Intern Med* 1998, 128:801–809.

9. Promislow JH, Goodman-Gruen D, Slymen DJ, Barrett-Connor E: Retinol intake and bone mineral density in the elderly: the Rancho Bernardo Study. *J Bone Miner Res* 2002, 17:1349–1358.

10. Michaelsson K, Lithell H, Vessby B, Melhus H: Serum retinol levels and the risk of fracture. *N Engl J Med* 2003, 348:287–294.

11. Feskanich D, Singh V, Willett WC, Colditz GA: Vitamin A intake and hip fractures among postmenopausal women. *JAMA* 2002, 287:47–54.

12. Melhus H, Michaelsson K, Kindmark A, *et al.*: Excessive dietary intake of vitamin A is associated with reduced bone mineral density and increased risk for hip fracture. *Ann Intern Med* 1998, 129:770–778.

13. Bischoff-Ferrari HA, Dietrich T, Orav EJ, Dawson-Hughes B: Positive association between 25-hydroxy vitamin D levels and bone mineral density: a population-based study of younger and older adults. *Am J Med* 2004, 116:634–639.

14. Kiel DP, Zhang Y, Hannan MT, *et al.*: The effect of smoking at different life stages on bone mineral density in elderly men and women. *Osteoporos Int* 1996, 6:240–248.

15. Kanis JA, Johnell O, Oden A, *et al.*: Ten year probabilities of osteoporotic fractures according to BMD and diagnostic thresholds. *Osteoporos Int* 2001, 12:989–995.

16. Kanis JA, Johnell O, Oden A, *et al.*: Smoking and fracture risk: a meta-analysis. *Osteoporos Int* 2005, 16:155–162.

17. Felson DT, Zhang Y, Hannan MT, *et al.*: Alcohol intake and bone mineral density in elderly men and women: the Framingham Study. *Am J Epidemiol* 1995, 142:485–492.

18. Kanis JA, Johansson H, Johnell O, *et al.*: Alcohol intake as a risk factor for fracture. *Osteoporos Int* 2005, 16:737–742.

19. Ott SM, Lipkin EW, Newell-Morris L: Bone physiology during pregnancy and lactation in young macaques. *J Bone Miner Res* 1999, 14:1779–1788.

20. Black AJ, Topping J, Durham B, *et al.*: A detailed assessment of alterations in bone turnover, calcium homeostasis, and bone density in normal pregnancy. *J Bone Miner Res* 2000, 15:557–563.

21. Sowers M, Crutchfield M, Jannausch M, *et al.*: A prospective evaluation of bone mineral change in pregnancy. *Obstet Gynecol* 1991, 77:841–845.

22. Sowers M, Corton G, Shapiro B, *et al.*: Changes in bone density with lactation. *JAMA* 1993, 269:3130–3135.

23. Sowers M, Eyre D, Hollis BW, *et al.*: Biochemical markers of bone turnover in lactating and nonlactating postpartum women. *J Clin Endocrinol Metab* 1995, 80:2210–2216.

24. Kalkwarf HJ, Specker BL, Bianchi DC, *et al.*: The effect of calcium supplementation on bone density during lactation and after weaning. *N Engl J Med* 1997, 337:523–528.

25. Kalkwarf HJ, Specker BL, Ho M: Effects of calcium supplementation on calcium homeostasis and bone turnover in lactating women. *J Clin Endocrinol Metab* 1999, 84:464–470.

26. More C, Bhattoa HP, Bettembuk P, Balogh A: The effects of pregnancy and lactation on hormonal status and biochemical markers of bone turnover. *Eur J Obstet Gynecol Reprod Biol* 2003, 106:209–213.

27. Naylor KE, Iqbal P, Fledelius C, *et al.*: The effect of pregnancy on bone density and bone turnover. *J Bone Miner Res* 2000, 15:129–137.

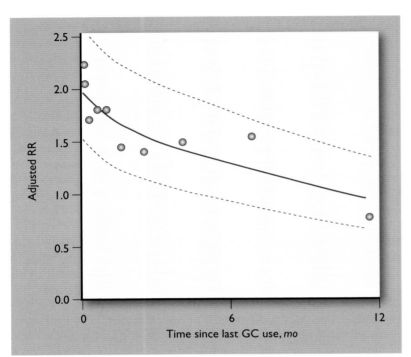

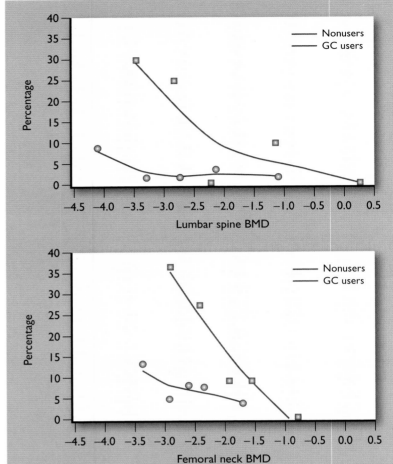

Figure 8-7. Relative risk (RR) of fracture in patients receiving high-dose (≥ 15 mg/d) oral glucocorticoids (GCs) according to the amount of time since discontinuation. This study from the General Practice Research Database also analyzed the duration of offset of the adverse fracture effects of oral GCs. It was found that the risk of fracture was not increased in patients who had stopped receiving high-dose oral GCs more than 12 months previously. (*Data from* de Vries *et al.* [14].)

Figure 8-8. Incidence of vertebral fracture in glucocorticoid (GC) users (*green line*) and nonusers (*red line*) by baseline lumbar spine (*top*) and femoral neck (*bottom*) bone mineral density (BMD). The individual data points correspond to the incidence in subgroups of the GC and nonuse populations, as based on quintiles of baseline BMD; the lines represent a curve smoothing these individual estimates.

This study used data from the placebo groups of randomized clinical trials in fracture prevention. In patients using oral GCs, the rate of incident vertebral fractures was higher at each level of BMD in women using oral GCs as compared to women in other trials not using oral GCs. This study supports earlier findings that the BMD threshold for fracture risk appears to be different in oral GC users. (*Data from* van Staa *et al.* [15].)

Figure 8-9. Risk of hip fracture associated with the ever-increasing use of glucocorticoids (GCs) according to age, with and without bone mineral density (BMD). Kanis *et al.* [7] analyzed data from seven large prospectively studied cohorts and found that previous oral GC use was associated with a significantly increased risk of fracture, including hip fracture. Adjusting for BMD did not change the results substantially. There was no difference in the relative risk (RR) of fracture between men and women, but there was a trend for higher RRs in younger users. The authors concluded that oral GCs confer an increased risk of fracture that is of substantial importance beyond what is explained by BMD. (*Data from* Kanis *et al.* [7].)

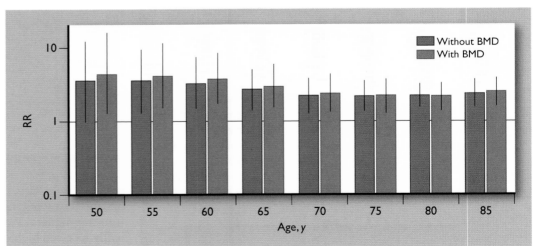

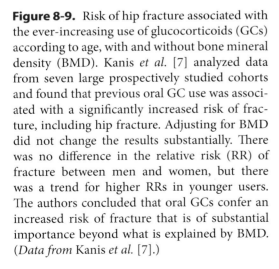

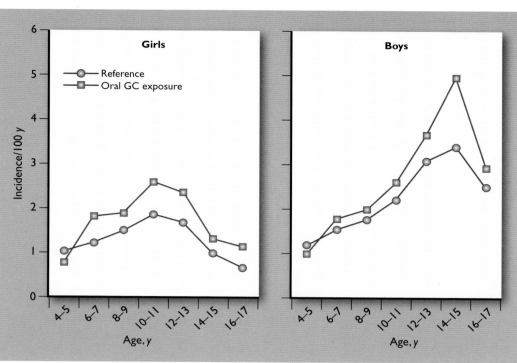

Figure 8-10. Incidence of fractures in children using oral glucocorticoids (GCs) and control children stratified by age and gender [16]. Children frequently use oral GCs, often at high doses for short periods of time (> 1% of the children in the United Kingdom receive a course of GC therapy during any 1-year period). A large study in the General Practice Research Database found that the risk of fracture was increased in children with a history of frequent use of oral GCs; children who received four or more courses of oral GCs had an adjusted odds ratio for fracture of 1.32 (95% CI: 1.03–1.69). Children who stopped taking oral GCs had a comparable risk of fracture to those in the control group. van Staa et al. [16] concluded that children who require more than four courses of oral GC as treatment for underlying disease are at increased risk of fracture. It is reassuring, to some extent, that the sporadic use of high doses of oral GCs was not associated with an increased risk of fracture in children and that children who stopped using oral GCs also sustained no increased risk. However, children who used oral GCs regularly had an increased risk of fracture and it is this group that probably needs attention with respect to the adverse effects on the bone. (*Data from* van Staa et al. [16].)

Figure 8-11. Overview of the data available from studies on the impact of inhaled glucocorticoids on bone mineral density (BMD) [2]. The objective of this meta-analysis was to analyze the effects of inhaled glucocorticoids (GCs) on BMD, fracture risk, and bone turnover markers, including a systematic search for randomized trials or observational studies. It was found that patients using inhaled GCs had lower BMD as compared to controls. These effects were found both in studies that compared inhaled GC users with respiratory disease to healthy controls, as well as those comparing them to diseased control patients. This review was not just limited to randomized trials, but also included epidemiological studies. One of the challenges of epidemiological research is to find a comparable control group. This review clearly found that inhaled GC users have lower BMD. But is this finding related to the direct systemic effects of inhaled GCs or to underlying disease severity? BDP—beclomethasone dipropionate; BUD—budesonide; FN—femorral neck; FN TCA—femoral neck triamcinolone acetonide; LS—lumbar spine; LS FLU—lumbar spine fluticasone; LS TCA—lumbar spine triamcinolone acetonide; troch—trochanter. (*Data from* Richy et al. [2].)

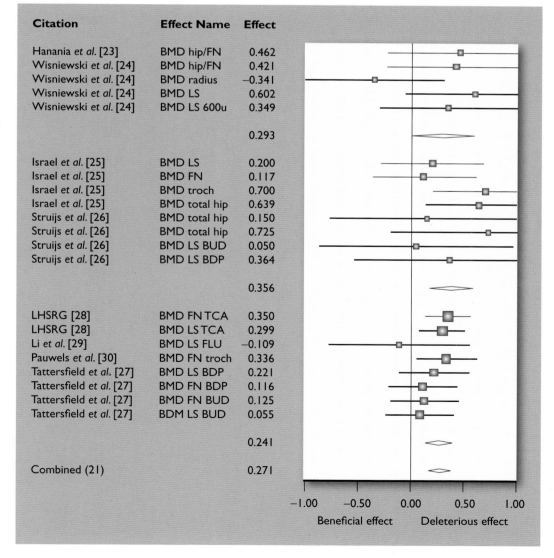

Citation	Effect Name	Effect
Hanania et al. [23]	BMD hip/FN	0.462
Wisniewski et al. [24]	BMD hip/FN	0.421
Wisniewski et al. [24]	BMD radius	−0.341
Wisniewski et al. [24]	BMD LS	0.602
Wisniewski et al. [24]	BMD LS 600u	0.349
		0.293
Israel et al. [25]	BMD LS	0.200
Israel et al. [25]	BMD FN	0.117
Israel et al. [25]	BMD troch	0.700
Israel et al. [25]	BMD total hip	0.639
Struijs et al. [26]	BMD total hip	0.150
Struijs et al. [26]	BMD total hip	0.725
Struijs et al. [26]	BMD LS BUD	0.050
Struijs et al. [26]	BMD LS BDP	0.364
		0.356
LHSRG [28]	BMD FN TCA	0.350
LHSRG [28]	BMD LS TCA	0.299
Li et al. [29]	BMD LS FLU	−0.109
Pauwels et al. [30]	BMD FN troch	0.336
Tattersfield et al. [27]	BMD LS BDP	0.221
Tattersfield et al. [27]	BMD FN BDP	0.116
Tattersfield et al. [27]	BMD FN BUD	0.125
Tattersfield et al. [27]	BDM LS BUD	0.055
		0.241
Combined (21)		0.271

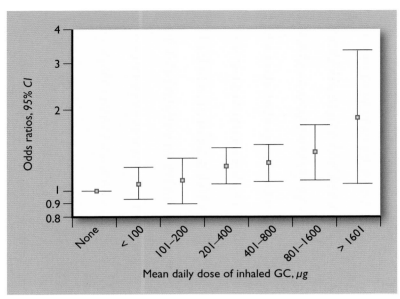

Figure 8-12. Association between the average daily dose of inhaled glucocorticoids (GCs) and the risk of hip fracture [17]. This large case-control study used the medical records of general practitioners in England and Wales. The risk of hip fracture was increased in patients using inhaled GCs as compared to those not using inhaled GCs. There was a strong dose-response relationship between inhaled GC use and hip fracture even after adjusting for the annual number of courses of oral GCs. The authors concluded that the use of inhaled GCs is associated with a dose-related increase in hip fracture in older subjects. The dose response in this study was similar to that reported in an earlier study that used the same data source [18]. Interestingly, the conclusions with respect to the cause of this increased risk differed between the two studies. The earlier study had found that patients who used other asthma drugs (such as β-agonists) also had increased risks of fracture and that, overall, there was no difference between users of inhaled GC and other asthma drugs [18]. (*Data from* Hubbard *et al.* [17].)

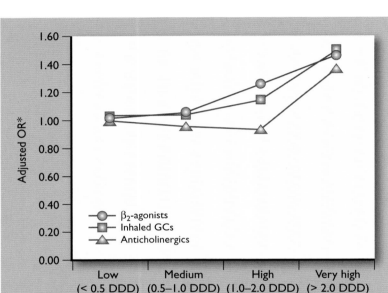

Figure 8-13. Risk of hip fracture among current users of β_2-agonists, inhaled glucocorticoids (GCs), or inhaled anticholinergics stratified by the average daily dose. The defined daily dose (DDD) of 1 is equivalent to 800 μg inhaled salbutamol, 800 μg inhaled beclomethasone dipropionate, or 120 μg ipratropriumbromide.

A Dutch case-control analysis of over 6700 patients hospitalized for hip fracture [19] found that patients using higher doses of β_2-agonists had increased risks of hip fracture (crude odds ratio [OR] 1.94 [95% CI 1.41–2.66]) for daily dosages of ≥ 1600 μg salbutamol equivalent. The excess fracture risk was reduced after adjustment for disease severity (adjusted OR 1.46; 95% CI, 1.02–2.08) and after the exclusion of oral GC users (adjusted OR 1.31; 95% CI, 0.80–2.15). Interestingly, the dose response with hip fracture was similar between inhaled GCs, β_2-agonists, and anticholinergics. These findings suggest the severity of the underlying disease, rather than the use of β_2-agonists or inhaled GCs, may play an important role in the etiology of hip fractures. (*Data from* de Vries *et al.* [19].)

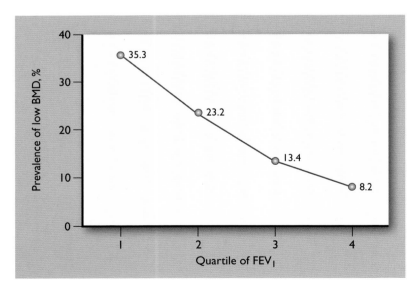

Figure 8-14. Prevalence of low bone mineral density (BMD) stratified by quartile of forced expiratory volume in 1 second (FEV_1). In this cross-sectional study [20], the relationship between hip BMD and respiratory function was examined in women from the general community, including 4830 women 45 to 76 years old. Hip BMD was significantly and positively correlated with respiratory function (FEV_1). This association was independent of age, weight, height, smoking habit, history of respiratory diseases, and use of hormone replacement therapy and oral glucocorticoids (GCs). Women in the lowest quartile as compared to the top quartile of respiratory function had about double the risk of low BMD. There are various plausible mechanisms that may be responsible for an increased risk of osteoporosis and fractures in patients with obstructive airway disease. Patients with obstructive airway disease may have reduced physical activity. Cigarette smoking could also explain this relation, as it is a major cause of airway disease and may also have negative effects on BMD. The adverse effects of hypoxia and of the ongoing inflammatory processes may also play a role. (*Adapted from* Lekamwasam *et al.* [20].)

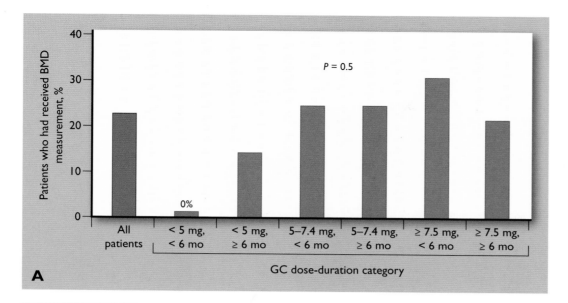

A

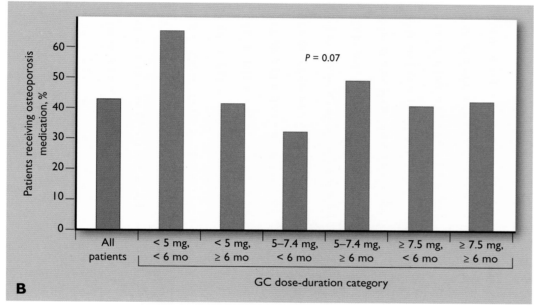

B

Figure 8-15. Management of corticosteroid-induced osteoporosis: is there room for improvement? The study by Solomon *et al.* [21] examined the medical charts of patients in a United States academic rheumatology practice who were taking oral glucocorticoids (GCs). **A,** The rates of bone densitometry during the 2-year study period for patients in each dosage-duration category are shown. Overall, 23% of the patients underwent bone densitometry. **B,** Rate of prescription medication use. Less than half the patients were prescribed a medication for osteoporosis, including hormone therapy. These data support other literature, which suggest suboptimal management of GC-induced osteoporosis. Although the quality of care may be improving, more recently the challenge has been to further improve the prevention of GC-induced fractures and to find the best way to do so. (*Data from* Solomon *et al.* [21].)

Challenges for Improving Osteoporosis Care for Long-Term Glucocorticoid Users

Variable	Intervention group	Control group	Rate difference (95% CI)	P Value
BMD testing	19	21	−2 (−8 to 4)	0.48
Bisphosphonate prescribing	25	22	3 (−2 to 8)	0.28
Any osteoporosis medication prescribing†	32	29	3 (−3 to 9)	0.34
BMD testing or osteoporosis medication prescribing	49	50	−1 (−8 to 5)	0.72

Data are given as a percentage unless otherwise indicated.
†Includes bisphosphonates, estrogens, calcitonin, raloxifene hydrochloride, and tenparatide.

Figure 8-16. Challenges in improving the quality of osteoporosis care for long-term glucocorticoid users. The results of a randomized trial comparing educational intervention with no intervention are shown [22]. This study was conducted to improve the widespread undertreatment for GC-induced osteoporosis. Physicians frequently prescribing oral GCs were identified and randomized to receive a Web-based training course specific for GC-induced osteoporosis or a control course focusing on chronic illness in general. It was found that training in GC-induced osteoporosis had no effect on the rate of bone mineral testing or osteoporosis medication prescribing. Innovative strategies that promote appropriate management of GC-induced osteoporosis continue to be needed to improve the quality of osteoporosis care. BMD—bone mineral density.

References

1. Jones A, Fay JK, Burr M, *et al.*: Inhaled corticosteroid effects on bone metabolism in asthma and mild chronic obstructive pulmonary disease (Cochrane review). In *The Cochrane Library,* issue 3. Oxford, UK: Update Software; 2003.

2. Richy F, Bousquet J, Ehrlich GE: Inhaled corticosteroids effects on bone in asthmatic and COPD patients: a quantitative systematic review. *Osteoporos Int* 2003, 14:179–190.

3. American College of Rheumatology Ad Hoc Committee on Glucocorticoid-Induced Osteoporosis: Recommendations for the prevention and treatment of glucocorticoid-induced osteoporosis. *Arthritis Rheum* 2001, 44:1496–1503.

4. Royal College of Physicians: *Glucocorticoid-Induced Osteoporosis: Guidelines for Prevention and Treatment*. London: Royal College of Physicians; 2002.

5. van Staa TP: Glucocorticoid-induced osteoporosis. *Calcif Tissue Int* 2006, 79:129–137.

6. van Staa TP, Leufkens HGM, Abenhaim L, *et al.*: Use of oral corticosteroids and risk of fractures. *J Bone Miner Res* 2000, 15:993–1000.

7. Kanis JA, Johansson H, Oden A, *et al.*: A meta-analysis of prior corticosteroid use and fracture risk. *J Bone Miner Res* 2004, 19:893–899.

8. Steinbuch M, Youket TE, Cohen S: Oral glucocorticoid use is associated with an increased risk of fracture. *Osteoporos Int* 2004, 15:323–328.

9. van Staa TP, Leufkens HGM, Cooper C: The epidemiology of corticosteroid-induced osteoporosis: a meta-analysis. *Osteoporos Int* 2002, 13:777–787.

10. Vestergaard P, Olsen ML, Paaske Johnsen S, *et al.*: Corticosteroid use and risk of hip fracture: a population-based case-control study in Denmark. *J Intern Med* 2003, 254:486–493.

11. van Staa TP, Geusens P, Pols HA, *et al.*: A simple score for estimating the long-term risk of fracture in patients using oral glucocorticoids. *QJM* 2005, 98:191–198.

12. Ton FN, Gunawardene SC, Lee H, Neer RM: Effects of low-dose prednisone on bone metabolism. *J Bone Miner Res* 2005, 20:464–470.

13. Laan RFJM, van Riel PLCM, van de Putte LBA, *et al.*: Low-dose prednisone induses rapid reversible axial bone loss in patients with rheumatoid arthritis. *Ann Intern Med* 1993, 119:963–968.

14. de Vries F, Bracke M, Leufkens HG, *et al.*: Fracture risk with intermittent high-dose oral glucocorticoid therapy. *Arthritis Rheum* 2007, 56:208–217.

15. van Staa TP, Laan RF, Barton I, *et al.*: Predictors and bone density threshold for vertebral fracture in patients using oral glucocorticoids. *Arthritis Rheum* 2003, 48:3224–3229.

16. van Staa TP, Cooper C, Leufkens HGM, *et al.*: Children and the risk of fractures caused by oral corticosteroids. *J Bone Miner Res* 2003, 18:913–918.

17. Hubbard RB, Smith CJP, Smeeth L, *et al.*: Inhaled corticosteroids and hip fracture: a population-based case-control study. *Am J Respir Crit Care Med* 2002, 166:1563–1566.

18. van Staa TP, Leufkens HGM, Cooper C: Use of inhaled corticosteroids and risk of fractures. *J Bone Miner Res* 2001, 3:581–588.

19. de Vries F, Pouwels S, Bracke M, *et al.*: Use of beta-2 agonists and risk of hip/femur fracture: a population-based case-control study. *Pharmacoepidemiol Drug Saf* 2007, 16:612–619.

20. Lekamwasam S, Trivedi DP, Khaw KT: An association between respiratory function and bone mineral density in women from the general community: a cross sectional study. *Osteoporos Int* 2002, 13:710–715.

21. Solomon DH, Katz JN, Jacobs JP, *et al.*: Management of glucocorticoid-induced osteoporosis in patients with rheumatoid arthritis. *Arthritis Rheum* 2002, 46:3136–3142.

22. Curtis JR, Westfall AO, Allison J, *et al.*: Challenges in improving the quality of osteoporosis care for long-term glucocorticoid users. *Arch Intern Med* 2007, 167:591–596.

23. Hanania NA, Chapman KR: Dose-related decrease in bone density among asthmatic patients treated with inhaled corticosteroids. *J Allergy Clin Immunol* 1996, 5:571–579.

24. Wisniewski AF, Lewis AS, Green DJ, *et al.*: Cross-sectional investigation of the effects of inhaled corticosteroids on bone density and bone metabolism in patients with asthma. *Thorax* 1997, 52:853–860.

25. Israel E, Banerjee TR, Fitzmaurice GM, *et al.*: Effects of inhaled glucocorticoids on bone density in premenopausal women. *N Engl J Med* 2001, 345:941–947.

26. Struijs A, Mulder H: The effects of inhaled glucocorticoids on bone mass and biochemical markers of bone homeostasis: a 1-year study of beclomethasone dipropionate. *Nederlands J Med* 1997, 50:233–237.

27. Tattersfield AE, Town GI, Johnell O, *et al.*: Bone mineral density in subjects with mild asthma randomized to treatment with inhaled corticosteroids or non-corticosteroid treatment for two years. *Thorax* 2001, 56:272–278.

28. The Lung Health Study Research Group: Effect of inhaled triamcinolone on the decline in pulmonary function in chronic obstructive pulmonary disease. *N Engl J Med* 2000, 343:1902–1909.

29. Li JTC, Ford LB, Chervinsky P, *et al.*: Fluticasone propionate powder and lack of clinically significant effects on hypothalamic–pituitary–adrenal axis and bone mineral density over 2 years in adults with mild asthma. *J Allergy Clin Immunol* 1999, 103:1062–1068.

30. Pauwels RA, Löfdahl CG, Laitinen LA, *et al.*: Long-term treatment with inhaled budesonide in persons with mild chronic obstructive pulmonary disease who continue smoking. *N Engl J Med* 1999, 340:1948–1953.

Transplantation and Bone Disease

Dina E. Green and Sol Epstein

9

Organ transplantation has become an increasingly common procedure in recent decades to treat a variety of forms of organ failure. Transplantation has achieved increasing success in large part due to improved surgical technique and immunosuppressant regimens. With this enhanced success, organ-transplant recipients are now living long enough to experience chronic medical diseases including posttransplantation bone disease.

The etiologies of posttransplantation bone disease vary considerably and are partly related to the underlying condition that prompted the transplantation. Importantly, the type of immunosuppressant regimen used, most notably glucocorticoids and calcineurin inhibitors, each exhibit deleterious effects on bone homeostasis.

There presently is limited data on the treatment of posttransplantation bone disease. Treatment modalities largely revolve around calcium and vitamin D supplementation; the use of bisphosphonates; and, more recently, the potential use of recombinant human parathyroid hormone (teriparatide). This chapter delineates the prevalence and etiologies of, as well as treatment options for, bone disease in the transplant population.

Transplantation and Osteoporosis

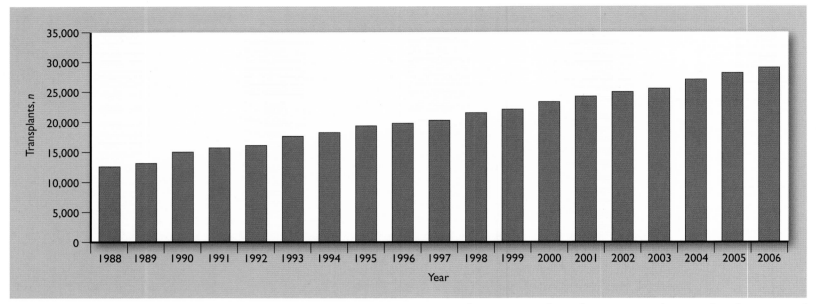

Figure 9-1. Increasing prevalence of organ transplantation in the United States. There has been a progressive rise in the number of organs transplanted in the past two decades. This is related to recent successes in transplantation resulting from improved surgical techniques and immunosuppressant regimens. (*Adapted from* UNOS [1].)

Prevalence of Osteoporosis and Fractures Posttransplant

Type of Transplant	Osteoporosis Prevalence	Fracture Prevalence
Bone marrow	4%–15%	5%
Kidney	11%–56%	3%–29%
Heart	25%–50%	22%–35%
Liver	30%–46%	29%–47%
Lung	57%–73%	42%

Figure 9-2. Prevalence of osteoporosis and fractures posttransplant. Prevalences vary among the different types of transplant in part due to the underlying pathology associated with each form of organ failure. For example, liver transplantation is associated with significant pretransplant vitamin D malabsorption in part due to cholestasis and jaundice; renal transplantation is associated with the unique pathology of renal osteodystrophy, a cascade of events related to secondary hyperparathyroidism; lung transplantation is typically associated with pretransplant steroid use; and cardiac transplant patients tend to be at substantial risk because of immobility and debility prior to transplantation. (*Data from* Cohen and Shane [2].)

Transplantation Drugs: Glucocorticoids

Glucocorticoids (GCs) continue to play a salient role in immunosuppressive regimens despite the increasing emphasis on nonsteroid immunomodulators. GCs have well-established deleterious effects on bone homeostasis.

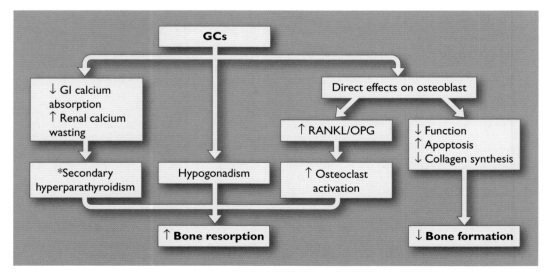

Figure 9-3. Effect of glucocorticoids (GCs) on bone loss. GCs work through a number of mechanisms to exert deleterious effects on bone. The direct effects on osteoblasts include a combination of apoptosis as well as decreased cellular functionality. GCs also upregulate osteoblast–osteoclast signaling through receptor activator for the nuclear factor κB ligand/osteoprotegerin (RANKL/OPG) system, causing increased osteoclast activation. Finally, GCs in substantial doses can result in hypogonadism, which further potentiates bone resorption. *Although GCs may cause a secondary hyperparathyroidism, this mechanism likely does not contribute substantially to bone loss. GI—gastrointestinal. (*Adapted from* Maalouf and Shane [3].)

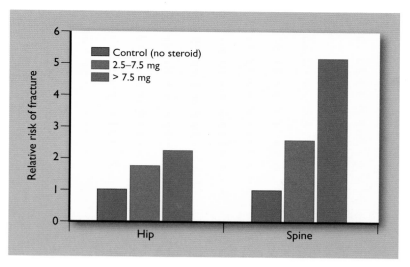

Figure 9-4. Increasing relative risk of fracture by steroid dose. The bone loss induced by chronic glucocorticoid (GC) use translates into an increased fracture risk. Data from a retrospective cohort study of over 200,000 oral corticosteroid users looking at the risk of fracture based on GC dose is summarized. GCs were found to increase the risk of both hip and vertebral fractures at doses of 2.5–7.5 mg daily with a greater risk at daily doses above 7.5 mg. In this same study, fracture risk was found to decline toward baseline after cessation of GC therapy. (*Data from* van Staa *et al.* [4].)

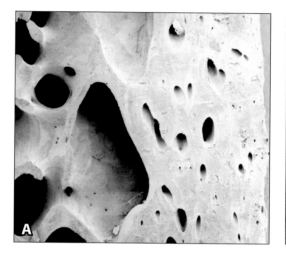

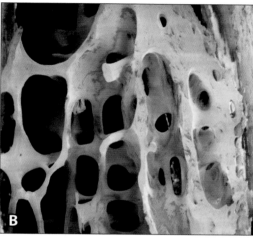

Figure 9-5. Bone structure in glucocorticoid-induced osteoporosis (GIO). Histomorpho-metry of normal bone (**A**) and bone affected by GIO (**B**). Bone affected by GIO is characterized by thinning and low connectivity as well as disorganization of the trabecular network. These findings are likely related in part to the reduction in the number and activity of osteoblasts. As a result, there is a reduced synthesis of bone matrix and a reduction in the amount of bone replaced in each remodeling cycle. (*From* D. Dempster, PhD, *with permission.*)

Management of Glucocorticoid-Induced Osteoporosis

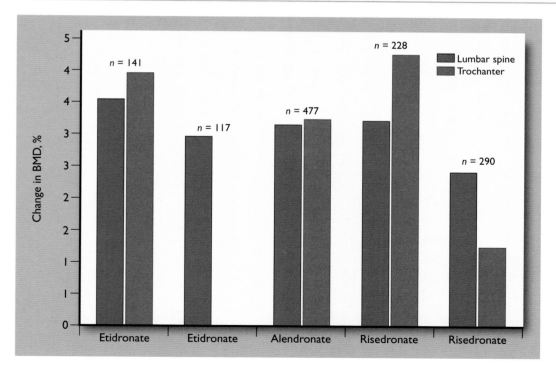

Figure 9-6. Data on the management of glucocorticoid-induced osteoporosis (GIO) with bisphosphonates. Bisphosphonate therapy of patients receiving glucocorticoids results in an increase in lumbar spine and trochanter bone mineral density (BMD). In some trials, the subjects were already receiving GCs when the bisphosphonate was begun, while in others the glucocorticoid and bisphosphonate were started simultaneously. The management of GIO largely involves the use of bisphosphonates and, more recently, recombinant human parathyroid hormone. A summary of these trials of bisphosphonates in patients on chronic glucocorticoid therapy is provided. Results from these five large randomized trials provide evidence that bisphosphonates are effective in both the prevention and treatment of GIO. The most significant increases in BMD were observed in the lumbar spine. (*Data from* American College of Rheumatology Ad Hoc Committee on Glucocorticoid-Induced Osteoporosis [5].)

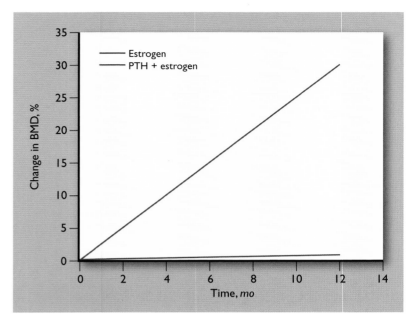

Figure 9-7. Effect of parathyroid hormone (PTH) and estrogen therapy on bone mineral density (BMD) in glucocorticoid-induced osteoporosis (GIO). Recombinant human PTH has recently become an attractive option to treat a variety of forms of osteoporosis, including GIO. In this trial, 51 postmenopausal women with inflammatory conditions treated with glucocorticoids were randomized to PTH + estrogen versus estrogen alone for 12 months. The spine BMD by dual energy x-ray absorptiometry measurement increased significantly in the PTH-treated group (11%) with no significant change in BMD observed in the estrogen-only group. (*Data from* Lane *et al.* [6].)

Transplantation Drugs: Nonsteroid Immune Modulators

Nonsteroid immune modulators are a relatively new class of drugs that capitalize on the role of T and B lymphocytes as mediators of immune function. The two major classes of drugs within this category are the calcineurin inhibitors (CIs), tacrolimus and cyclosporine, and the non-CIs, including sirolimus (rapamycin)

and mycophenolate mofetil (CellCept; Roche, Nutley, NJ). Both CIs have been found to have adverse effects on bone, while rapamycin and CellCept at therapeutic doses have a minimal effect. The following figures depict the interaction between the nonsteroid immune modulators and bone homeostasis.

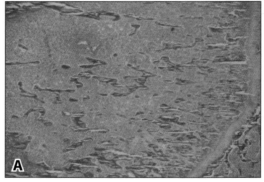 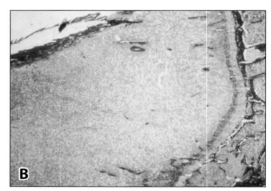

Figure 9-8. Calcineurin inhibitors: effect of cyclosporine A (CsA) on bone. CsA causes acute, rapid, and severe bone loss [7,8]. In a rat model, the administration of immunosuppressive doses of CsA produced significant losses of trabecular and cortical bone within weeks, which was dose dependent and reversible after use of the drug was discontinued. This figure shows the effect of cyclosporine on the tibial metaphyses of rats after

tetracycline labeling and histomorphometric examination. The control (**A**) shows the trabecular bone islands (*darker blue*), whereas bone sections of treated animals (**B**) show a severe loss of trabecular bone.

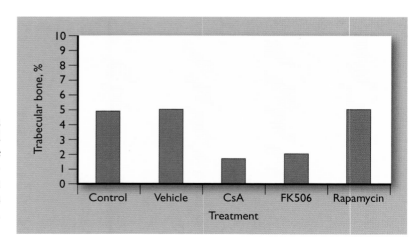

Figure 9-9. Comparison of the effect of immunosuppressive agents on bone loss. In contrast to the calcineurin inhibitors (CIs), other nonsteroid immune modulators including sirolimus (rapamycin) and mycophenolate mofetil (CellCept; Roche, Nutley, NJ) have not been shown to be deleterious to bone at therapeutic doses. A comparison of the in vivo effect on trabecular bone of the CIs versus rapamycin is shown; rapamycin causes no significant change in trabecular volume as compared to the vehicle. CsA— cyclosporine A; FK506—tacrolimus.

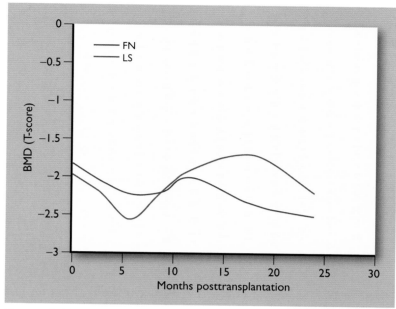

Figure 9-10. Timing of bone loss after liver transplantation. Twelve patients were followed with serial bone mineral density (BMD) measurements for 24 months following orthotopic liver transplantation. The average baseline BMD T-score is low at both the lumbar spine (LS) and the femoral neck (FN), then decreases significantly by 3 months posttransplantation at the LS and by 6 months posttransplantation at the FN. BMD at both the LS and the FN begins to increase at 6 months posttransplantation. LS BMD values approached baseline values approximately 12 months posttransplantation. (*Data from* Crosbie *et al.* [9].)

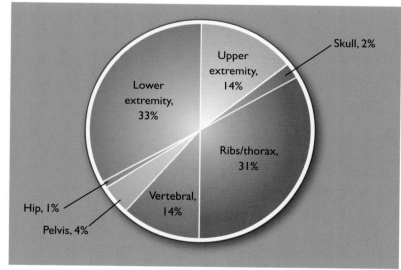

Timing of Bone Loss Following Cardiac Transplantation				
Year		1	2	3
BMD Δ	FN	−10%	−1%	+2%
	LS	−7.3%	−2.3%	−3%

Figure 9-11. Timing of bone loss following cardiac transplantation. Seventy-seven patients who underwent cardiac transplantation were treated with calcium and vitamin D alone. Bone loss at both the lumbar spine (LS) and femoral neck (FN) was substantial in the first year after transplantation. Rates of bone loss declined significantly during the second year. LS bone density increased modestly in the third year, while no further change occurred in FN bone density. BMD—bone mineral density. (*Data from* Shane *et al.* [10,11].)

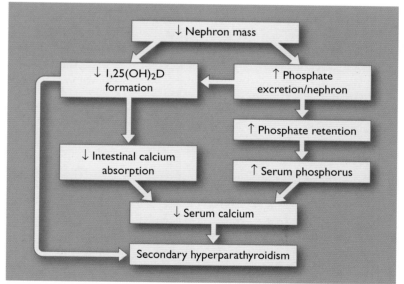

Figure 9-12. Pathophysiology of bone loss prior to renal transplantation/renal osteodystrophy. Osteoporosis is common in postrenal transplant patients, affecting between 10% and 40%. Bone disease in this population is related, in part, to pre-existing alterations in bone homeostasis, termed *renal osteodystrophy*. The pathophysiology of renal osteodystrophy is detailed in this schematic: it is related to secondary hyperparathyroidism from both rising serum phosphorus levels as well as reduced calcium absorption.

Figure 9-13. Relative sites of fracturing in renal transplant recipients. A retrospective cohort study of long-term fracture risk among 86 renal transplant recipients is shown. In this cohort, 117 fractures were observed during 33 years of followup. Transplant recipients experienced both an increased short-term as well as long-term fracture risk with a 3-fold increased risk at 15 years posttransplant. Unique to renal transplantation is the distribution of the type of fracture with both vertebral and lower limb fractures predominating, as depicted. Diabetes was identified as an independent predictor of lower limb fractures in this analysis. (*Data from* Vautour *et al.* [12].)

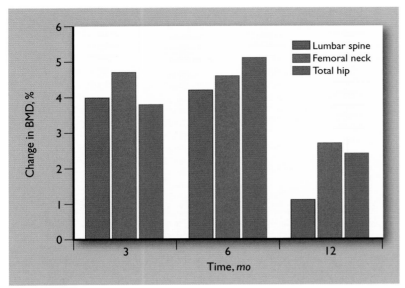

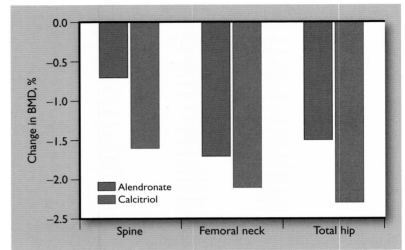

Figure 9-14. Treatment of osteoporosis following liver transplantation. In a randomized controlled trial, 62 orthotopic liver transplant patients were treated with high-dose intravenous zoledronic acid (4 mg) at 0, 1, 3, 6, and 9 months posttransplantation. In both the lumbar spine and the femoral hip, significant differences from baseline bone mineral density (BMD) were observed between the treated and untreated groups at 3 and 6 months. The difference from the baseline BMD at the spine was no longer significant at 12 months. The zoledronic acid group experienced more hypocalcemia and secondary hyperparathyroidism as compared to placebo. The study suggests a role for early treatment with bisphosphonates, but also is notable in revealing the degree of spontaneous recovery of BMD in the placebo group. (*Data from* Crawford *et al.* [13].)

Figure 9-15. Treatment of osteoporosis following cardiac transplantation. In a randomized controlled trial, 149 cardiac transplant patients were treated with calcitriol (0.5 mg/d) versus alendronate (10 mg/d) for 1 year posttransplantation. Both were compared to a reference group of untreated patients. There were no statistically significant differences observed at any site between calcitriol- and alendronate-treated patients, although both groups exhibited greater bone mineral density (BMD) as compared to the reference group. The calcitriol-treated patients experienced hypercalciuria more frequently than those patients treated with alendronate. (*Data from* Shane *et al.* [10,11].)

Treatment with Bisphosphonates After Renal Transplant: RR

Outcome	Trials, *n*	RR (95% CI)
All-cause mortality	5 (192)	0.94 (0.27, 3.24)
Fracture at any site	5 (219)	0.62 (0.33, 1.19)

A

Treatment with Bisphosphonates After Renal Transplant: Weighted Mean Difference

Outcome	Trials, *n*	Weighted mean difference (95% CI)
Percent change in BMD at the lumbar spine	8 (270)	7.66 (4.82, 10.5)
Percent change in BMD at the femoral neck	4 (149)	7.18 (6.22, 8.13)

B

Figure 9-16. Treatment of osteoporosis with bisphosphonates after renal transplantation. The decision to treat renal transplant patients with bisphosphonates is complicated. Renal transplant recipients suffer from bone disease in part from pre-existing renal osteodystrophy, as well as from the use of transplant medication. They are known to experience higher short- and long-term fracture risks. Bisphosphonates are a potential treatment, but they also carry a potential risk. Renal transplant patients may have pre-existing adynamic bone disease, in large part secondary to overexuberant treatment of secondary hyperparathyroidism. Treatment of such patients with an antiresorptive agent could theoretically worsen bone disease. The data on bisphosphonate use after renal transplantation largely consists of multiple small trials, few of which are adequately powered to assess fracture risk. Nevertheless, in the single meta-analysis depicted, there appears to be a benefit to bisphosphonate treatment. **A,** Relative risk (RR). **B,** Weighted mean difference. BMD—bone mineral density. (*Data from* Palmer *et al.* [14].)

In November 2007, a randomized trial was published of over 400 glucocorticoid-treated individuals treated with daily alendronate versus teriparatide for 18 months. The teriparatide group experienced superior increases in bone density at the spine and hip, and sustained fewer new vertebral fractures compared to the alendronate group. There had previously been a paucity of head-to-head data comparing teriparatide to alendronate. This finding suggests that teriparatide may potentially play an important role in the management of glucocorticoid-treated posttransplant patients [15].

References

1. UNOS (United Network for Organ Sharing): Available at http://www.optn.org/latestData/rptData.asp

2. Cohen A, Shane E: Osteoporosis after solid organ and bone marrow transplantation. *Osteoporos Int* 2003, 14:617–630.

3. Maalouf NM, Shane E: Osteoporosis after solid organ transplantation. *J Clin Endocrinol Metab* 2005, 90:2456–2465.

4. van Staa TP, Leufkens HGM, Abenhaim L, *et al.*: Use of oral corticosteroids and risk of fractures. *J Bone Miner Res* 2000, 15:993–1000.

5. American College of Rheumatology Ad Hoc Committee on Glucocorticoid-Induced Osteoporosis: Recommendations for the prevention and treatment of glucocorticoid induced osteoporosis. *Arthritis Rheum* 2001, 44:1496–1503.

6. Lane NE, Sanchez S, Modin GW, *et al.*: Parathyroid hormone treatment can reverse corticosteroid-induced osteoporosis. *J Clin Invest* 1998, 102:1627–1633.

7. Movsowitz C, Epstein S, Fallon M, *et al.*: Cyclosporin-A in vivo produces severe osteopenia in the rat: effect of dose and duration of administration. *Endocrinology* 1988, 123:2571–2577.

8. Movsowitz C, Epstein S, Ismail F, *et al.*: Cyclosporin A in the oophorectomized rate: unexpected severe bone resorption. *J Bone Miner Res* 1989, 4:393–398.

9. Crosbie OM, Freaney R, McKenna MJ, *et al.*: Predicting bone loss following orthotopic liver transplantation. *Gut* 1999, 44:430–434.

10. Shane E, Addesso V, Namerow PB, *et al.*: Alendronate versus calcitriol for the prevention of bone loss after cardiac transplantation. *N Engl J Med* 2004, 350:767–776.

11. Shane E, Rivas M, McMahon DJ, *et al.*: Bone loss and turnover after cardiac transplantation. *J Clin Endocrinol Metab* 1997, 82:1497–1506.

12. Vautour LM, Melton LJ, Clarke BL, *et al.*: Long term fracture risk following renal transplantation: a population-based study. *Osteoporos Int* 2004, 15:160–167.

13. Crawford BAL, Kam C, Pavlovic J, *et al.*: Zolendronic acid prevents bone loss after liver transplantation: a randomized, double blind, placebo controlled trial. *Ann Intern Med* 2006, 144:239–248.

14. Palmer SC, McGregor DO, Strippoli GFM: Interventions for preventing bone disease in renal transplant recipients: a systematic review of randomized controlled trials. *Cochrane Database Syst Rev* 2007, 2:1–61.

15. Saag KG, Shane E, Boonen S, *et al.*: Teriparatide or alendronate in glucocorticoid induced osteoporosis. *N Eng J Med* 2007, 357:2028–2029.

Estrogen-Deficiency–Associated Bone Loss and Osteoporosis

10

Diana Antoniucci and Deborah E. Sellmeyer

The relationship between estrogen deficiency and osteoporosis was first formally described in the 1940s. Since then, the biologic relationship between estrogen deficiency and bone loss has been explored in detail. With the onset of estrogen deficiency, increased activation of bone remodeling is seen at the bone histomorphometric level, with a consequential increase in biochemical markers of bone turnover in blood and urine. Bone loss occurs most rapidly in the first 5 years after overt menopause, especially at cancellous bone sites, but estrogen-dependent bone loss continues throughout life. Although estrogen deficiency is most often due to natural menopause, there are a number of conditions, discussed in this chapter, which lead to estrogen deficiency in premenopausal women.

Mechanisms of estrogen-deficiency–associated bone loss include the increased monocyte and osteoblast production of a variety of cytokines, including tumor necrosis factor (TNF), interleukin (IL)-1, IL-6, and the receptor activator of nuclear factor κB ligand, among others, all of which promote osteoclastogenesis and osteoclast activity, which is the first event in the remodeling process. Estrogen deficiency also leads to a global rise in IL-7 production that, along with an increase in TNF concentrations, directly suppresses osteoblast activity and, therefore, blunt bone formation. It is the resultant imbalance between bone formation and resorption that leads to a net loss of bone during each remodeling cycle.

Consistently, it has been shown in randomized controlled trials that estrogen administration to postmenopausal women reduces biochemical markers and histomorphometric evidence of bone remodeling as well as improves bone mass at all skeletal sites. For many years, the evidence of the ultimate impact of estrogen and hormone administration on fractures was observational, with only a few small prospective clinical trials in agreement. Several years ago, the results of the Heart and Estrogen/Progestin Replacement Study shed some doubt on estrogen's effect on fracture occurrence. However, the results of the Women's Health Initiative now confirm that hormone-replacement therapy reduces the risk of all osteoporosis-related fractures in postmenopausal women of average age 62 years whose osteoporosis status is unknown. However, other systemic risks of hormone therapy have been confirmed and constitute important limitations to a more widespread use of hormone therapy.

This chapter highlights the most important data concerning the biology of estrogen deficiency, the effects of estrogen intervention on intermediate markers (bone mass and bone turnover) and fractures, and the importance of estrogen for the skeletal status of men.

Biology of Estrogen Deficiency

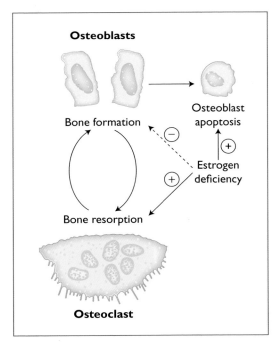

Figure 10-1. Overview of the effects of estrogen deficiency on bone turnover and architecture. Estrogen deficiency leads to a net loss of bone over each remodeling cycle via several different mechanisms. It has an overall negative impact on bone formation by increasing osteoblast apoptosis and decreasing the number of mature osteoblasts. Estrogen deficiency also augments bone resorption by increasing osteoclast formation and by decreasing osteoclast apoptosis, which is associated with a prolonged resorption phase. (*Adapted from* Postgraduate Institute for Medicine [1].)

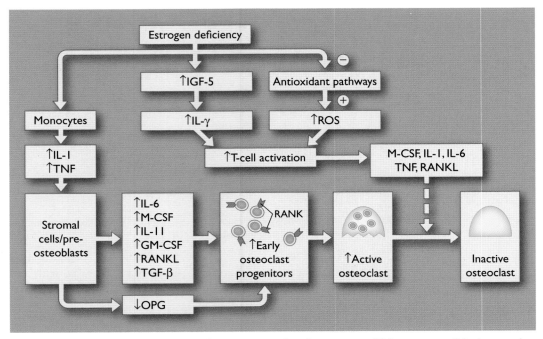

Figure 10-2. Influence of various cytokines on osteoclast formation and lifespan, one of the key mechanisms by which estrogen causes increased bone resorption and remodeling [2–12]. In the absence of estrogen, the production of tumor necrosis factor (TNF) by monocytes increases and cells of the stromal/osteoblastic lineage become more sensitive to interleukin (IL)-1. IL-1 and TNF stimulate stromal cells and preosteoblasts to release IL-6, macrophage colony-stimulating factor (M-CSF), IL-11, granulocyte-macrophage colony-stimulating factor (GM-CSF), transforming growth factor-beta (TGF-β), and receptor activator of NF-κB ligand (RANKL), all of which are factors that stimulate the proliferation of osteoclast precursors or osteoclastogenesis. Receptor activator of NF-κB (RANK) is expressed by osteoclast progenitors and promotes osteoclastogenesis when it binds to RANKL. With estrogen deficiency, there is also a global increase in IL-7 production and a downregulation of antioxidant pathways, with a resultant increase in reactive oxygen species (ROS). The increases in ROS and IL-7 result in T-cell activation, which in turn lead to an increase in RANKL and TNF release. TNF and RANKL, along with M-CSF, IL-1, TNF, and IL-6, inhibit osteoclast apoptosis, thereby increasing the lifespan of osteoclasts. In addition, estrogen deficiency may negatively influence osteoprotegerin (OPG). Lower levels of OPG, a soluble decoy receptor for RANKL, result in more RANKL available to bind to RANK and stimulate osteoclast activity. By similar mechanisms, estrogen deficiency also leads to increased osteoblastogenesis and to reduced lifespans of osteoblasts and osteocytes, all of which contribute to postmenopausal osteoporosis (these effects are not depicted in this figure). IGF-5—insulin-like growth factor 5.

Figure 10-3. Evaluation of the effects of menopause as well as osteoporosis and estrogen replacement by measuring levels of pyridinoline (PYD) and deoxypyridinoline (DPD) in four groups of women [13]. Mean urinary concentrations of the hydroxypyridinium cross-links PYD (**A**) and DPD (**B**) in postmenopausal (Post) healthy women and untreated (UTO) and estrogen-treated (ETO) women with postmenopausal osteoporosis compared with premenopausal (Pre) healthy women. *Column inserts* denote the percentage change of mean value compared with normal premenopausal controls. *Bars* represent the standard error of the mean. *Asterisks* indicate *P* values greater than 0.01. Levels of both PYD and DPD were 53% to 58%

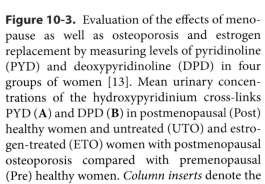
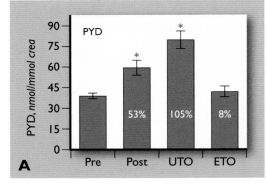
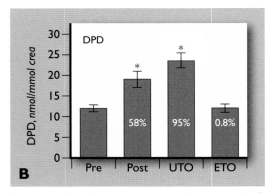

higher in postmenopausal women than in premenopausal women. Both PYD and DPD were significantly higher in the UTO group than in the postmenopausal group (*P* < 0.01). Crea—creatine.

Effects of Estrogen Treatment on Intermediate Markers (Bone Mass and Turnover)

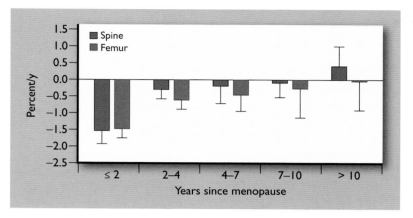

Figure 10-4. The importance of early bone loss and its association with estrogen deficiency is shown in these data associating years since menopause and rates of bone loss [14]. Longitudinal data for spontaneous loss of lumbar and femoral neck bone mineral density (BMD) in women receiving placebo ($n = 71$; mean age 56.3 ± 4.4 y) are combined from two randomized, controlled trials. The highest rates of bone loss occurred in women close to menopause. A significant relationship between years since menopause and BMD loss was observed at the spine ($r = 0.34$; $P < 0.01$) and femoral neck ($r = 0.25$; $P < 0.001$). (*Adapted from* Bjarnason *et al.* [14].)

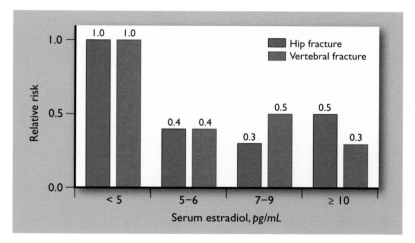

Figure 10-5. Lower serum estradiol concentrations are associated with an increased risk of hip and vertebral fractures in postmenopausal women. The risk of hip or vertebral fracture associated with baseline serum estradiol concentrations was analyzed in a cohort of community-dwelling women 65 years or older, who were not taking hormone-replacement therapy. There were 317 women in the hip-fracture analysis (228 controls and 89 who had hip fracture) and 282 women in the vertebral-fracture analysis (186 controls and 96 who had vertebral fracture). After adjustment for weight and age, the women with the lowest serum estradiol concentrations had the highest risk of hip and vertebral fracture. The investigators estimated that an undetectable serum estradiol concentration was associated with an attributable risk of 33% for hip fractures and 32% for vertebral fractures. (*From* Cummings *et al.* [15]; with permission.)

Causes of Premenopausal Estrogen Deficiency

Hypogonadotropic hypogonadism
  Low weight
  Eating disorders
  Excessive exercise
  Hyperprolactinemia
  Hypopituitarism
Premature ovarian failure
  Autoimmune
  Idiopathic
  Secondary to chemotherapy for cancer
GnRH agonist therapy
  Used to treat endometriosis
Aromatase inhibitor therapy
  Used to treat breast cancer or endometriosis
Turner's syndrome

Figure 10-6. Conditions associated with estrogen deficiency in premenopausal women. There are a number of conditions that can lead to estrogen deficiency and its associated bone loss in premenopausal women. Some of the more common conditions are listed. GnRH—gonadotrophin-releasing hormone.

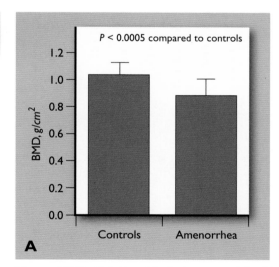

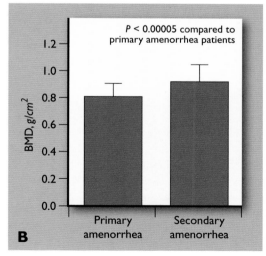

Figure 10-7. Relationship between vertebral bone mineral density (BMD) and amenorrhea in premenopausal women. Vertebral BMD was measured in 57 healthy controls and in 200 women of reproductive age with a past or current history of amenorrhea (defined as no menses for at least 6 months) of varying etiology. **A,** Vertebral BMD was significantly lower in the amenorrheic women than in the controls (0.89 vs 1.05 g/cm², $P < 0.0005$). **B,** Further, women with primary amenorrhea had significantly lower BMD than those with secondary amenorrhea, irrespective of diagnosis (0.81 vs 0.92 g/cm², $P < 0.00005$). In the same study, vertebral BMD was shown to be inversely and significantly correlated to the duration of amenorrhea ($r = -0.474$, $P < 0.00005$). BMD was also significantly correlated with serum concentrations of 17β-estradiol. These data suggest that the estrogen deficiency associated with amenorrhea also leads to bone loss. (*Adapted from* Davies *et al.* [16].)

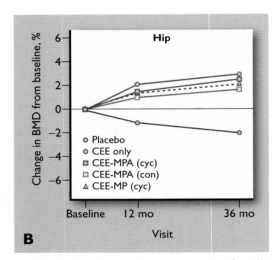

Figure 10-8. Estrogen prevents or slows bone loss and may modestly increase bone mineral density, whenever it is initiated, as demonstrated in the landmark study by Lindsay *et al.* [17]. This prospective, double-blind trial investigated the effects of long-term treatment with estrogen-replacement therapy (24.8 µg mestranol, an estrogen formulation that is no longer widely used in postmenopausal women) or placebo in 120 women who began therapy 2 months, 3 years, or 6 years after oophorectomy for benign pelvic disease in their late 40s. In a further analysis of the data from the original trial, long-term (> 10 y) estrogen-replacement therapy significantly reduced the rate of loss of metacarpal bone mineral content. The earlier treatment was begun, the more beneficial was its effect on bone loss, since bone that was already lost could not be replaced to any significant extent. These results indicate that estrogen-replacement therapy should be initiated as soon as possible after the onset of menopause in order to maximize its beneficial long-term effects. (*Adapted from* Lindsay *et al.* [17].)

Figure 10-9. Results of the Postmenopausal Estrogen/Progestin Intervention (PEPI) Trial. In this 3-year, double-blind, placebo-controlled, multicenter trial, 875 women aged 45 to 64 years of age were randomly assigned to one of five treatment groups: 1) conjugated equine estrogen (CEE) 0.625 mg/d; 2) CEE 0.625 mg/d plus medroxyprogesterone acetate (MPA) 10 mg/d for 12 d/mo; 3) CEE 0.625 mg/d plus MPA 2.5 mg/d; 4) CEE 0.625 mg/d plus 200 mg micronized progesterone (MP) 12 d/mo; or 5) placebo. **A** and **B**, By 36 months, women who were compliant with the placebo regimen had lost an average of 2.8% of spinal bone mineral density (BMD) and 2.2% of hip BMD, whereas those found to be compliant with any active regimen had gained approximately 4% in the spine and 2% in the hip. There was a significant increase in hip and spine BMD in each active treatment group from baseline to the 12-month visit, and for each active treatment group from the 12- to 36-month visit. Among the patients compliant with therapy, results of all active regimens were significantly different from placebo, but no active treatment was significantly different from other active treatments. (**B** *adapted from* Writing Group for the PEPI Trial [18].)

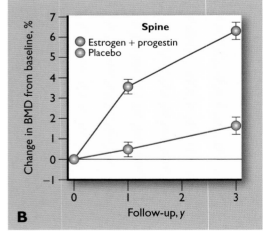

Figure 10-10. Mean percentage change in total hip and spine bone mineral density (BMD) during 3 years of treatment with estrogen plus progestin as compared to a placebo in the Women's Health Initiative (WHI). In the estrogen-plus-progestin therapy arm of the WHI, postmenopausal women were randomly assigned to receive 0.625 mg/d of conjugated equine estrogen with 2.5 mg/d of medroxyprogesterone acetate (*n* = 8506) or placebo (*n* = 8102). **A** and **B**, By 3 years, in women on active treatment, BMD had increased by 3.7% at the total hip and by 6.1% at the lumbar spine, as compared to increases of 0.14% and 1.5%, respectively, in the women on placebo treatment. Differences in 3-year BMD changes were statistically significant at both the hip and spine. Analyses were limited to women adherent to therapy and revealed larger increases in BMD in the women on treatment. (*From* Cauley *et al.* [19]; with permission.)

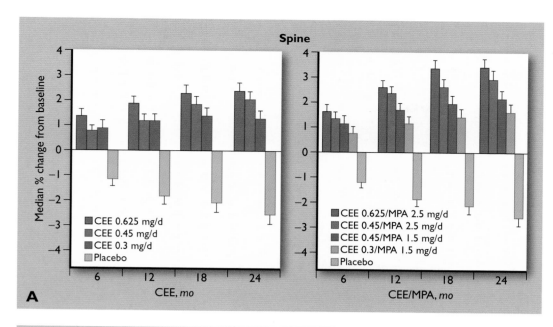

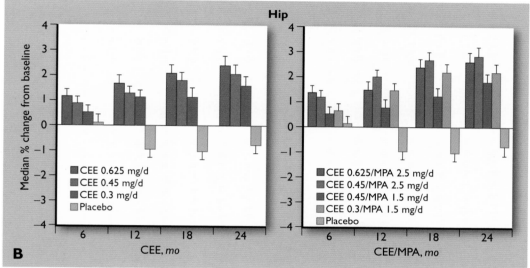

Figure 10-11. There is evidence that doses of hormone-replacement therapy (HRT) lower than those most commonly prescribed may be effective in preventing bone loss in older women; however, the effects of lower doses of HRT in early postmenopausal women have not been well studied. The Women's Health, Osteoporosis, Progestin, Estrogen (Women's HOPE) Trial was a prospective, randomized, double-blind, placebo-controlled, multicenter trial that investigated the efficacy and safety of lower doses of conjugated equine estrogen (CEE) alone and with continuous medroxyprogesterone acetate (MPA) in early postmenopausal women (who were within 4 years of their last menstrual period) [20]. The 2-year bone substudy used a subpopulation of the Women's HOPE Trial (*n* = 822) to evaluate the skeletal effects of lower doses of CEE and CEE/MPA. The substudy included the following groups: CEE 0.625 mg; CEE 0.45 mg; CEE 0.3 mg; CEE 0.625 mg/MPA 2.5 mg; CEE 0.45 mg/MPA 2.5 mg; CEE 0.45 mg/MPA 1.5 mg; CEE 0.3 mg/MPA 1.5 mg; and placebo. These graphs include data from the intent-to-treat population, which consisted of all women randomized to treatment who recorded taking at least one dose of the study drug and had at least one bone mineral density (BMD) measurement after baseline.

After 2 years, women assigned to all of the active treatment groups had significant gains from baseline (*P* < 0.001) in spine BMD (**A**). These changes were statistically different from those in the placebo group. In addition, adding 2.5 mg MPA to 0.625 mg or 0.45 mg CEE significantly increased spine BMD relative to CEE alone (*P* < 0.05). These data demonstrate that lower doses of CEE and CEE/MPA effectively prevent bone loss in the spine in early postmenopausal women. All estrogen and estrogen/progestin dose combinations also increased BMD in the hip (**B**) and total body. Moreover, estrogen and hormone therapy in all doses reduced the biochemical markers of bone turnover.

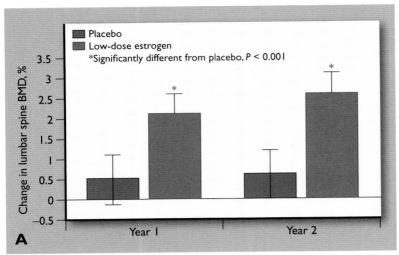

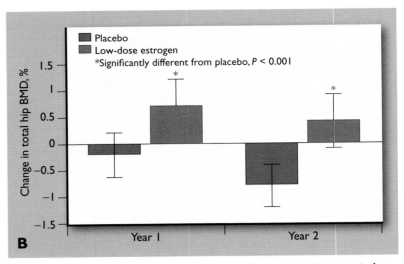

A   **B**

Figure 10-12. In response to concerns of risks associated with standard-dose hormone-replacement therapy after the Women's Health Initiative results, a 2-year randomized controlled trial of ultra-low–dose transdermal estrogen compared to placebo was conducted in 417 postmenopausal women with intact uterus. The study found that the ultra-low–dose transdermal patch significantly increased plasma estradiol from 4.8 pg/mL at baseline to 8.6 pg/mL at 2 years, whereas plasma estradiol did not change in the placebo group. **A** and **B** depict the mean percentage of bone mineral density (BMD) change from the baseline with 95% CIs and a significance

level. The treatment group experienced a significant 2-year increase in lumbar spine BMD of 2.6% as compared to 0.6% in the placebo group and a 0.4% increase in total hip BMD, whereas the placebo group experienced a 0.8% decline. Bone turnover markers also were significantly lower in the treatment group as compared to the placebo group. The study also found no increase in the rate of endometrial hyperplasia development in the treatment group as compared to the placebo group. These data suggest that ultra-low–dose transdermal estrogen therapy may be an option to consider in postmenopausal women. (*Adapted from* Ettinger *et al.* [21].)

Figure 10-13. Vertebral bone mineral content (BMC) changes induced by transdermal estrogen are dose dependent. A 2-year randomized double-blind, placebo-controlled trial investigated the bone turnover and bone-mass response to three dosages of transdermally administered 17β-estradiol in 127 postmenopausal women. The change from baseline in vertebral BMC, measured by single-photon absorptiometry after 12 and 24 months of therapy with increasing doses of transdermal estrogen, is shown. Similar to the results of the Health, Osteoporosis, Progestin, Estrogen (HOPE) trial, it was found that suppression of bone turnover markers was dose dependent, as was the response of vertebral BMC. *Significantly different from placebo, $P < 0.05$; †significantly different from placebo, $P < 0.01$; ‡significantly different from placebo, $P < 0.001$; §significantly different from estradiol 0.025 mg (comparison only made at 24 months). (*Adapted from* Field *et al.* [22].)

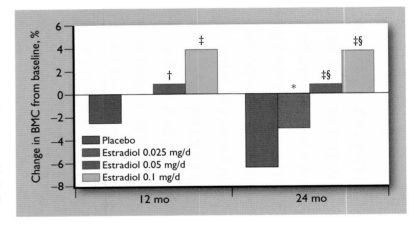

Figure 10-14. A and **B,** A 3-year randomized prospective study (STOP IT) was conducted in 489 postmenopausal women 65 to 77 years old to test the efficacy of 3 years of treatment with estrogen-replacement therapy (ERT)/hormone-replacement therapy (HRT)—conjugated equine estrogen 0.625 mg/d alone or with medroxyprogesterone acetate 2.5 mg/d in women with an intact uterus. At the end of 3 years of treatment, therapy was discontinued and the women were asked to volunteer for 2 years of follow-up. Analyses were performed in the 178 women who completed the fifth year of the study. Discontinuing ERT/HRT in these older post-

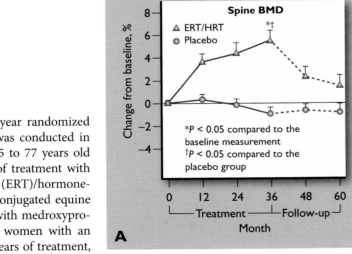

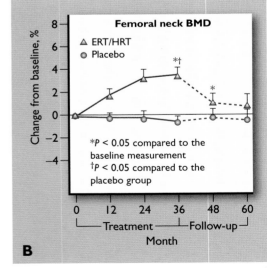

A   **B**

menopausal women resulted in rapid bone loss—almost 6% in the spine and about 2% in the femoral neck. BMD—bone mineral density. (*Adapted from* Gallagher *et al.* [23].)

Effects of Estrogen Intervention on Fracture Occurrence

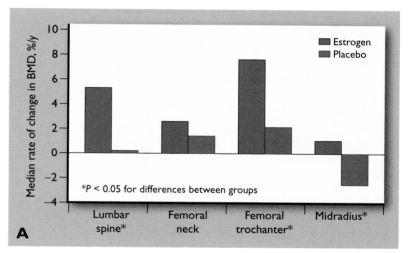

Figure 10-15. A number of case-control and cohort studies have provided epidemiologic evidence that estrogen-replacement therapy (ERT)/hormone-replacement therapy (HRT) reduces the risk of hip fracture. These studies suggested that hip fractures may be reduced by 20% to 60% in ERT/HRT users as compared with nonusers [24–31].

Estrogen and Vertebral Fractures

Long-term study of ERT in oophorectomized women
100 women treated with either estrogen or placebo
Followed for 9.5 y
Radiographs at conclusion of the study
Significantly fewer vertebral deformities
Less height loss in estrogen-treated women

Figure 10-16. The first randomized, controlled clinical trial data suggesting that estrogen-reduced fracture risk came from the study by Lindsay *et al.* [32], who in a small population of ovariectomized women showed that estrogen could reduce the appearance of new vertebral fractures. ERT—estrogen-replacement therapy.

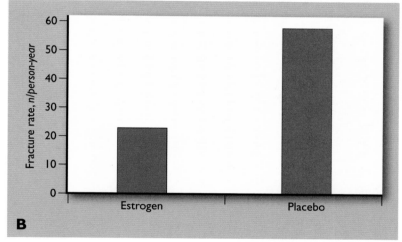

Figure 10-17. A and **B**, Estrogen's effects are not dependent on the route of administration. Lufkin *et al.* [33] demonstrated in a small 1-year study that transdermal estrogen could also increase bone mass and reduce the risk of vertebral fracture. BMD—bone mineral density. (*Adapted from* Lufkin *et al.* [33].)

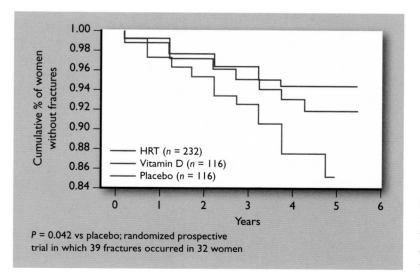

P = 0.042 vs placebo; randomized prospective trial in which 39 fractures occurred in 32 women

Figure 10-18. More recently, we have seen the accumulation of data suggesting that estrogen can reduce the risk of nonvertebral fracture. Komulainen *et al.* [34] showed that fewer nonvertebral fractures occurred over 5 years in early postmenopausal women (*n* = 232) treated with hormone-replacement therapy (HRT).

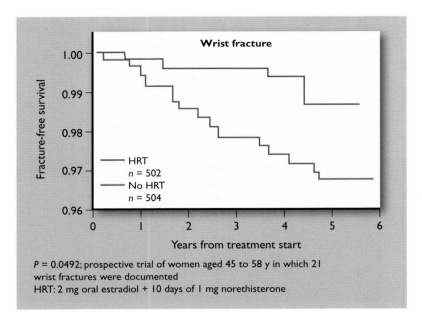

P = 0.0492; prospective trial of women aged 45 to 58 y in which 21 wrist fractures were documented
HRT: 2 mg oral estradiol + 10 days of 1 mg norethisterone

Figure 10-19. The Danish Osteoporosis Prevention Study was the first large randomized prospective study that assessed the preventive effects of hormone-replacement therapy (HRT) on fracture rates in 2016 recently postmenopausal women 45 to 58 years old. After 5 years of treatment, the women receiving HRT experienced statistically significant reductions in the relative risk (RR) of Colles' fracture (RR, 0.45; 95% CI, 0.22–0.90) and borderline statistically significant reductions in overall nonvertebral fracture risk (RR, 0.73; 95% CI, 0.50–1.05). However, when the analysis was restricted to women who adhered to the regimen, significant risk reductions were seen in overall fracture risk (RR, 0.61; 95% CI, 0.39–0.97) and in the risk of Colles' fracture (RR, 0.24; 95% CI, 0.09–0.69). (*Adapted from* Mosekilde *et al.* [35].)

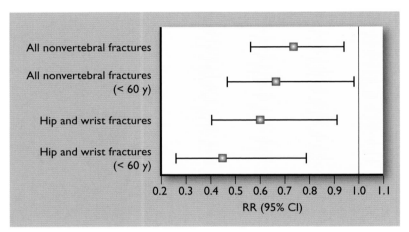

Figure 10-20. These results are from recent meta-analysis of all randomized trials of hormone-replacement therapy (HRT) that have reported or collected information on nonvertebral fracture, although most did not focus on fracture prevention. This meta-analysis reported a 27% reduction in the relative risk (RR) of nonvertebral fractures (RR, 0.73; 95% CI, 0.56–0.94). Greater reductions in the RR of nonvertebral fracture were observed in women with a mean age younger than 60 years (RR, 0.67%; 95% CI, 0.46–0.98). In women 60 years of age and older, HRT appeared to have less effect on nonvertebral fracture (RR, 0.88%; 95% CI, 0.71–1.08).

The effectiveness of HRT appeared more marked for hip and wrist fractures alone (RR, 0.60; 95% CI, 0.40–0.91), especially for women younger than 60 years of age (RR, 0.45; 95% CI, 0.26–0.79). This meta-analysis confirmed the significant benefits of HRT in preventing nonvertebral fractures, particularly in younger women. Initiating therapy early in menopause may be necessary to maximize the benefit of HRT in preventing fracture. (*Adapted from* Torgerson and Bell-Syer [36].)

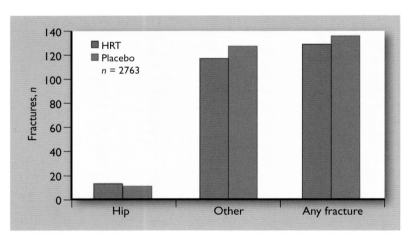

Figure 10-21. The Heart Estrogen/Progestin Replacement Study, which evaluates hormone-replacement therapy (HRT) for secondary prevention of heart disease, could find no evidence of fracture reduction in 2763 women with established coronary heart disease. The osteoporosis status of the majority of these women was unknown and they were followed for a median of 5.3 years. Results indicated that HRT produced an increased risk of coronary heart disease, particularly in the first year, and no overall reduction in the risk of cardiovascular disease. Moreover, there was no reduction in the risk of any clinical fracture (spine or hip) or of all fractures in women receiving HRT versus those receiving placebo. (*Adapted from* Hulley *et al.* [37].)

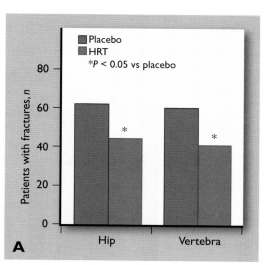

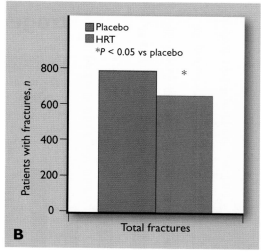

Figure 10-22. The largest clinical trial of hormone-replacement therapy (HRT) ever conducted is the HRT portion of the Women's Health Initiative [38], a large complex clinical trial evaluating HRT, estrogen, low-fat diet, and calcium and vitamin D supplementation. **A** and **B**, In the HRT arm of the study, some 16,600 postmenopausal women were randomized to receive placebo or HRT–conjugated equine estrogen 0.625 mg/d + medroxyprogesterone acetate 2.5 mg/d. The multiple outcomes evaluated included heart disease; stroke; venous thromboembolism; and breast, uterine, and colon cancer, as well as fractures, which did not include those of the ribs, chest/sternum, skull/face, fingers, toes, and cervical vertebrae. Such fractures are more difficult to confirm or are often not osteoporotic in etiology.

Forty-four patients (0.10%) receiving HRT experienced hip fractures, compared with 62 receiving placebo (0.15%), 41 patients (0.09%) receiving HRT and 60 patients (0.15%) receiving placebo experienced clinical vertebral fractures, and 650 women (1.47%) receiving HRT and 780 women (1.91%) receiving placebo experienced other types of fractures. The use of HRT reduced the rates of observed hip and clinical vertebral fractures by 34% and reduced the risk of all other fractures compared with placebo by 24%. This reduction was nominally significant for all fractures. In terms of absolute risk, 10,000 women taking HRT compared with placebo might experience five fewer hip fractures over 1 year. These data confirm the overwhelming body of data on the biologic impact of estrogen deficiency on the skeleton, the previous small clinical trials, and the observational studies that make the Heart and Estrogen/Progestin Replacement Study trial the one outstanding negative study of estrogen and fracture outcomes.

WHI Results: Absolute and Relative Risk or Benefit of CEE/MPA

| Health Event | Overall Hazard Ratio | CI | | Increased Absolute Risk per 10,000 Women/Y | Increased Absolute Benefit per 10,000 Women/Y |
		Normal 95%	Adjusted 95%		
CHD	1.29	1.02–1.63*	0.85–1.97	7	
Strokes	1.41	1.07–1.85*	0.86–2.31	8	
Breast cancer	1.26	1.00–1.59	0.83–1.92	8	
VTED	2.11	1.58–2.82*	1.26–3.55*	18	
Colorectal cancer	0.63	0.43–0.92*	0.32–1.24		6
Hip fractures	0.66	0.45–0.98*	0.33–1.33		5
Total fractures	0.76	0.69–0.85*	0.63–0.92*		44

Figure 10-23. For the clinical outcomes listed here, the overall hazard ratios at 5.2 years for conjugated equine estrogen (CEE)/medroxyprogesterone acetate (MPA) users versus placebo are shown in the second column from the left. For each of these ratios, two different CIs were calculated—nominal and adjusted (based on multiple comparisons)—and the intervals that reached statistical significance (that is, those that did not cross 1.0) are indicated with *asterisks*. Reporting on both types of CIs in the same publication is rare, as they tend to make interpretation of the data difficult. The nominal CI for coronary heart disease (CHD) and the adjusted CI for stroke indicate statistically significant increases in risk among CEE/MPA users. Both the nominal and adjusted CIs for venous thromboembolic disease (VTED—the combination of deep vein thrombosis and pulmonary embolism) indicate a statistically significant, more than twofold, increase in risk among CEE/MPA users. Both the nominal and adjusted CIs for total fractures indicate statistically significant decreased risk among CEE/MPA users. The nominal CIs for colorectal cancer and hip fracture indicate statistically significant decreases in risk among CEE/MPA users [38].

The risk of breast cancer was increased by 26%, just missing statistical significance. The absolute excess risk or benefit attributable to CEE/MPA was low. The Women's Health Initiative (WHI) findings predict that over 1 year, 10,000 women taking CEE/MPA, compared with placebo, might be expected to experience seven more CHD events, eight more strokes, eight more invasive breast cancers, 18 more thromboembolic events, six fewer colorectal cancers, five fewer hip fractures, and 44 fewer total fractures. All these numbers must be multiplied by years of use, however, in order to fully estimate the absolute risk of all these diseases.

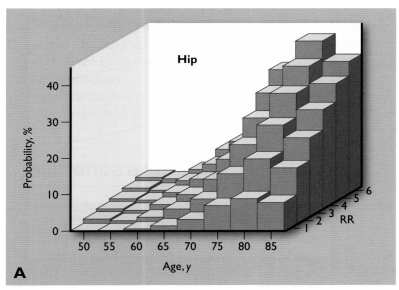

A

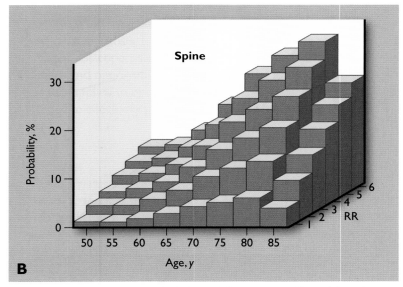

B

Figure 11-5. Probability of fracture [10]. The relationship between the 10-year probability of hip (**A**) and spine (**B**) fracture to increasing age and relative risk (RR) in men is shown. The 10-year probability of fracture is heavily dependent on the subject's age and RR of fracture; the RR changes as the clinical situation varies (*eg*, in the presence of smoking or a positive family history of fracture) and it is useful to observe how much the probability of fracture is affected by changes in age and relative risk. Data from the Swedish population were used to model these relationships. In this model, an 85-year-old man with an RR greater than 4 (*eg*, low bone mineral density, increased fall risk, and positive family history) has a 10-year probability of hip fracture of over 20%.

Factors Associated with Hip Fractures in Men	
Metabolic Disorders	**Disorders of Movement and Balance**
Thyroidectomy	Hemiparesis/hemiplegia
Gastrectomy	Parkinsonism
Pernicious anemia	Other neurologic diseases
Chronic respiratory diseases	Vertigo
Low body mass	Alcoholism
	Anemia
	Blindness
	Use of cane or walker
	Inactivity
	Dementia

Figure 11-6. Factors associated with hip fractures in men. As in women, there is overlap between bone density in men with and without fracture, indicating that bone density is not the sole determinant of osteoporotic fracture risk. Fracture is a somewhat chance event, and the propensity to fall is an important variable. In men, few prospective data exist that directly relate fall propensity to subsequent fractures, but a variety of factors indirectly related to the risk of falling have been related to hip fracture. Many of these factors suggest a body habitus and lifestyle more conducive to falls and injury, as well as the possibility of other interacting risk factors (nutritional deficiencies and comorbidities). In this retrospective study of conditions associated with hip fracture, increased risk was related to increased age, leanness, increased height, a history of previous fracture, and osteoporosis. In addition, a number of metabolic and neurologic diagnoses were more often found in the medical histories of men who experienced a hip fracture [11].

Bone Mass

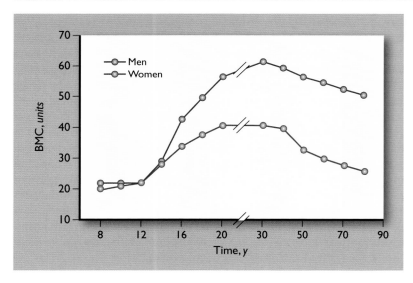

Figure 11-7. Changes in bone mass with growth and aging in men and women. Both men and women exhibit a dramatic increase in bone mass that begins during adolescence and is almost complete when puberty ends. A peak is reached in both men and women at about 20 to 30 years. By the fourth or fifth decade, men and women begin an age-related process of gradual bone loss that continues throughout the remainder of life and results from an excess of bone resorption over bone formation, the causes of which are not well understood. Women experience an accelerated phase of bone loss that lasts 5 to 15 years, which is the result of the relatively abrupt decline in gonadal function occurring with menopause. In contrast with the clearly demarcated event of menopause in women, the reproductive changes that take place in men as they age are more subtle. Acceleration occurs in the rate of bone loss in elderly men (> 50 years), which in part is the result of reductions in sex steroid levels. At any given time, bone mass depends on the peak bone mass achieved in adolescence and subsequent bone loss. BMC—bone mineral content. (*Adapted from* Nevitt [12].)

Figure 11-8. Determinants of peak bone mass in men. Peak bone mass may be a major determinant of osteoporotic fracture risk up to the age of approximately 60 to 65 years, when factors such as age-related bone loss become relatively more important. Hence, the failure to achieve optimal peak bone mass is an important pathogenetic mechanism in osteoporosis in both men and women. Heredity, dietary components (calcium and protein), endocrine factors (sex steroids, calcitriol, and insulin-like growth factor-I), and mechanical forces (physical activity and body weight) all may have an influence. As in women, a prominent determinant appears to be genetically related, but the precise genes involved remain to be elucidated.

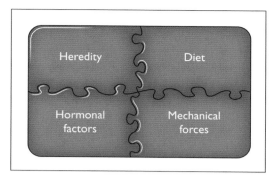

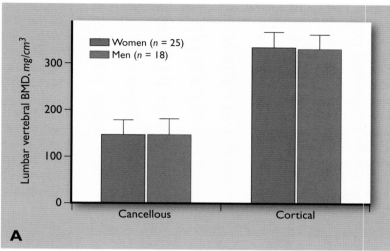

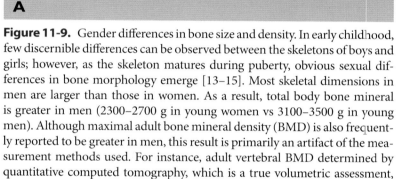

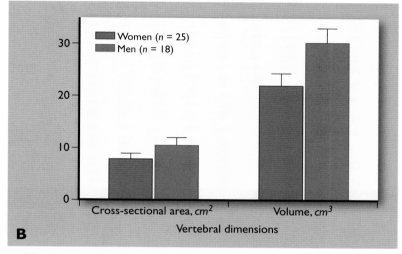

Figure 11-9. Gender differences in bone size and density. In early childhood, few discernible differences can be observed between the skeletons of boys and girls; however, as the skeleton matures during puberty, obvious sexual differences in bone morphology emerge [13–15]. Most skeletal dimensions in men are larger than those in women. As a result, total body bone mineral is greater in men (2300–2700 g in young women vs 3100–3500 g in young men). Although maximal adult bone mineral density (BMD) is also frequently reported to be greater in men, this result is primarily an artifact of the measurement methods used. For instance, adult vertebral BMD determined by quantitative computed tomography, which is a true volumetric assessment, is alike in men and women (**A**). Although vertebral density by measures of area (eg, dual-photon absorptiometry or dual-energy x-ray absorptiometry) appears to reach slightly higher levels in men, this apparent advantage disappears (or is even slightly reversed) once those values are corrected for differences in vertebral dimensions. From the time of puberty on, mean vertebral cross-sectional area is 15% to 25% greater in men and tubular bones exhibit greater total and cortical widths in early adulthood (**B**). The larger size of bones in men adds greatly to their strength and the sex differences in peak bone mass, and, in part, size underlies the differences in fracture patterns that emerge later in life. (*Adapted from* Gilsanz *et al.* [15].)

Figure 11-10. Gender differences in age-related changes in cortical bone. Bone loss occurs with aging in men as it does in women; however, gender differences in the pattern of age-related bone loss affect eventual fracture risk. Both men and women experience an increase in cortical porosity, although the rate is somewhat slower in men. This increase results in a reduction in density and mechanical strength, thereby increasing fracture risk. However, the decrease in mass is compensated, to some extent, by changes in cortical dimensions. An age-related increase in total cortical width occurs in men and women. This change is beneficial because fracture resistance is dependent on geometry. However, periosteal apposition is somewhat greater in men and endocortical loss somewhat less, mitigating the loss of thickness and overall mass [16,17]. The typical pattern of age-related change observed in cross-sections of long bones is depicted. Men and women experience cortical thinning; however, men may undergo compensatory increases in section breadth to a greater degree than do women. The tensile resistance of a long bone to fracture is exponentially related to its diameter; thus, the morphologic changes are in accord with the fracture patterns observed in the elderly, in whom the rate of appendicular fractures is less in men than in women. (*Adapted from* Beck *et al.* [16].)

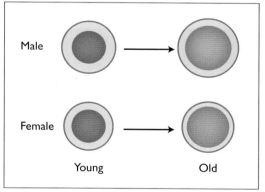

Figure 11-22. The history, physical examination, and routine biochemical profile can be very helpful in directing a focused evaluation of a man with low bone mass. At this stage of the evaluation, emphasis is placed on determining the specific diagnosis (what is the cause of the low bone mass, osteoporosis, or osteomalacia?) and identifying contributing factors in the genesis of the disorder. Risk factors for osteoporosis are explored, including family history, ethnic background, tobacco and alcohol use, lifelong dietary habits, and physical activity. A history of gastrointestinal or renal disease is elicited and information on a loss of height and fracture histories are also obtained. Medications that cause bone loss are identified. A history of fall frequency is obtained and factors that increase the propensity to fall are reviewed. The systems review focuses on conditions that cause secondary osteoporosis (*eg*, endocrinopathies, immobilization, and malabsorption). The physical examination begins with an accurate measurement of height and includes a detailed examination of the spine and hip. The object of the laboratory examination is to find secondary causes of osteopenia. Routine tests, including levels of serum creatinine, albumin, calcium, phosphorus, alkaline phosphatase, and liver function tests, as well as a complete blood count, should be carried out.

Assessing a Man with Low Bone Mass

History	Pharmacologic
Genetic	Glucocorticoids
Family history	Anticonvulsants
Ethnic background	Thyroid hormone
Nutrition	Heparin
Calcium	Physical examination
Vitamin D intake	Height
Malnutrition	Spine anatomy (degree of dorsal kyphosis and lumbar lordosis)
Environmental factors	Hip anatomy
Exercise	Gait
Fall frequency	Testicular examination
Smoking	Laboratory studies
Alcohol	Serum creatinine, albumin, calcium, phosphorus, alkaline phosphatase, liver function tests
Medical	Complete blood count
Hypogonadism	Serum 25(OH) vitamin D
Gastrointestinal disease	Serum testosterone
Renal disease	24-h urine calcium, creatinine

If, on the basis of these tests, there is evidence for medical conditions associated with bone loss (*eg*, alcoholism, hyperparathyroidism, malignancy, Cushing's syndrome, thyrotoxicosis, or malabsorption), a definitive diagnosis should be pursued with appropriate testing.

Figure 11-23. Causes of osteoporosis in men with vertebral fracture. A secondary cause of osteoporosis will be identified in approximately half of men with vertebral fracture. Of these, excessive alcohol ingestion, exogenous use of corticosteroids, and hypogonadism will account for more than half [30].

Evaluation of the Male Patient with Idiopathic Osteoporosis

24-h urine cortisol

Immunological testing for sprue

Serum level of thyroid-stimulating hormone

Serum protein electrophoresis, in those > 50 y to exclude multiple myeloma

Biochemical marker of bone remodeling, to determine whether a cause of high bone turnover is present

Figure 11-24. In men with reduced bone mass in whom no clear pathophysiology is identified by the routine methods listed, it has been considered appropriate to be aggressive diagnostically, primarily because the potential for occult "secondary" causes of osteoporosis is perceived to be high. However, the incidence of occult causes of osteoporosis in men is poorly studied. The diagnostic yield and cost effectiveness of extensive biochemical studies in men with apparently "idiopathic" osteoporosis is unknown. Nevertheless, in the absence of this information, a reasonable evaluation of men for whom the cause of osteoporosis is unknown is outlined.

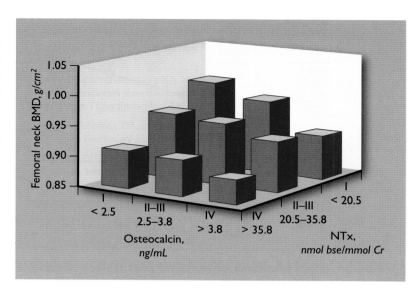

Figure 11-25. Correlation of bone remodeling markers with bone density. Aging in healthy men is associated with detectable appendicular and substantial axial bone loss. The cause of age-related bone loss in men is unknown but has been speculated to be related to an accelerator in bone turnover. Specific biochemical markers of skeletal metabolism, such as serum levels of osteocalcin and urinary excretion of N-telopeptide cross-links (NTx), correlate well with overall remodeling rates in patients with overt metabolic bone disorders and may also be of use in predicting bone mineral density (BMD) in healthy persons. In a study of 273 healthy men aged 65 to 87 years, Krall *et al.* [31] found both serum osteocalcin and urinary NTx levels to be inversely related to BMD. The difference between the femoral neck BMD of persons in the low-osteocalcin low-NTx group and those in the high-osteocalcin high-NTx group was 11%. The strength of the relationship between BMD and biochemical markers of turnover is similar to previous findings in women. These observations raise the possibility that biochemical markers of bone turnover could be used as indicators of current bone status in men.

Therapy

Figure 11-26. Approach to the treatment of reduced bone mass in men. In any man in whom osteoporosis has developed or is considered a clinically important possibility, efforts should be made to improve bone strength and prevent bone loss. Such efforts are the foundation on which a successful treatment plan is based and should always be a part of the prevention of and therapy for osteoporosis, regardless of the other causes of bone disease that may also be present. Calcium supplements are safe and may slow bone loss. Based on suggestive but not definitive data, a recent National Institutes of Health Consensus Development Conference recommended a calcium intake of 1000 mg/d in young men and 1500 mg/d in men older than 65 years of age. Vitamin D deficiency should be suspected in all elderly persons and, if present, treated with daily vitamin D supplements. Available data strongly suggest an effect of weight and mechanical force on the skeletons of men. In view of the decrease in physical activity and muscle strength with aging, senile bone loss in men may be related partly to a diminution of the trophic effects of mechanical force on skeletal tissues. However, a specific exercise prescription is difficult to generate with currently available information. At present, general guidelines include the use of weight-bearing exercise to the extent it can be safely undertaken and the avoidance of situations that might materially increase the risk of trauma and fracture. Measures designed merely to prevent further age-related bone loss may be insufficient in men with moderate or severe osteopenia (these men are at high risk for bone loss because of coexisting and unremediable conditions) and those in whom sustained bone loss has been demonstrated. In these situations, additional pharmacologic therapies should be considered.

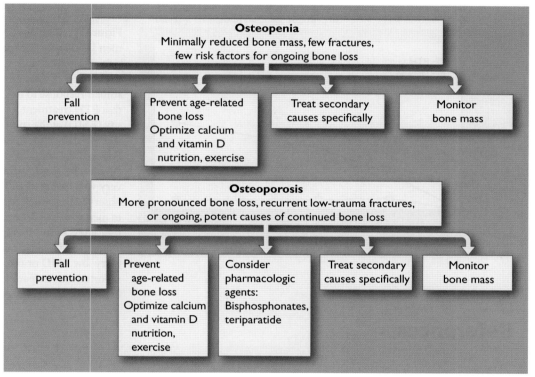

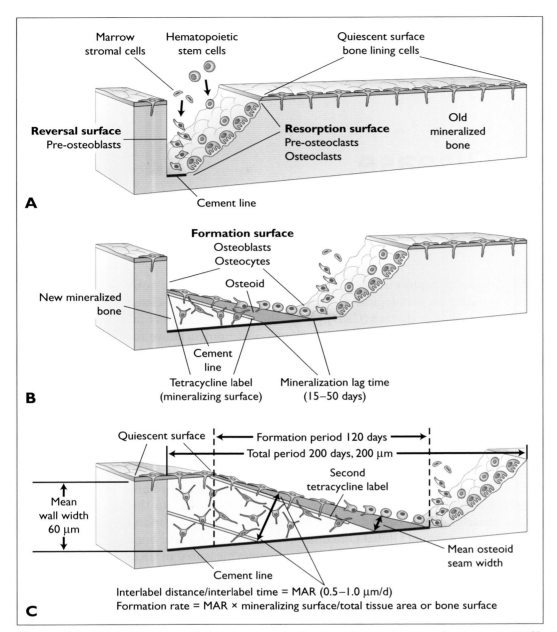

Figure 12-1. Normal bone remodeling. As shown in **A**, remodeling begins with osteoclastic bone resorption that carves out a resorption cavity and ends with the formation of a cement line. As shown in **B**, remodeling continues with osteoblasts depositing nonmineralized bone that then becomes mineralized. The deposition of a new calcification front and mineralizing surface is represented by the tetracycline label (*blue line*). The mineralization lag time is the period from the end of the first tetracycline label to the end of the cement line. In **C**, mineralization is complete and the mineral apposition and bone formation rates are calculated from the distance between the first and second tetracycline label. MAR—mineral apposition rate.

Figure 12-2. Bone remodeling. Normal bone turnover (**A**), low bone turnover due to osteomalacia (**B**), no bone turnover due to adynamic bone disease (**C**), and high bone turnover due to hyperparathyroidism (osteitis fibrosa; **D**) are shown.

In normal bone remodeling states, the amount of bone resorbed matches the amount of bone formed and bone balance is equal. In osteomalacia, there is a mineralization (calcification) defect related to many different etiologies (such as vitamin D deficiency, chronic hypophosphatemia, chronic metabolic acidosis, and excess fibroblast growth factor 23). Osteoid accumulates on most bone surfaces due to a defect in mineralization.

Adynamic bone disease is a form of very low bone turnover bone disease that also has modifiable as well as nonmodifiable etiologies [15,16]. Hyperparathyroid is a form of high bone turnover bone disease often related to hyperparathyroidism. The severity of the high bone turnover is highly correlated to the height of the serum parathyroid hormone.

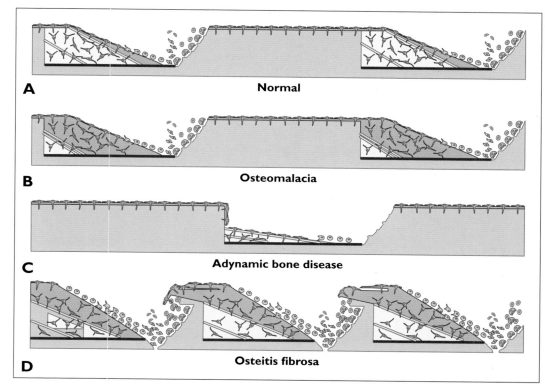

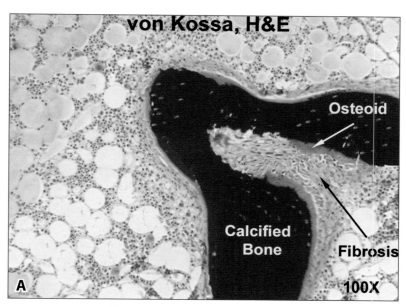

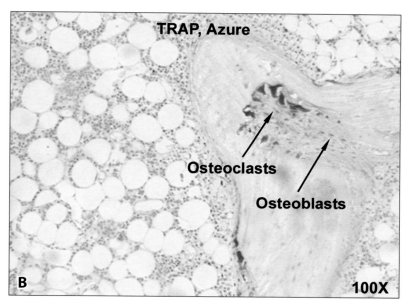

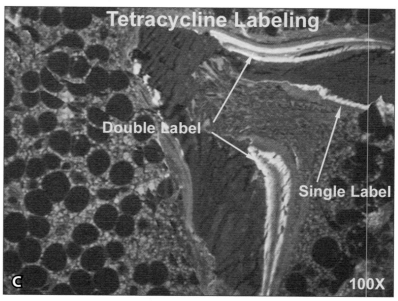

Figure 12-3. Tunneling resorption (high bone turnover from excess parathyroid hormone [PTH]). Osteitis fibrosa cystica (hyperparathyroid bone disease): with progressive chronic kidney disease (CKD), PTH levels rise. The highest PTH levels ever seen in human biology are in patients with severe or stage 5 CKD: a glomerular filtration rate less than 15 mL/min or end-stage renal disease CKD. Even though there is some element of end-organ (bone) resistance to PTH such that these patients rarely become hypercalcemic, the bone histology often reflects the activity of high PTH values. In the biopsy shown, there is evidence of high bone turnover, increased mineralization as reflected by active tetracycline incorporation into bone, increased resorption and formation surfaces, and abundant osteoclasts and osteoblasts. In severe hyperparathyroidism there is tunneling resorption where the resorption front drills into the deeper portion of the bone and there is marrow fibrosis. **A,** Normal bone remodeling. **B,** Osteomalacia where bone turnover is reduced and there is an accumulation of wide and abundant osteoid surfaces. **C,** Osteitis fibrosa cystica where there is high bone remodeling, many osteoclasts, and marrow fibrosis. H&E—hematoxylin and eosin; TRAP—tartrate-resistant acid phosphatase. (*From* Miller and Huffer [4]; with permission.)

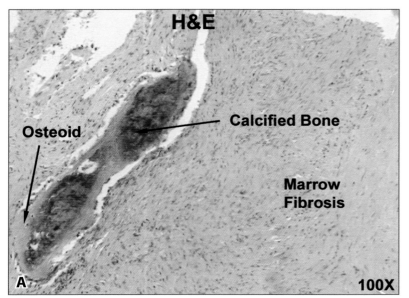

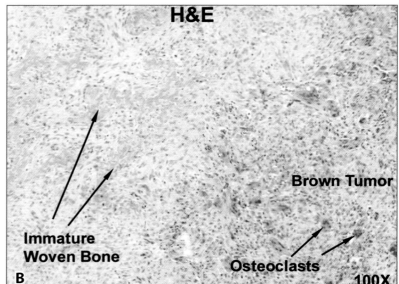

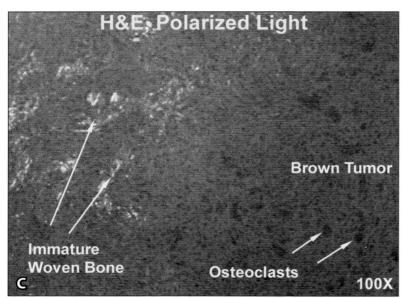

Figure 12-4. Osteitis fibrosa cystica: severe secondary hyperparathyroidism. **A,** Abundant marrow fibrosis with more severe hyperparathyroidism is shown. **B,** A "brown tumor," a collection of mesenchymal giant cells due to excess parathyroid hormone, is shown. **C,** The same brown tumor is shown using polarized light. H&E—hematoxylin and eosin. (*From* Miller and Huffer [4]; with permission.)

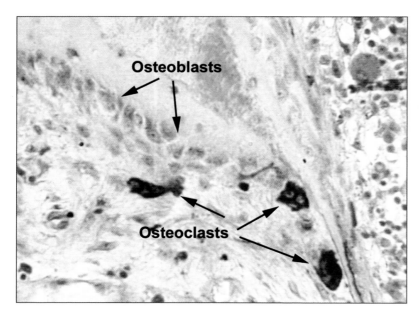

Figure 12-5. Hyperparathyroidism demonstrating a high number of osteoblasts and osteoclasts per millimeter of bone surface is shown. In hyperparathyroidism, both cell lines have increases in activity and number. (*From* Miller and Huffer [4]; with permission.)

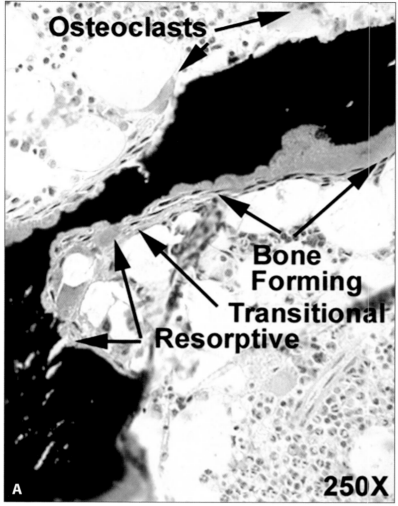

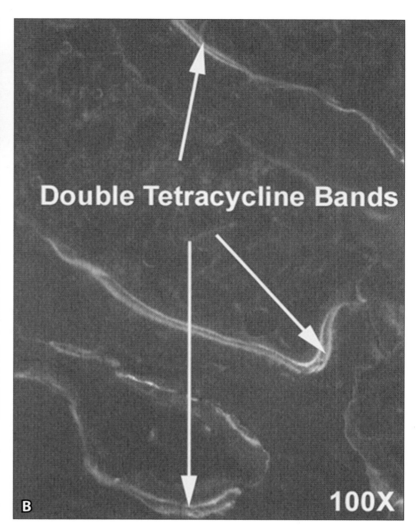

Figure 12-6. High bone turnover possibly due to cyclosporin, a calcineurin inhibitor. The calcineurin inhibitors used to reduce the risk of transplant rejection may independently induce high bone remodeling [17].

A, Abundant osteoclasts and resorptive surfaces. **B,** Abundant double-tetracycline bands, indicating increased mineralization. (*From* Miller and Huffer [4]; with permission.)

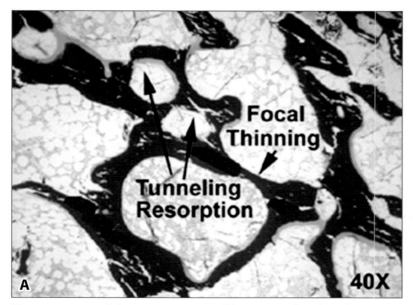

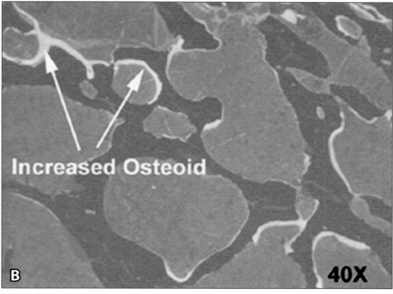

Figure 12-7. High bone turnover possibly associated with cyclosporin, a calcineurin inhibitor. These four panels show the high bone turnover commonly seen with use of the antirejection drug cyclosporine. **A,** Thinning of

the trabeculae and tunneling resorption. **B,** Increased osteoid that accompanies many high bone turnover states.

Continued on the next page

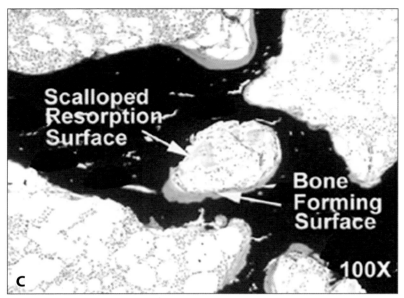

C

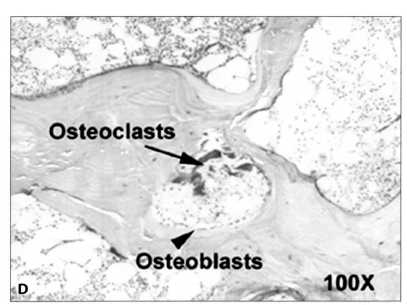

D

Figure 12-7. *(Continued)* **C,** Scalloped resorptive surfaces and **D,** abundant osteoclasts and osteoblasts that are also seen in high bone turnover states. These histological changes may also be seen with severe hyperparathyroidism. (*From* Miller and Huffer [4]; with permission.)

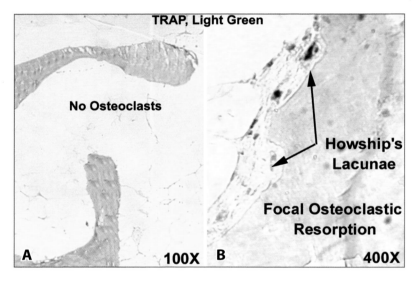

A   B

Figure 12-8. A, Tartrate-resistant acid phosphatase (TRAP) stain showing no osteoclasts on trabecular surfaces or in Howship's Lacunae. **B,** TRAP stain showing no osteoclasts, a characteristic of adynamic bone disease (no bone turnover). (*From* Miller and Huffer [4]; with permission.)

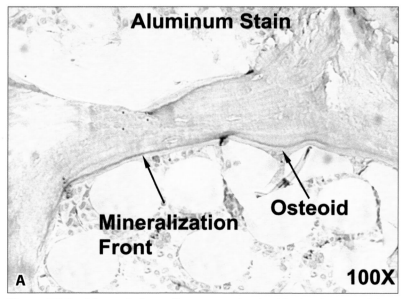

A

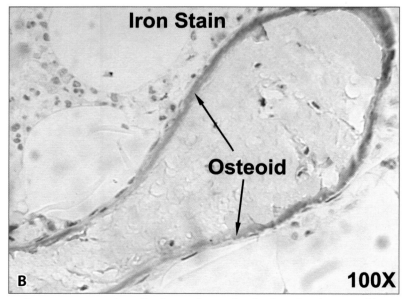

B

Figure 12-9. Adynamic bone disease associated with aluminum and iron accumulation at the osteoid surface. Two of the modifiable etiologies of low bone turnover bone disease is either aluminum or iron accumulation on the osteoid surfaces. The presence of these metals, which can attach to the bone surfaces, prevents mineralization and can also lead to the absence of bone formation (no tetracycline labels) and represents the most severe end of the spectrum of low bone turnover disorders (adynamic bone disease). **A,** On the mineralization front there is abundant aluminum (*light blue lines*).

Continued on the next page

Figure 12-9. *(Continued)* **B,** Aluminum bone disease is also associated with the accumulation of osteoid (matrix) in *blue* due to the inhibition of mineralization of osteoid caused by the presence of aluminum (*From* Miller and Huffer [4]; with permission.)

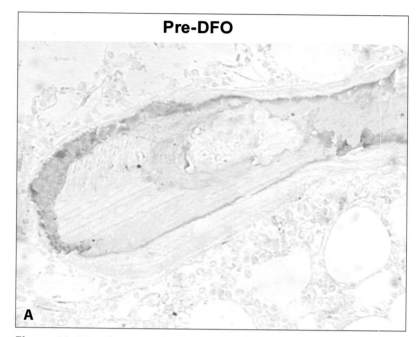

Pre-DFO

A

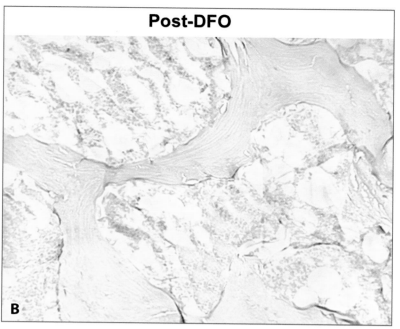

Post-DFO

B

Figure 12-10. Aluminum bone disease. Low bone turnover is associated with aluminum deposition and removal with desferrioxamine (DFO) chelation. Aluminum bone disease, a form of low bone turnover bone disease, is less common since nonaluminum phosphate binders have been used to control hyperphosphatemia in chronic kidney disease (CKD). However, its presence is still found since aluminum is ubiquitous in the environment and patients with severe CKD cannot excrete aluminum, which binds by a physiochemical mechanism to the calcification front (**A**). DFO can remove aluminum (**B**), which is best documented by repeat bone biopsy. (*From* Miller and Huffer [4]; with permission.)

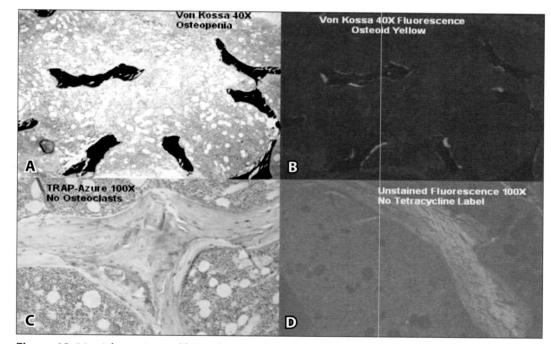

Figure 12-11. Adynamic renal bone disease. These four panels show clear evidence of renal adynamic bone disease. **A,** A scant amount of bone (few trabeculae) and **B,** scant osteoid. **C,** No osteoclasts in the tartrate-resistant acid phosphatase (TRAP) stain. **D,** Hallmark of adynamic bone disease—absent tetracycline labels that are indicative of no mineralization.

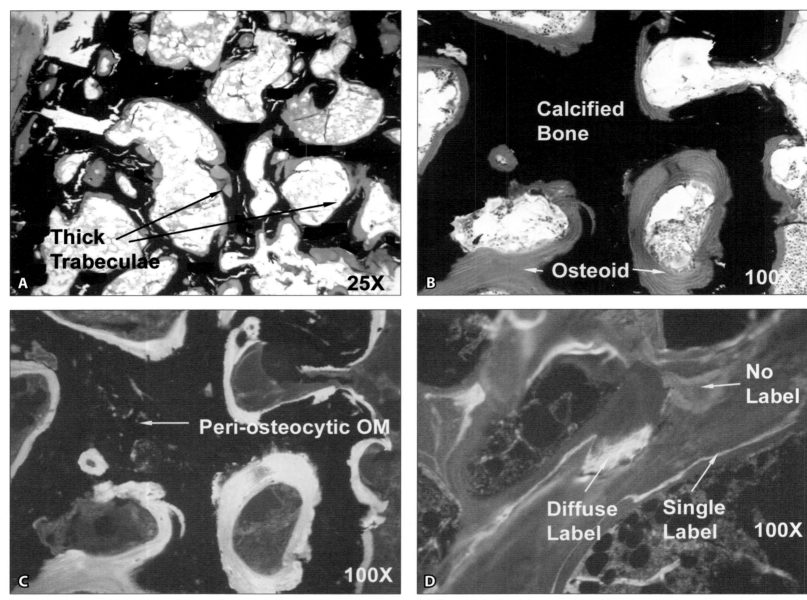

Figure 12-12. Osteomalacia. Osteomalacia has very specific quantitative histomorphometric criteria. **A** and **B** show the calcified bone (*black*) and the abundant noncalcified bone (*pink* and *yellow*). There must be more than 80% of the total bone surface covered by osteoid and the osteoid thickness must be greater than 14 μm. Since osteomalacia is a low bone turnover state, there are few tetracycline labels seen and in some cases the labels are "smudged," suggestive of the altered mineralization that is seen. **C,** Osteomamalca (OM) is characterized by abundant (> 80% of the trabecular surfaces covered by osteoid), thick (< 14 microns) osteoid, and a prolonged mineralization lag time. **D,** OM is a low bone turnover state and the mineralization (shown in *yellow* with tetracycline labels) is disorderly and not linear. (*From* Miller and Huffer [4]; with permission.)

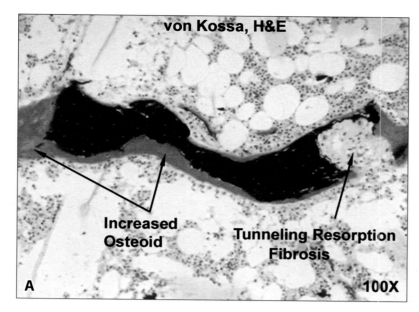

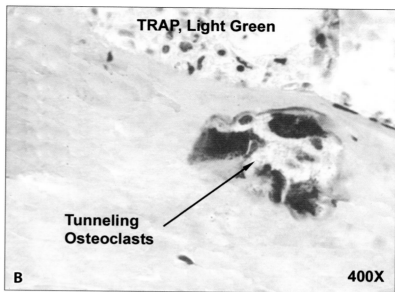

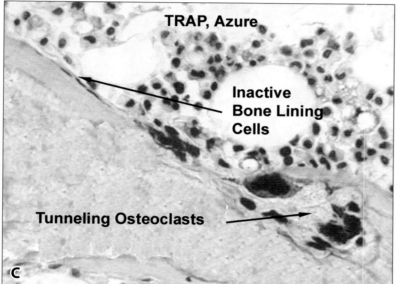

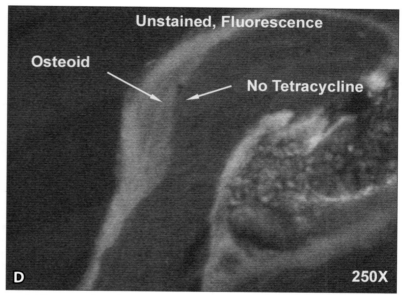

Figure 12-13. Mixed renal bone disease: osteitis fibrosa and osteomalacia. In some cases of renal bone disease, a "mixed" histology is seen; *ie*, a combination of high bone turnover with what appears to be areas of "low" bone turnover. In fact, most of these cases are really not a combination of osteitis fibrosa cystica (hyperparathyroid bone disease) and osteomalacia (low bone turnover), but situations in which there is predominately high bone turnover and osteoid (nonmineralized bone) accumulates because mineralization rates cannot keep up with the high bone resorption and osteoid production.

A, There are abundant osteoids, but areas of tunneling bone resorption are characteristic of severe hyperparathyroid bone disease. **B,** Tunneling osteoclasts are also a feature of severe hyperparathyroidism. **C,** Tunneling osteoclasts and areas of osteoid are shown; inactive bone cells are seen as well. **D,** The absence of tetracycline labels (mineralization) is suggestive of low bone turnover areas in the bone section. However, the high bone turnover may lead to areas where osteoid accumulates so quickly that mineralization cannot keep up. These cases do not represent a true biological combination of hyperparathyroid bone disease and osteomalacia. (*From* Miller and Huffer [4]; with permission.)

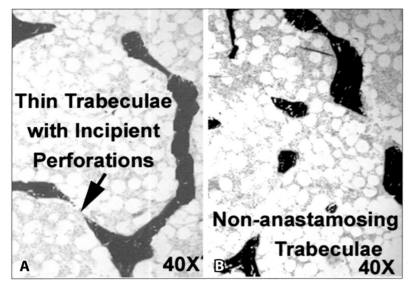

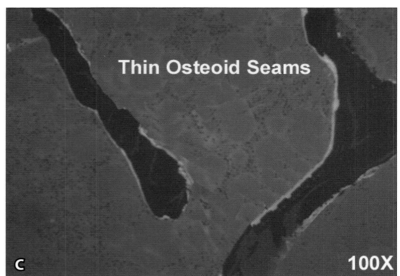

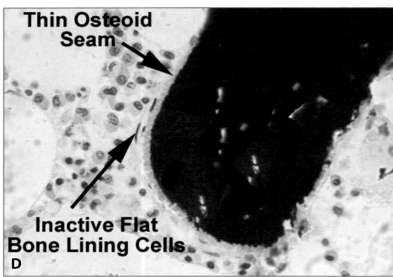

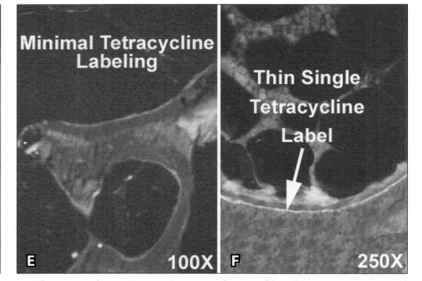

Figure 12-14. Low bone turnover renal bone disease. These six panels show histological features of low bone turnover but not true adynamic bone disease since there are some, albeit few, tetracycline labels. In **A, B,** and **D,** Von Kossa hematoxylin and eosin microscopy was used. In **C, E,** and **F,** fluorescent microscopy was used. In **A** and **B,** there are scant trabeculae and in **D** the osteoid seam is thin, suggesting that matrix formation is reduced. These osteoid seams are shown again in **C. E** shows the minimal tetracycline labels.

There may be an increasing prevalence of low bone turnover renal bone disease. There is a renal working group (Kidney Disease Improving Global Outcomes) that has developed a new concept in renal bone disease classification, metabolic bone disease–chronic kidney disease, to link the abnormalities in bone turnover that accompany chronic kidney disease to the systemic calcification of blood vessels and the subsequent cascade of cardiovascular events [8–9]. (*From* Miller and Huffer [4]; with permission.)

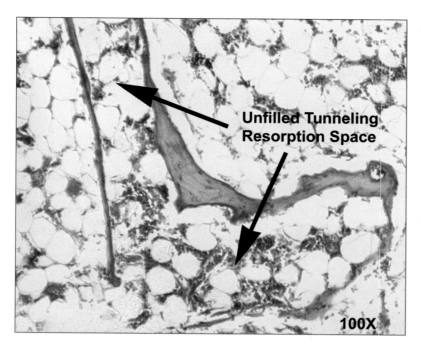

Unfilled Tunneling
Resorption Space

100X

Figure 12-15. Steroid-induced osteoporosis. Osteoporosis is defined as a systemic skeletal disease with microarchitectural deterioration of bone and disrupted and thin trabeculae, which leads to poor bone strength. A secondary cause of osteoporosis is shown with sparse trabeculae and unfilled tunneling and resorption space. Glucocorticoids lead to poor bone formation [18]. (*From* Miller and Huffer [4]; with permission.)

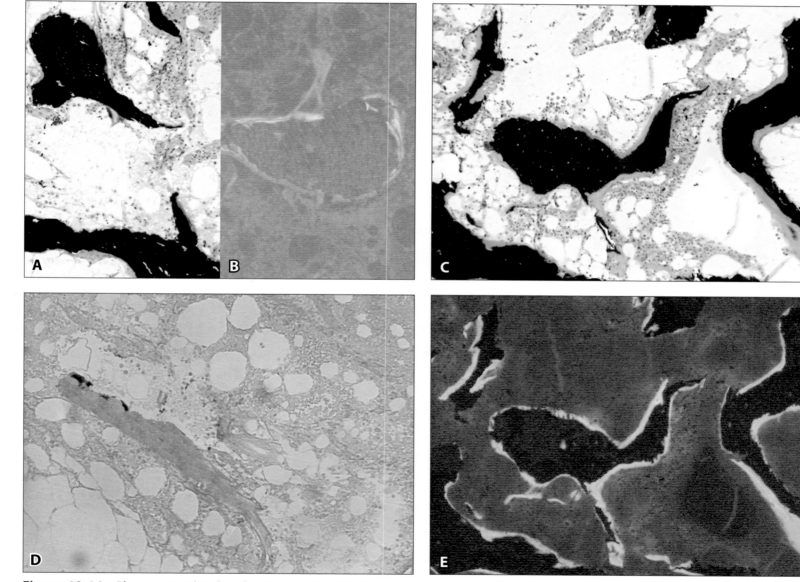

Figure 12-16. Glucocorticoid-induced osteoporosis with low bone formation, resorption, and mineralization and focal hyperosteoidosis. **A,** Both a hematoxylin and eosin stain and **B,** a polarized light show thin disrupted trabeculae. **C** shows the focal bone resorption (*scalloping* *of trabeculae*) and focal osteoid accumulation (*pink areas*) that are also demonstrated in **E** under polarized light. **D** shows the sparse trabeculae in bone in this osteoporotic state. (*From* Miller and Huffer [4]; with permission.)

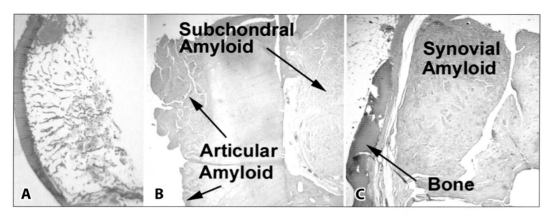

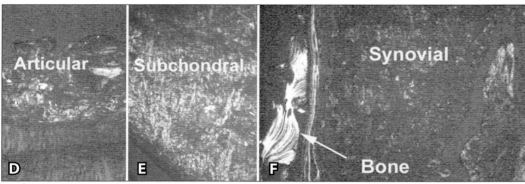

Figure 12-17. Amyloid bone disease. Amyloid (β-2 microglobulin) can accumulate in joints and soft tissue in chronic kidney disease and lead to articular and joint disease. Synovial amyloid is seen in both the hematoxylin and eosin (**A–C**) and congo red, polarized light stains (**D–F**). (*From* Miller and Huffer [4]; with permission.)

References

1. Hruska KA, Teitelbaum SL: Renal osteodystrophy. *N Engl J Med* 1995, 333:166–172.

2. Goodman WG, Coburn JW, Slatopolsky E, Salusky I: Renal osteodystrophy in adults and children. In *Primer on the Metabolic Bone Diseases and Disorders of Mineral Metabolism*, edn 4. Edited by Favus MJ. Philadelphia: Lippincott-Raven; 1999:347–363.

3. Sherrard DJ, Hercz G, Pei Y, *et al.*: The spectrum of bone disease in end-stage renal failure—an evolving disorder. *Kidney Int* 1993, 43:436–442.

4. Miller PD, Huffer W: Renal osteodystrophy. In *Essential Atlas of Nephrology and Hypertension*, edn 2. Edited by Schrier RW, Bennett W. Philadelphia: Current Medicine; 2006:261–276.

5. Parfitt AM, Drezner MK, Glorieux FH, *et al.*: Bone histomorphometry: standardization of nomenclature, symbols, and units. *J Bone Miner Res* 1987, 2:595–610.

6. Massry SG, Coburn JW: K/DOQI clinical practice guidelines for bone metabolism and disease in chronic kidney disease. *Am J Kid Dis* 2003, 42:S10–S135.

7. Moe S, Drueke T, Cunningham J, *et al.*: Definition, evaluation, and classification of renal osteodystrophy: a position statement from Kidney Disease: Improving Global Outcomes (KDIGO). *Kidney Int* 2006, 69:1945–1953.

8. Hruska K: New concepts in renal osteodystrophy. *Nephrol Dial Transplant* 1998, 13:2755–2760.

9. Moe SM: Vascular calcification and renal osteodystrophy relationship in chronic kidney disease. *Eur J Clin Invest* 2006, 36:51–62.

10. WHO Study Group: *Assessment of Fracture Risk and Its Application to Screening for Postmenopausal Osteoporosis*. Geneva, Switzerland: World Health Organization; 1994.

11. NIH Consensus Development Panel on Osteoporosis Prevention, Diagnosis, and Therapy: March 7–29, 2000: highlights of the conference. *South Med J* 2001, 94:569–573.

12. Miller PD: Treatment of osteoporosis in chronic kidney disease and end-stage renal disease. *Curr Osteoporos Rep* 2005, 3:5–12.

13. Cunningham J, Sprague SM, Cannata-Andia J, *et al.*: Osteoporosis in chronic kidney disease. *Am J Kidney Dis* 2004, 43:566–571.

14. Gal-Moscovici A, Sprague S: Osteoporosis and chronic kidney disease. *Semin Dial* 2007, 20:423–430.

15. Coen G: Adynamic bone disease: an update. *J Nephrol* 2005, 18:117–122.

16. Salusky IB, Goodman WG: Reversible and non-reversible adynamic renal bone disease. *J Am Soc Nephrol* 2001, 12:1978–1985.

17. Epstein S: Post-transplantation bone disease: the role of immunosuppressive agents on the skeleton. *J Bone Miner Res* 1996, 11:1–7.

18. Canalis E, Mazziotti G, Giustina A, Bilezikian JP: Glucocorticoid-induced osteoporosis: pathophysiology and therapy. *Osteoporos Int* 2007, 18:1319–1328.

Radiology of Osteoporotic Fracture

13

Jan E. Vandevenne, Carl S. Winalski, and Philipp K. Lang

Osteoporosis is characterized by a decrease in the bone mineral density (BMD) of structurally normal bone: the dynamic equilibrium between bone resorption and bone formation is perturbed in favor of bone resorption, resulting in osteopenia. Decreased BMD undermines the structural integrity of bone. The elastic range of osteopenic bone is decreased and deformative stress on these bones more readily results in microfractures. Continued and progressive stress on osteoporotic bone may lead to structural failure [1–6]. For this reason, insufficiency fractures as well as fractures after minor trauma occur more frequently in the osteopenic skeleton of the patient who has osteoporosis [7–9]. Osteoporotic fractures are seen mainly in older white women, but osteoporosis induced by any other condition, eg, hyperparathyroidism, cortisone treatment, and pregnancy, can lead to fractures [10–13]. Healing of osteoporotic fractures may be slow and difficult, and nonunion of fractures can result.

Insufficiency fractures due to osteoporosis and fractures from minor traumatic events tend to involve certain locations of the axial and appendicular skeleton. Typically, the thoracic and lumbar vertebrae and the hip, wrist, and proximal humerus are the areas involved. Thoracic and lumbar vertebrae may show collapse and spontaneous fractures frequently occur in the pelvic girdle, especially in the sacral wings, pubic symphysis, and supra-acetabular region [14]. Femoral neck insufficiency fractures may occur spontaneously but are more often related to trauma. A fall on an outstretched hand is the most frequent cause of fracture of the distal radius and the proximal humerus. Less frequently, osteoporotic fractures are seen in the calcaneus, talus, proximal tibia, and ribs. This chapter provides an overview of osteoporotic fractures and their characteristic locations.

Vertebral Compression Fractures

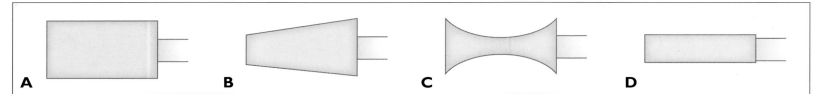

Figure 13-1. Vertebral deformity after vertebral fracture can be classified into three groups. Normal vertebrae have parallel endplates (**A**). On the lateral view, most collapsed vertebrae are wedge shaped or biconcave. A wedge-shaped deformity is most frequently seen in thoracic vertebrae that sustain more compression anteriorly than posteriorly (**B**). Biconcave (or "fish") vertebrae have concave depressions of the upper and sometimes also the lower endplates, and are more common in the lumbar spine (**C**). The completely collapsed or crushed vertebrae demonstrate a flattened or "pancake" appearance (**D**).

A practical and commonly used way to estimate the severity of a compression fracture, in addition to the description as either a wedge-shaped, biconcave, or crush fracture, is the semiquantitative method proposed by Genant *et al.* [15]. A loss of vertebral height by up to 25% is considered to be a minor compression fracture (grade 1), while between 26% and 40% is moderate (grade 2) and more than 40% is a severe compression fracture (grade 3) [15]. With approximately 700,000 cases in the United States each year, vertebral fractures account for nearly half of all osteoporotic fractures and are at least twice as common as hip fractures [16]. The identification of vertebral fractures has a vital role in the prognosis and management of patients with osteoporosis [17–26]. Patients who have a vertebral fracture have a five-fold higher risk of further vertebral fractures and a two-fold higher risk of hip fracture [27]. A patient with vertebral fracture and low bone mineral density is at a 25-fold increased risk for subsequent vertebral fracture compared to a patient with no fracture and high bone density [28,29]. Mild vertebral fractures are a risk factor for subsequent vertebral and nonvertebral fracture in postmenopausal women with osteoporosis: one of four patients with an incident mild vertebral fracture in the last 2 years will fracture again within the 2 next years [30].

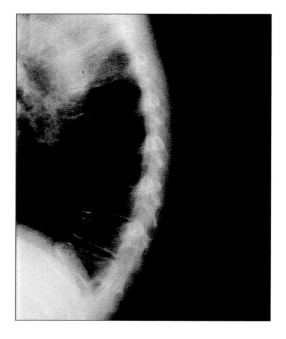

Figure 13-2. Two compression fractures of the vertebrae in the lower thoracic and upper lumbar spine as seen on the lateral chest view of a 91-year-old woman. General osteopenia of the spine is evident, with decreased density of the vertebrae and thinning of the cortical and subchondral bone. In some cases of early osteopenia, the relatively more pronounced decrease in density of the trabecular bone compared with the cortical and subchondral bone may give the erroneous impression of increased bone density in the cortical and subchondral bone. In this patient, weight-bearing forces have overmatched the structural integrity of the osteopenic vertebral bodies at the thoraco-lumbar level of the spine, which resulted in anterior collapse of the twelfth thoracic and the first lumbar vertebral body, showing a wedge-shaped deformity in these vertebrae. Vertebral collapse is frequently seen at the point of transition between the thoracic kyphosis and the lumbar lordosis.

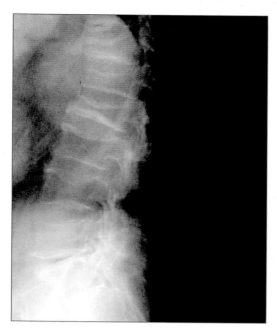

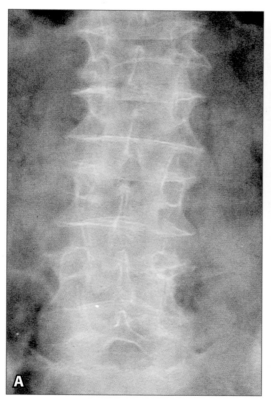

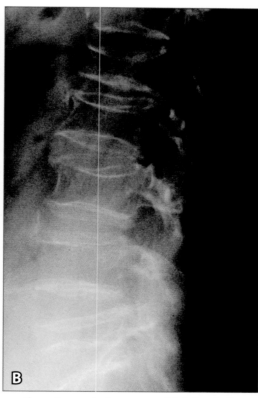

Figure 13-3. Multiple compression fractures of the lumbar spine of a 55-year-old man who received prolonged cortisone treatment. Decreased density of the vertebrae results from drug-induced demineralization. Compression fractures with decreased vertebral height are seen in the twelfth thoracic vertebra, and the first, second, and third lumbar vertebrae. Biconcave collapse of the fourth lumbar vertebra is seen. Note that the disk spaces are not narrowed and even appear to be enlarged, owing to the collapse of the vertebrae. Prolonged cortisone treatment may induce pronounced osteopenia and lead to multiple compression fractures of the spine.

Figure 13-4. Multiple compression fractures, as seen on the anteroposterior (**A**) and lateral (**B**) views of the lumbar spine of a 76-year-old woman. Note the generalized osteopenia with increased translucency of the vertebral bodies and thinning of the cortical and subchondral bone. Vertebral collapse has occurred at multiple levels. Severe compression of the fifth lumbar vertebra has resulted in a flattened vertebra. Partial collapse with loss of height and biconcave deformity is seen in the twelfth thoracic and the first three lumbar vertebrae. The height of the fourth lumbar vertebra is unchanged.

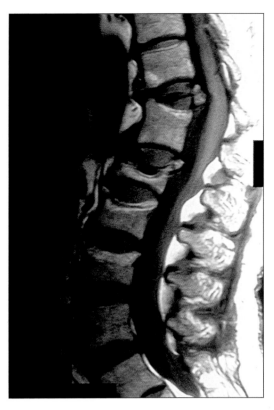

Figure 13-5. MRI of compression fractures in the spine is useful in demonstrating the compression of important structures, such as spinal nerves and the spinal cord. MRI is also used to exclude other causes of back pain and may help to differentiate osteoporotic compression fractures from pathologic fractures. This T1-weighted MR image was obtained after an intravenous injection of a gadolinium-chelated MR contrast agent, in a 48-year-old woman. It confirmed the presence of a concave compression fracture of the upper endplate of the first lumbar vertebra. A bone fragment extending posteriorly into the epidural space can be seen. The T12 vertebral body is completely collapsed, demonstrating low signal intensity on this sequence. There is a second larger bone fragment in the epidural space located posteriorly at this level. Depression of the superior endplates of the second and third lumbar vertebrae is also seen. The spinal cord compression by the collapsed vertebral bodies represents clinically important information in this patient [31,32]. Although spinal canal compromise due to fracture fragments is often considered to be a contra-indication to perform vertebroplasty, a recent series described no major complications after vertebroplasty in these patients [33].

MRI can be used to exclude the presence of a neoplastic process as the underlying cause of compression fractures, *eg*, by the absence of a mass lesion. Specific sequences or the injection of gadolinium contrast agent can be used to demonstrate a neoplastic mass within the collapsed vertebra [34,35]. When malignancy is suspected for clinical reasons and MR cannot exclude a neoplastic process, biopsy should be performed.

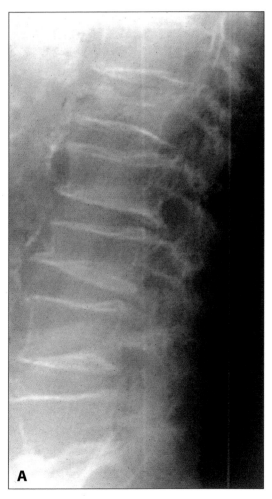

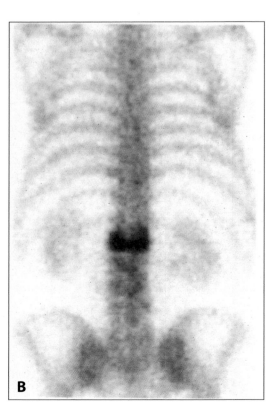

Figure 13-6. Lateral radiograph (**A**) and bone scan (**B**) of the lumbar spine in a patient with multiple compression fractures of thoracic and lumbar vertebrae. A generalized decrease in bone density is noted as well, which represents bone demineralization and thinning of the bony trabeculae and the cortical bone. The lateral view of the lumbar spine shows several compression fractures, whereas the bone scan is positive in only the L1 vertebral body. This finding suggests an acute process in the L1 vertebral body and makes the fractures of the other vertebral bodies likely to be older ones.

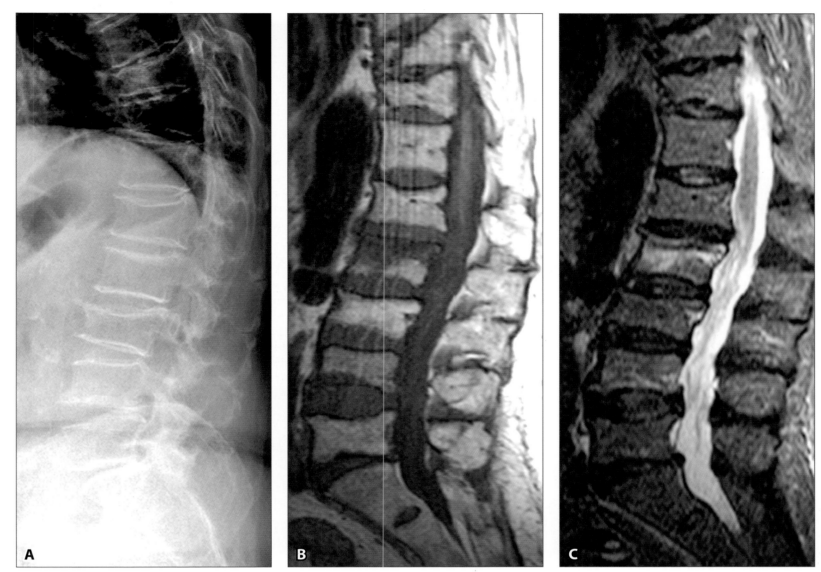

Figure 13-7. Lateral radiograph (**A**) and MRIs (**B** and **C**) of the dorsolumbar spine of a 74-year-old woman who has persistent lower back pain. Compression fractures of multiple vertebra are seen on the radiograph and height loss is most notable at levels D10, D11, L1, L3, and L4. Back pain is less likely to be related to older healed vertebral compression fractures, and differentiation between older and more recent fractures is important to plan minimally invasive interventions such as vertebroplasty. T1-weighted (**B**) and short time-to-invert inversion recovery (STIR) (**C**) MR sequences, respectively, are most useful to demonstrate bone marrow edema. Edema in the vertebral bodies is revealed as dark areas in T1-weighted sequences (**B**) and light areas in STIR sequences (**C**). In this patient, the L2 vertebra surprisingly demonstrated marked bone marrow edema, suggestive of a recent insuffuciency fracture. Note also some bone marrow edema adjacent to the inferior endplate of L4. Both L2 and L4 are considered to have unhealed fractures and to be responsible for persistent low back pain. Vertebroplasty may be performed at these levels. No bone marrow edema is seen in the other vertebrae with height loss and these fractures are considered to be healed.

Figure 13-8. Vertebroplasty performed in a 71-year-old woman as demonstrated on the antero-posterior (**A**) and lateral (**B**) views of the lumbar spine. These radiographs show osteopenia of the lumbar spine, moderate to severe compression deformity of the L3 vertebral body, and a biconcave compression fracture of the L4 vertebral body. Two needles are placed in the L4 vertebral body via a bilateral transpedicle approach. Cement is injected bilaterally in order to achieve an even distribution of the material in the vertebral body. The vertebroplasty of the L3 vertebral body has already been completed.

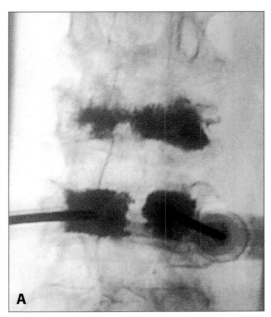
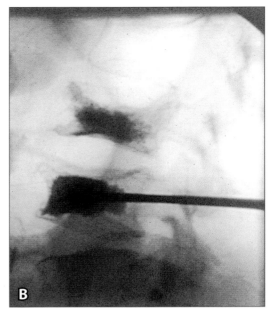

Percutaneous vertebroplasty [35–50] is a therapeutic procedure in which polymethylmethacrylate is injected under continuous radiologic guidance into a diseased vertebra. The aim of this procedure in osteoporotic vertebral lesions is to stabilize the vertebra in order to relieve pain and to prevent further deterioration of the vertebra in a patient whose pain and clinical symptoms are not responding to conservative treatment.

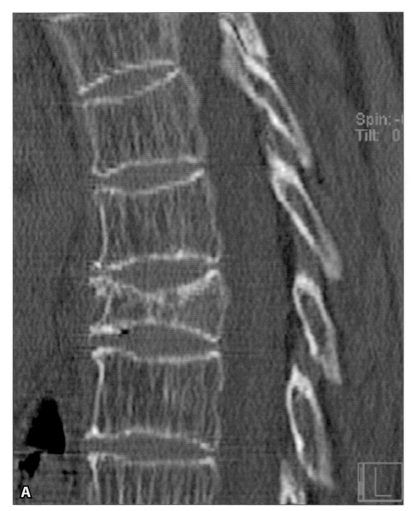
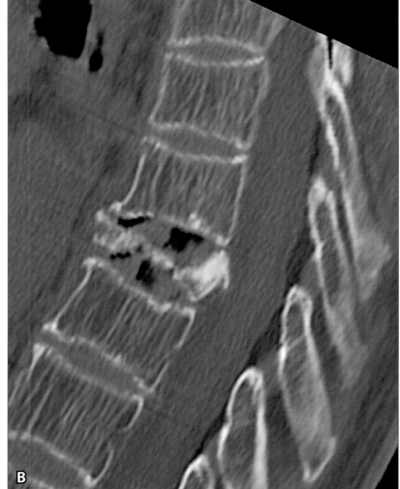

Figure 13-9. CT scan of a 79-year-old woman at the time of a vertebral compression fracture (**A**) and at followup 3 months later (**B**). Osteopenia may be inferred from the thinned cortical bone and the sparse bone trabecula present in all vertebrae. At presentation (**A**), a moderate to severe crush-type fracture of D8 is present and conservative medical treatment with relative rest was used. At followup (**B**), further collapse of this vertebra is seen, demonstrating a flattened "pancake" appearance. These imaging findings illustrate that vertebral compression fractures may not heal easily, particularly in the presence of osteopenia. In such cases, further vertebral collapse may occur and potentially compression of nerve roots or spinal cord may result. Complete vertebral collapse could be prevented by performing vertebroplasty.

Hip Fractures

Figure 13-10. Femoral neck fracture in the left hip of a 66-year-old woman. Note the presence of a fracture in the femoral neck at the transition between the neck and the femoral head. The distal fracture fragment (femoral shaft) is displaced in a superior direction and rotated externally. Overall, decreased density of the hip is indicative of osteopenia. In a normal hip, specifically arranged groups of bony trabeculae, vertically directed (compressive) and horizontally directed (tensile) groups, run through the obliquely oriented femoral neck and connect the femoral shaft with the femoral head. Bone demineralization secondary to osteoporosis decreases the loading capacity of the obliquely oriented femoral neck; as a result, fractures may occur after minor trauma. In this patient, a fall with the leg externally rotated caused the femoral neck fracture. Fractures that occur as a consequence of osteopenia in patients suffering from osteoporosis are most frequently seen in the spine, followed by the hip (the proximal portion of the femur). However, hip fractures are clinically more significant and may lead to permanent disability or death, *eg*, from pulmonary embolism.

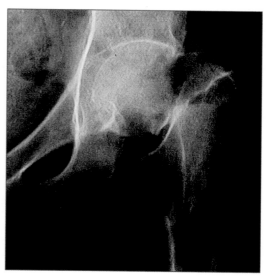

Figure 13-11. Cervical fracture of the left hip of a 73-year-old woman. Note the decreased bone mineral density in the hip and pelvic bones. No definite fracture line can be seen and no displacement of fracture fragments is present. However, the foreshortening of the femoral neck and the presence of a linear area of increased density perpendicular to the normal direction of the bone trabeculae indicate an impaction fracture. Classification of hip fractures by anatomic location includes subcapital, cervical, basicervical, intertrochanteric, and subtrochanteric types. Intracapsular fractures (subcapital and cervical fractures) are often classified according to the degree of displacement, as described in the Garden system [51]. Type I fractures are incomplete or impacted in nature; type II fractures are complete without osseous displacement; type III fractures are complete with partial displacement of the fracture fragments; and type IV fractures are complete with total displacement of the fracture fragments. Intracapsular hip fractures with displacement of the fracture fragments often cause avascular necrosis of the femoral head because the disrupted capsule contains the most important vessels that supply blood to the femoral head. The cervical fracture in this patient was classified as type I according to the Garden system.

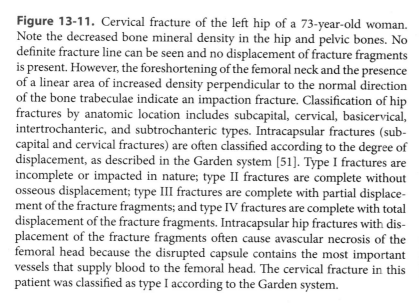

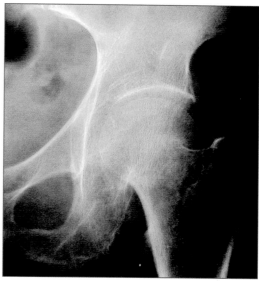

Figure 13-12. Combined subtrochanteric and intertrochanteric fracture of the left hip of a 74-year-old woman after a fall. A transverse fracture line is present inferior to the lesser and the greater trochanters, both of which have been avulsed. Note the varus position of the proximal fracture fragment (femoral neck) and proximal shift of the distal fracture fragment (femoral shaft). Generalized osteopenia is seen in all pelvic bones, related to osteoporosis [52,53].

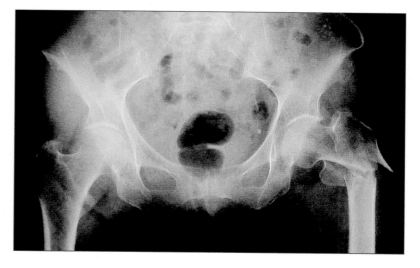

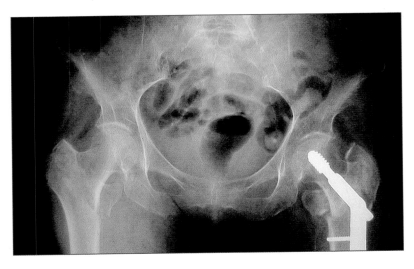

Figure 13-13. Intertrochanteric fracture of the right hip in the same patient as in Figure 13-11, 6 weeks later. Note the presence of a complete fracture through the lesser and greater trochanters of the right hip without displacement of the fracture fragments. The fracture of the left hip has been treated surgically, using a dynamic hip screw and plate device to fixate the femoral neck to the femoral shaft. Three weeks after her release from the hospital, the patient fell again and fractured her right hip. Elderly patients tend to fall more often for a variety of reasons, which can contribute substantially to their increased incidence of hip fractures.

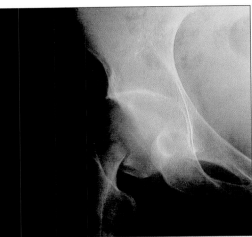

Figure 13-14. Subcapital fracture of the right hip of a patient a few weeks after the delivery of her second child. Thinning and obscuration of the subchondral cortex and decreased density of the bony trabeculae in the femoral head suggest extensive bone demineralization in the femoral head, whereas bone mineralization remains normal in the adjacent acetabulum. This radiologic image in a young woman in the postpartum period strongly suggests the presence of "transient osteoporosis of the hip." Although this condition does not usually lead to fracture, it has resulted in a subcapital fracture in this patient. The cause of pregnancy-related transient osteoporosis is unknown, and various joints and bones may be affected [12,13]. Pregnancy-related osteoporotic fractures are rare, but they may be seen in the hip and thoracic spine. Transient osteoporosis of the hip occurs in young and middle-aged adults, more frequently in men. It starts with spontaneous hip pain without previous trauma, which progresses in a few weeks and usually subsides in 2 to 6 months. Radiographically progressive marked osteoporosis of the femoral head is seen several weeks after the onset of the hip pain and restoration of the normal bone density follows clinical recovery. MRI is currently the most sensitive technique for early detection of the bone marrow edema that may indicate transient osteoporosis of the hip: extensive diffuse increased signal intensity of the femoral neck and head is seen on fat-suppressed T2-weighted MR images.

Pelvic Insufficiency Fractures

Figure 13-15. Pelvic insufficiency fractures in a 72-year-old woman. Note the overall osteopenic aspect of the pelvic bones. The pubic bones have a mixed osteosclerotic and osteolytic appearance, with irregular areas of increased and decreased density seen in the trabecular bone. The cortical bone at the symphysis is not well defined, which is indicative of an insufficiency fracture of the symphysis pubis. Bilateral areas of mixed osteosclerosis and osteolysis are typically seen in insufficiency fractures of the symphysis pubis and may represent areas of microfractures and areas of bone regrowth. In some cases, bone tumors, such as chondrosarcoma, can mimic this radiologic presentation, particularly when the pathology is unilateral [54]. The sacrum appears very osteopenic and the arcuate lines (*arrow*) outlining the sacral neuroforamina are indistinct. This radiologic appearance, together with the patient's clinical complaints of pain posteriorly at the pelvic girdle, raises the suspicion of sacral pathology, *eg*, sacral insufficiency fracture (*see* Fig. 13-14). Additionally, a step-off is noted at the inferior aspect of the left sacrum adjacent to the sacroiliac joint.

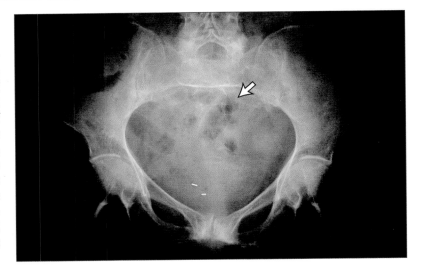

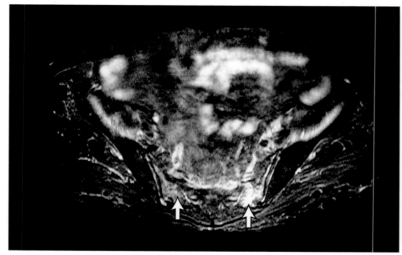

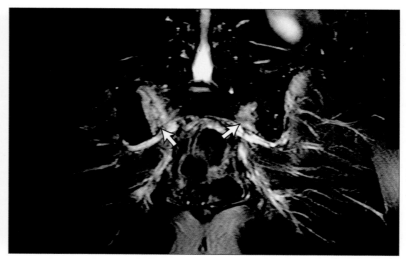

Figure 13-16. MRI of sacral insufficiency fracture in the same patient shown in Figure 13-15. In this axial fat-saturated T2-weighted MR image, all structures with high water content have a bright signal. For example, the small intestines superiorly in the image are filled with fluid and have a bright signal (*white*). Note the normal low signal (*black*) of the bone marrow in the iliac bones. However, increased signal (*white*) is seen in the sacrum bilaterally (*arrows*), which indicates increased water content of the bone marrow (*bottom center of image*). This pattern of bone marrow edema in elderly osteopenic patients is highly suggestive of bilateral sacral insufficiency fractures [21]. Bone tumors and metastases can simulate this condition, but tend to be unilateral and asymmetric, while the bone marrow edema of insufficiency fractures is usually bilateral and decreases with adequate treatment. Also, a fracture line with low signal intensity on both TI- and T2-weighted images may be visualized.

Figure 13-17. Coronal T2-weighted MR image of an insufficiency fracture of the sacrum of a 67-year-old woman. This patient was previously treated with radiotherapy for ovarian carcinoma. No metastatic lesions were diagnosed at the time of treatment. Recently, the patient complained of pain at the sacrum and bone metastasis of ovarian carcinoma was suspected on clinical grounds. The MR examination, however, demonstrated the presence of bilateral sacral insufficiency fractures. The bone marrow edema associated with sacral insufficiency fractures is characterized by increased (*white*) signal (*arrows*) in the normally dark bone marrow of the sacral wings on fat-saturated T2-weighted MR images. No definite tumoral lesion is seen. Note the thin, irregular, black line in the middle of the bone marrow edema (on the *left* side of the image), which represents the fracture line.

Treatment options include conservative medical treatment (immobilization in a wheelchair), sacroplasty, or screw fixation. Sacroplasty is a recently developed, minimally invasive technique analogous to vertebroplasty that consists of polymethylmetacrylate "cement" injections to stabilize the fracture components and to reduce pain [55,56].

Wrist Fractures

Figure 13-18. Colles' fracture as seen on the posteroanterior and lateral views of the left wrist of an 83-year-old woman. A Colles' fracture usually occurs in older individuals after a fall on an outstretched hand. Note the decreased bone mineralization. Clinically, a characteristic "dinner fork" or "bayonet" deformity is seen, owing to the dorsal angulation and shift of the distal fracture fragment and wrist. The fracture of the distal radius and the dorsal angulation are confirmed on the conventional radiographs. Additional findings may commonly include impaction and displacement of the fracture fragments of the radius and avulsion of the styloid process of the ulna. In this patient, widening of the normal space between the lunate and the scaphoid may represent scapholunar dissociation caused by axial stress of the capitate at this articulation at the time of trauma. Treatment of uncomplicated Colles' fractures consists mainly of a (closed) reduction of the fracture fragments to reestablish the normal volar tilt of the radial articular surface and stabilization of the fracture fragments by casting. Note the extensive osteoarthritic changes at the first carpometacarpal joint.

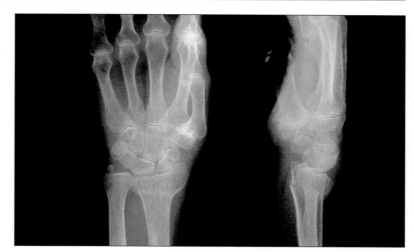

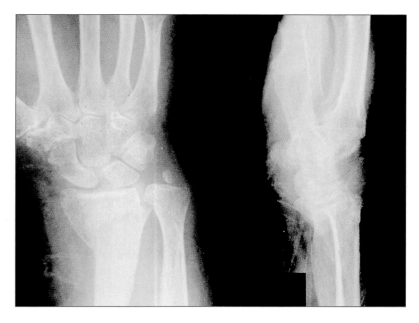

Figure 13-19. Smith's fracture of the wrist of an 84-year-old woman. On the posteroanterior view on the *left*, a fracture of the distal radius is seen. Volar angulation or displacement is characteristic of Smith's fracture, as seen on the *right*. Smith's fracture is much less common than Colles' fracture and is called Barton's fracture when it involves the articular surface of the distal radius. Smith's fracture may result from a (backward) fall on the wrist in dorsiflexion with the forearm supinated. Note the concomitant avulsion of the styloid process of the ulna and the osteoarthritic changes at the first carpometacarpal joint. Fractures of the distal radius are both a consequence of osteoporosis and of the patient's falls [57].

Fractures of the Proximal Humerus

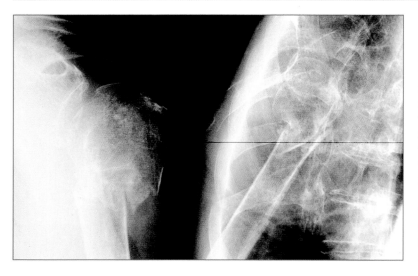

Figure 13-20. Fracture of the left proximal humerus of a 66-year-old man, as seen on the anteroposterior view (*left*) and on the transthoracic view (*right*). Note the overall decreased bone mineralization. A fracture is present at the surgical neck level of the humerus. The humeral head is well centered over the glenoid (*see* the transthoracic view) and is therefore not dislocated. The distal fracture fragment (humeral shaft) is displaced anteriorly and medially as a result of traction of the pectoralis major muscle. A fracture of the greater or lesser tuberosities is not seen and the fracture of this patient may be classified as a two-part fracture of the proximal humerus according to the Neer classification [51]. Rotator cuff tears may be associated with fractures of the greater tuberosity. Fractures of the proximal humerus in patients who have osteoporosis are less common than vertebral, hip, and wrist fractures and most often result from a fall on an outstretched hand. Closed and rarely open reduction of the fracture may sometimes be required.

Other Insufficiency Fractures

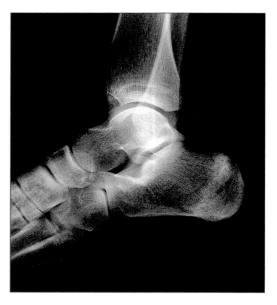

Figure 13-21. Insufficiency fracture of the right calcaneus of a 62-year-old woman. A linear area of radiodensity in the posterior part of the calcaneus is present and aligned perpendicular to the direction of the bony trabeculae. This represents bone sclerosis and healing of a cancellous bone insufficiency fracture of the calcaneus. Calcaneal stress fractures may also be seen in healthy runners or in patients with diabetes. Decreased bone mineralization, as in patients with osteoporosis, results in a decreased elastic capacity of the bones and microfractures occur more easily. Although these fractures occur less frequently in patients with osteoporosis, a predilection for certain anatomic locations is known and includes the posterior third of the calcaneus, the medial portion of the proximal tibia, and the third and fourth metatarsal bones [11,12]. Cancellous bone stress fractures, such as in the calcaneus, may not be visible on initial radiographs, but if a radiograph is repeated 2 weeks later a linear area of bone sclerosis is often readily visible. Early diagnosis of insufficiency fractures may be enhanced with radionuclide scanning or MRI.

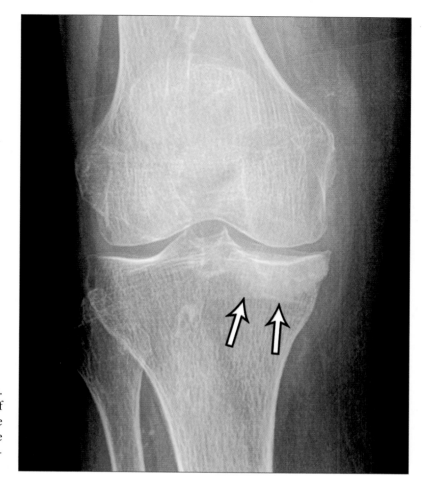

Figure 13-22. Insufficiency fracture of the tibia of an 89-year-old man. The patient was referred to the radiology department with complaints of medial knee pain for several weeks. Note the bandlike area of dense bone immediately underlying the articular surface of the medial tibial condyle (*arrows*): this represents bone sclerosis and endosteal callus formation several weeks after an insufficiency fracture [58].

Figure 13-23. Plot showing the age-specific incidence rate of hip, forearm, humerus, and pelvic fracture per 1000 women per year in the United States [59]. The incidence of fractures in the appendicular skeleton increases with age over 50 years. Pelvic and humerus fracture incidences gradually increase to 3 and 4, respectively, per 1000 women who are 80 years of age or older. Forearm fracture incidence increases relatively quickly after the age of 50 years and reaches a plateau of 8 per 1000 women who are between the ages of 60 and 80 years old. Above the age of 80, there is a decrease in forearm fracture incidence. On the other hand, hip fractures are not frequent before the age of 60 years. After the age of 60 years, there is a very steep increase in hip fractures, reaching over 20 per 1000 in women older than 80 years. High mortality and morbidity is associated with hip fractures in the elderly. Maintaining body weight, walking for exercise, avoiding long-acting benzodiazepines, minimizing caffeine intake, and treating impaired visual function to prevent falls are among the steps that may decrease the risk of hip fracture in white women [60].

Most fractures after the age of 50 years are related to low bone density (osteoporosis). Other factors, such as severe trauma or specific pathologic processes (*eg*, metastatic malignancies) causing fracture, are less common. The National Osteoporosis Foundation reported on the contribution of osteoporosis to specific types of fractures among different populations residing in the United States [61]. They estimated that 90% of hip fractures in white women between 65 and 84 years old were related to osteoporosis. The estimate for spine fractures (vertebral compression fractures) was 90% and that for wrist fractures was 70%. White women, in general, have the highest risk of osteoporotic fractures. Men are less at risk than women of the same race. Black individuals have the lowest risk and Asians have intermediate risk.

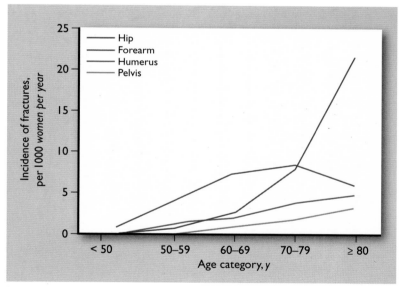

The chance of fracture has been calculated in numerous studies and includes estimations on lifetime risk, cumulative risk, and actuarial risk. Cumulative risk is the probability that a person of an exact age (*eg*, 65 years) will sustain a fracture at a later exact age (*eg*, 90 years). The actuarial risk takes into account the chance that a person can die from another disease during this period. Therefore, actuarial risks are lower than cumulative risks. In a study using data from a 5% sample of United States Medicare recipients, the actuarial risk for a 65-year-old white woman sustaining a fracture by age 90 was reported to be 16% for the hip, 9% for the distal forearm, and 5% for the proximal humerus [62]. (*Adapted from* Cummings *et al.* [59].)

References

1. Beaupied H, Lespessailles E, Benhamou CL: Evaluation of macrostructural bone biomechanics. *Joint Bone Spine* 2007, 74:233–239.

2. McDonnell P, McHugh PE, O'Mahoney D: Vertebral osteoporosis and trabecular bone quality. *Ann Biomed Eng* 2007, 35:170–189.

3. Seeman E, Delmas PD: Bone quality—the material and structural basis of bone strength and fragility. *N Engl J Med* 2006, 354:2250–2261.

4. Szulc P, Seeman E, Duboeuf F, *et al.*: Bone fragility: failure of periosteal apposition to compensate for increased endocortical resorption in postmenopausal women. *J Bone Miner Res* 2006, 21:1856–1863.

5. Diamant I, Shahar R, Masharawi Y, Gefen A: A method for patient-specific evaluation of vertebral cancellous bone strength: in vitro validation. *Clin Biomech* 2007, 22:282–291.

6. Augat P, Schorlemmer S: The role of cortical bone and its microstructure in bone strength. *Age Ageing* 2006, 35(Suppl 2):ii27–ii31.

7. Johnell O, Kanis JA, Oden A, *et al.*: Predictive value of BMD for hip and other fractures. *J Bone Miner Res* 2005, 20:1185–1194.

8. Damilakis J, Maris TG, Karantanas AH: An update on the assessment of osteoporosis using radiologic techniques. *Eur Radiol* 2007, 17:1591–1602.

9. Siris ES, Brenneman SK, Barrett-Connor E, *et al.*: The effect of age and bone mineral density on the absolute, excess, and relative risk of fracture in postmenopausal women aged 50–99: results from the National Osteoporosis Risk Assessment (NORA). *Osteoporos Int* 2006, 17:565–574.

10. Vanhoof J, Landewe S, Vandevenne J, Geusens P: An exceptional radiographic presentation of bilateral insufficiency fractures of the proximal tibia in a patient with rheumatoid arthritis. *Ann Rheum Dis* 2003, 62:277–279.

11. Alonso-Bartolome P, Blanco R, Canga A, Martinez-Taboada VM: Insufficiency fractures of the calcaneus: a diagnostic pitfall for ankle arthritis. *J Rheumatol* 2006, 33:1140–1142.

12. Clemetson IA, Popp A, Lippuner K, *et al.*: Postpartum osteoporosis associated with proximal tibial stress fracture. *Skeletal Radiol* 2004, 33:96–98.

13. Cohen I, Melamed E, Lipkin A, Robinson D: Transient osteoporosis of pregnancy complicated by a pathologic subcapital hip fracture. *J Trauma* 2007, 62:1281–1283.

14. Guggenbuhl P, Meadeb J, Chales G: Osteoporotic fractures of the proximal humerus, pelvis, and ankle: epidemiology and diagnosis. *Joint Bone Spine* 2005, 72:372–375.

15. Genant HK, Wu CY, van Kuijk C, Nevitt MC: Vertebral fracture assessment using a semiquantitative technique. *J Bone Miner Res* 1993, 8:1137–1148.

16. Cummings SR, Melton LJ: Epidemiology and outcomes of osteoporotic fractures. *Lancet* 2002, 359:1761–1767.

17. Delmas PD, van de Langerijt L, Watts NB, *et al.*: Underdiagnosis of vertebral fractures is a worldwide problem: the IMPACT study. *J Bone Miner Res* 2005, 20:557–563.

18. Cauley JA, Lui LY, Ensrud KE, *et al.*: Bone mineral density and the risk of incident nonspinal fractures in black and white women. *JAMA* 2005, 293:2102–2108.

19. Bessette L, Ste-Marie LG, Jean S, *et al.*: The care gap in diagnosis and treatment of women with a fragility fracture. *Osteoporos Int* 2008, 19:79–86.

20. Genant HK, Delmas PD, Chen P, *et al.*: Severity of vertebral fracture reflects deterioration of bone microarchitecture. *Osteoporos Int* 2007, 18:69–76.

21. Briggs AM, Greig AM, Wark JD: The vertebral fracture cascade in osteoporosis: a review of aetiopathogenesis. *Osteoporos Int* 2007, 18:575–584.

22. Kaptoge S, Armbrecht G, Felsenberg D, *et al.*: Whom to treat? The contribution of vertebral X-rays to risk-based algorithms for fracture prediction. Results from the European Prospective Osteoporosis Study. *Osteoporos Int* 2006, 17:1369–1381.

23. Gass M, Dawson-Hughes B: Preventing osteoporosis-related fractures: an overview. *Am J Med* 2006, 119(Suppl 1):S3–S11.

24. Blonk MC, Erdtsieck RJ, Wernekinck MG, Schoon EJ: The fracture and osteoporosis clinic: 1-year results and 3-month compliance. *Bone* 2007, 40:1643–1649.

25. Lentle BC, Brown JP, Khan A, *et al.*: Scientific Advisory Council of Osteoporosis Canada: Canadian Association of Radiologists. Recognizing and reporting vertebral fractures: reducing the risk of future osteoporotic fractures. *Can Assoc Radiol J* 2007, 58:27–36.

26. Sambrook P, Cooper C: Osteoporosis. *Lancet* 2006, 367:2070–2018.

27. Black DM, Arden NK, Palermo L, *et al.*: Prevalent vertebral fractures predict hip fractures and new vertebral fractures but not wrist fractures. Study of Osteoporotic Fractures Research Group. *J Bone Miner Res* 1999, 14:821–828.

28. Ross PD, Davis JW, Epstein RS, Wasnich RD: Pre-existing fractures and bone mass predict vertebral fracture incidence in women. *Ann Intern Med* 1991, 14:919–923.

29. Siris ES, Genant HK, Laster AJ, *et al.*: Enhanced prediction of fracture risk combining vertebral fracture status and BMD. *Osteoporos Int* 2007, 18:761–770.

30. Roux C, Fechtenbaum J, Kolta S, *et al.*: Mild prevalent and incident vertebral fractures are risk factors for new fractures. *Osteoporos Int* 2007, 18:1617–1624.

31. Demir SO, Akin C, Aras M, Koseoglu F: Spinal cord injury associated with thoracic osteoporotic fracture. *Am J Phys Med Rehabil* 2007, 86:242–246.

32. Weber M, Uehlinger K, Gerber H: Osteoporotic vertebral compression fracture causing neurologic deficit. *J Clin Rheumatol* 2002, 8:166–173.

33. Hiwatashi A, Westesson PL: Vertebroplasty for osteoporotic fractures with spinal canal compromise. *AJNR Am J Neuroradiol* 2007, 28:690–692.

34. Jung HS, Jee WH, McCauley TR, *et al.*: Discrimination of metastatic from acute osteoporotic compression spinal fractures with MR imaging. *Radiographics* 2003, 23:179–187.

35. Baur A, Huber A, Ertl-Wagner B, *et al.*: Diagnostic value of increased diffusion weighting of a steady-state free precession sequence for differentiating acute benign osteoporotic fractures from pathologic vertebral compression fractures. *AJNR Am J Neuroradiol* 2001, 22:366–372.

36. Diamond TH, Bryant C, Browne L, Clark WA: Clinical outcomes after acute osteoporotic vertebral fractures: a 2-year non-randomised trial comparing percutaneous vertebroplasty with conservative therapy. *Med J Aust* 2006, 184:113–117.

37. Voormolen MH, Mali WP, Lohle PN, *et al.*: Percutaneous vertebroplasty compared with optimal pain medication treatment: short-term clinical outcome of patients with subacute or chronic painful osteoporotic vertebral compression fractures. The VERTOS study. *AJNR Am J Neuroradiol* 2007, 28:555–560.

38. Koch CA, Layton KF, Kallmes DF: Outcomes of patients receiving long-term corticosteroid therapy who undergo percutaneous vertebroplasty. *AJNR Am J Neuroradiol* 2007, 28:563–566.

39. Cloft HJ, Jensen ME: Kyphoplasty: an assessment of a new technology. *AJNR Am J Neuroradiol* 2007, 28:200–203.

40. Deramond H, Saliou G, Aveillan M, *et al.*: Respective contributions of vertebroplasty and kyphoplasty to the management of osteoporotic vertebral fractures. *Joint Bone Spine* 2006, 73:610–613.

41. Lewis G: Percutaneous vertebroplasty and kyphoplasty for the stand-alone augmentation of osteoporosis-induced vertebral compression fractures: present status and future directions. *J Biomed Mater Res B Appl Biomater* 2007, 81:371–386.

42. Voormolen MH, Lohle PN, Lampmann LE, *et al.*: Prospective clinical follow-up after percutaneous vertebroplasty in patients with painful osteoporotic vertebral compression fractures. *J Vasc Interv Radiol* 2006, 17:1313–1320.

43. Lee WS, Sung KH, Jeong HT, *et al.*: Risk factors of developing new symptomatic vertebral compression fractures after percutaneous vertebroplasty in osteoporotic patients. *Eur Spine J* 2006, 15:1777–1783.

44. Heran MK, Legiehn GM, Munk PL: Current concepts and techniques in percutaneous vertebroplasty. *Orthop Clin North Am* 2006, 37:409–434, vii.

45. Ploeg WT, Veldhuizen AG, The B, Sietsma MS: Percutaneous vertebroplasty as a treatment for osteoporotic vertebral compression fractures: a systematic review. *Eur Spine J* 2006, 15:1749–1758.

46. Wilcox RK: The biomechanical effect of vertebroplasty on the adjacent vertebral body: a finite element study. *Proc Inst Mech Eng* 2006, 220:565–572.

47. Nakano M, Hirano N, Ishihara H, *et al.*: Calcium phosphate cement-based vertebroplasty compared with conservative treatment for osteoporotic compression fractures: a matched case-control study. *J Neurosurg Spine* 2006, 4:110–117.

48. Hochmuth K, Proschek D, Schwarz W, *et al.*: Percutaneous vertebroplasty in the therapy of osteoporotic vertebral compression fractures: a critical review. *Eur Radiol* 2006, 16:998–1004.

49. Singh AK, Pilgram TK, Gilula LA: Osteoporotic compression fractures: outcomes after single- versus multiple-level percutaneous vertebroplasty. *Radiology* 2006, 238:211–220.

50. Wagner AL: Vertebroplasty and the randomized study: where science and ethics collide. *AJNR Am J Neuroradiol* 2005, 26:1610–1611.

51. Weissman BN, Sledge CB: *Orthopedic Radiology.* Philadelphia: WB Saunders; 1986.

52. Lönnroos E, Kautiainen H, Karppi P, *et al.*: Incidence of second hip fractures. A population-based study. *Osteoporos Int* 2007, 18:1279–1285.

53. Patel SH, Murphy KP: Fractures of the proximal femur: correlates of radiological evidence of osteoporosis. *Skeletal Radiol* 2006, 35:202–211.

54. Peh WC, Khong PL, Yin Y, *et al.*: Imaging of pelvic insufficiency fractures. *Radiographics* 1996, 16:335–348.

55. Strub WM, Hoffmann M, Ernst RJ, Bulas RV: Sacroplasty by CT and fluoroscopic guidance: is the procedure right for your patient? *AJNR Am J Neuroradiol* 2007, 28:38–41.

56. Tsiridis E, Upadhyay N, Giannoudis PV: Sacral insufficiency fractures: current concepts of management. *Osteoporos Int* 2006, 17:1716–1725.

57. Nordvall H, Glanberg-Persson G, Lysholm J: Are distal radius fractures due to fragility or to falls? A consecutive case-control study of bone mineral density, tendency to fall, risk factors for osteoporosis, and health-related quality of life. *Acta Orthop* 2007, 78:271–277.

58. Prasad N, Murray JM, Kumar D, Davies SG: Insufficiency fracture of the tibial plateau: an often missed diagnosis. *Acta Orthop Belg* 2006, 72:587–591.

59. Cummings SR, Kelsey JL, Nevitt CN, O'Dowd KJ: Epidemiology of osteoporosis and osteoporotic fractures. *Epidemiol Rev* 1985, 7:178–208.

60. Cummings SR, Nevitt MC, Browner WS, *et al.*: Risk factors for hip fracture in white women. *N Engl J Med* 1995, 332:767–773.

61. Melton III LJ, Thamer M, Ray NF, *et al.*: Fractures attributable to osteoporosis: report from the National Osteoporosis Foundation. *J Bone Miner Res* 1997, 12:16–23.

62. Barret JA, Baron JA, Karagas MR, Beach ML: Fracture risk in the U.S. Medicare population. *J Clin Epidemiol* 1999, 52:243–249.

Laboratory Assessment of Skeletal Status

14

Richard Eastell

Bone turnover markers have been used in medicine for over 70 years. They have proved indispensable in the management of metabolic bone diseases such as Paget's disease of bone. The changes in bone turnover in osteoporosis are small; thus, markers that are not specific to bone were not very useful in investigating this disease. However, assays have recently been introduced that are more specific for bone. In this chapter, I consider the evidence for the use of these markers in the investigation of osteoporosis.

Bone Turnover Markers

Markers of Bone Formation and Resorption

Bone formation markers (products of the osteoblast)

Serum alkaline phosphatase (bone isoform), bone alkaline phosphatase
Serum osteocalcin
Serum C- and N-propeptides of type I collagen

Bone resorption markers (degradation products of type I collagen, enzymes)

Urinary excretion of pyridinium crosslinks of collagen, *eg*, deoxypyridinoline
Serum, or urinary excretion of, C- and N-telopeptides of type I collagen
Serum, or urinary excretion of, galactosyl hydroxylysine
Urinary excretion of hydroxyproline
Serum tartrate-resistant acid phosphatase

Figure 14-1. There is a wide choice of biochemical turnover markers. It is usual for a laboratory to establish a marker for bone resorption, *eg*, urinary N-telopeptides of type I collagen, and a marker of bone formation, *eg*, serum bone alkaline phosphatase. These measurements are useful for the initial evaluation of the patient, for providing additional information for the prediction of rapid bone losers or increased fracture risk, and to stimulate the further search for secondary osteoporosis.

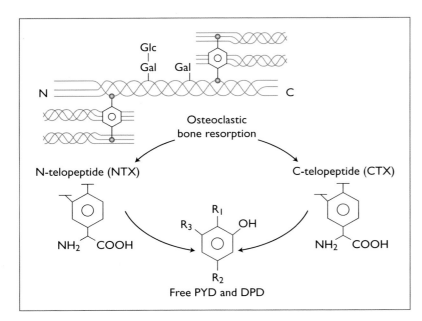

Figure 14-2. Type I collagen breakdown products as markers of bone resorption. Type I collagen is the most abundant protein in bone. It is a complex substance composed of three peptide chains that are held together by pyridinium crosslinks. The chains are released during bone resorption and are present in the serum and urine as free crosslinks (free pyridinoline [PYD] and deoxypyridinoline [DPD]) or as crosslinks bound to fragments from the N-terminus of collagen (N-telopeptides of type I collagen [NTX]) or the C-terminus (C-telopeptides of type I collagen [CTX]). These crosslinks were originally measured by high-performance liquid chromatography, but assays are now available for NTX, CTX, and free DPD in urine by immunoassay and for NTX and CTX in serum by immunoassay. Most recently, the assays for serum CTX, urinary NTX, and free DPD have been established on autoanalyzer devices, which are available in most clinical chemistry laboratories. Furthermore, point-of-care devices are being developed for the measurement of these bone resorption markers in urine.

Prediction of Bone Loss and Fractures with Bone Turnover Markers

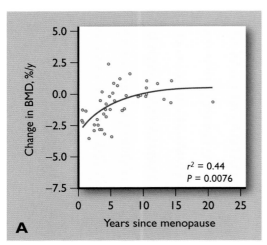

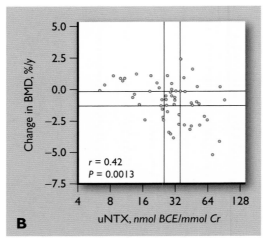

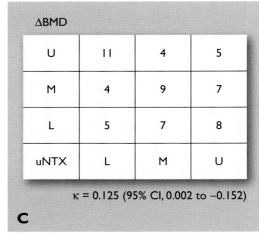

Figure 14-3. Relationship between change in bone mineral density (BMD) of the spine and bone turnover. A longstanding goal has been to use bone turnover markers to predict "fast losers" at the time of the menopause.

A, Change in BMD after menopause. Bone loss is most rapid in the first 5 years after menopause. **B,** The higher the rate of bone resorption (measured by N-telopeptides of type I collagen [NTX] in a second morning void urine sample and expressed as a ratio to creatinine), the greater the rate of bone loss. The *lines* represent the boundaries between tertiles. **C,** The ability of bone resorption markers to classify individuals into upper (U), middle (M), or lower (L) tertiles of bone loss is poor (κ score of < 0.2); thus, this approach is unsuitable for use in the individual [1]. (*Adapted from* Rogers et al. [2].)

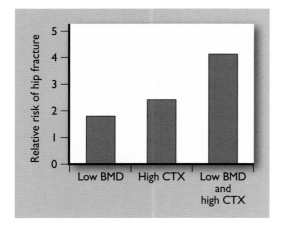

Figure 14-4. Results from the Epidimilogie de l'Osteoporose study. In older women, a high level of bone turnover has been associated with an increased risk of fracture. Results from bone turnover markers can be expressed in the same way as bone mineral density (BMD) results using T-scores. In this approach, a reference range is established in premenopausal women 30 to 50 years of age, with the results expressed in standard deviation units; the reference interval for young women, therefore, is –2 to +2. The risk of hip fracture is higher in women with low hip BMD (T < 2.5), high urinary C-telopeptides of type I collagen (CTX) (T > 2), and even higher with both low BMD (T < 2.5) and high urinary CTX (T > 2). (*Data from* Garnero et al. [3].)

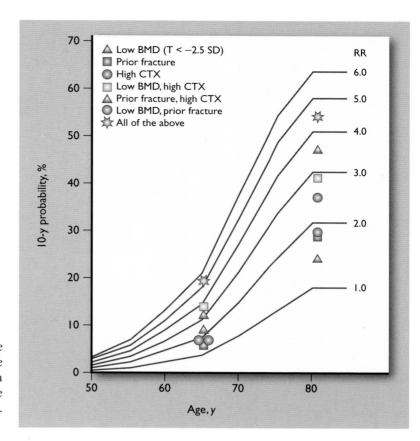

Figure 14-5. Fracture probability. The 10-year probability of a fracture increases with advancing age. The probability is further increased in the presence of low bone mineral density (BMD), a previous fracture, and high bone resorption markers (C-telopeptides of type I collagen [CTX]). The highest risk of fracture occurs in those with all three of these risk factors. RR—relative risk. (*Adapted from* Kanis *et al.* [4].)

Monitoring the Effect of Treatment on Bone Turnover Markers

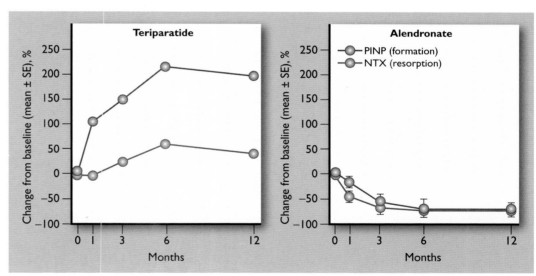

Figure 14-6. Treatments for osteoporosis can be either anabolic (such as teriparatide) or anti-catabolic (such as alendronate). This example shows the effect of teriparatide and alendronate on biochemical markers of bone formation (pro-collagen I N-terminal peptide [PINP]) and bone resorption (urinary N-telopeptides of type I collagen [NTX]). Teriparatide therapy is associated with an early and large increase in bone formation markers; the change is so large that most patients can be identified as responders in as early as 1 month. It is also associated with an increase in bone resorption, but this is smaller and later. Alendronate therapy is associated with an early and large decrease in bone resorption markers; the change is so large that most patients can be identified as responders in as early as 3 months. It is also associated with a decrease in bone formation, but this is smaller and later. (*Adapted from* Arlot *et al.* [5].)

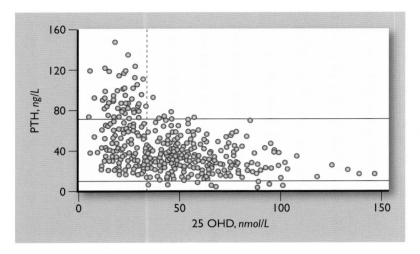

Figure 14-7. Vitamin D deficiency is common in association with osteoporosis and needs treatment before standard treatments for osteoporosis can be effective. In this United Kingdom study of women with vertebral osteoporosis, 39% had evidence of vitamin D deficiency (< 30 nmol/L or 12 ng/mL). A high level of parathyroid hormone (PTH) was identified in one-third of women with vitamin D deficiency and it was associated with higher levels of bone turnover markers and lower levels of bone mineral density. OHD—25-hydroxyvitamin D. (*Adapted from* Sahota *et al.* [6].)

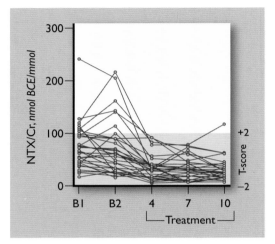

Figure 14-8. Bone resorption markers to monitor the response of the individual to antiresorptive treatments. In our practice, N-telopeptides of type I collagen (NTX) were measured in the second morning void urine sample in 49 patients with osteoporosis [7] on two occasions at baseline (B1 and B2) and then after 4, 7, and 10 months of treatment with hormone replacement therapy or bisphosphonates. Before starting treatment, the NTX level is usually within the reference interval for young women; in those with high values, the risk of fracture may be greater and they may be more likely to have secondary osteoporosis. Note that NTX does vary before starting treatment, which is why we make two collections and take the mean of these as our baseline. There is an early and marked decrease in NTX after starting treatment such that the maximum effect is seen by 4 months in most patients. Note that NTX is in the lower half of the premenopausal reference range (below a T-score of 0) in most subjects after 10 months of treatment.

Biochemical Evaluation of Osteoporosis: Secondary Osteoporosis

Recommended Initial Evaluation for Osteoporosis

Blood	24-H Urine
Complete blood count—hemoglobin, erythrocyte sedimentation rate	Calcium
Calcium, phosphate	Creatine
Alkaline phosphatase	
γ-Glutamyltranspeptidase	
Creatine	
Thyroid-stimulating hormone	
Testosterone (men)	
Protein electrophoresis (and urinary Bence Jones protein)	
Parathyroid hormone	
Serum CTX (or urine NTX)	
Bone alkaline phosphatase	

Figure 14-9. Recommended initial evaluation for osteoporosis. An underlying cause of osteoporosis may be found in about 20% of women and 40% of men with established osteoporosis. There are no guidelines on who should have a laboratory evaluation, but we consider it valuable to investigate all patients presenting with vertebral fracture and all patients who have a bone mineral density (BMD) value below the young adult reference range, a BMD below that expected for age (z < –2), or who have accelerated bone loss.

The choice of tests is based on our clinical experience and reports such as those shown in Figure 14-11. CTX—C-telopeptides of type I collagen; NTX—N-telopeptides of type I collagen.

Laboratory Investigation of Diseases Identified by Clinical Examination or Initial Evaluation

Osteomalacia	Repeat serum and urinary calcium and PTH
	25-OHD
	Phosphate threshold test
Primary hyperparathyroidism	Repeat serum and urinary calcium and PTH
Malabsorption syndrome	25-OHD
	Serum and urinary magnesium
	Antigliadin and antiendomysial antibodies
	Red cell folate, vitamin B12, ferritin
	Repeat serum and urinary calcium
Hyperthyroidism	Free tri-iodothyronine (T₃)
Cushing's disease	Overnight dexamethasone suppression test
Hypogonadism	Sex hormone–binding globulin
	Luteinizing hormone
	Follicle-stimulating hormone
	Prolactin
Chronic renal failure	Serum calcium, phosphate
	1,25-Dihydroxyvitamin D
Myeloma	Bone marrow biopsy
Hemochromatosis	Serum iron
	Total iron-binding capacity
	Ferritin
Primary biliary cirrhosis	Antimitochondrial antibody
	Immunoglobulins
	ALT, AST, bilirubin
Idiopathic hypercalciuria	Serum and urinary calcium (on low-calcium diet for 7 d), urinary sodium, serum uric acid
	Fasting urinary calcium and creatine, pH, and culture

Figure 14-10. Further laboratory investigation of diseases identified by clinical examination or the initial evaluation shown in Figure 14-9. Bone biopsy can be useful in patients with atypical forms of osteoporosis, osteomalacia, or renal osteodystrophy. ALT—alanine transaminase; AST—aspartate transaminase; 25-OHD—25-hydroxyvitamin D; PTH—parathyroid hormone.

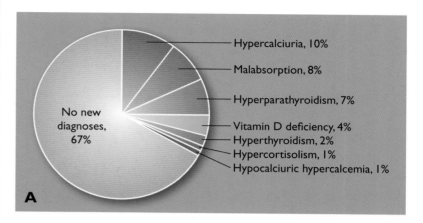

Secondary Contributors to Osteoporosis Identified in 173 Otherwise Healthy Women with Osteoporosis*

Disorder of Bone or Mineral Metabolism	Number
Hypercalciuria	17
Malabsorption	14
Hyperparathyroidism (primary and secondary)	12
Vitamin D deficiency (< 30 nmol/L)	7
Exogenous hyperthyroidism	4
Cushing's disease	1
Familial benign hypercalcemia	1
Total number of new diagnoses	56

*One patient had two unrelated diagnoses.

B

Figure 14-11. Secondary contributors to osteoporosis are identified in 173 otherwise healthy women with osteoporosis. The data are represented in schematic (**A**) and tabular (**B**) form. In patients who present to the clinic with low bone mineral density, a laboratory evaluation is useful in uncovering diagnoses that may be responsible for the osteoporosis, or that may affect the design of treatment. In this study, 173 women who had osteoporosis without obvious cause had laboratory measures including a complete blood count, chemistry profile, 24-hour urine calcium, 25-hydroxyvitamin D, and parathyroid hormone [8]. A substantial fraction was found to have secondary contributors to osteoporosis. (*Adapted from* Tannenbaum *et al.* [8].)

References

1. Delmas PD, Eastell R, Garnero P, *et al.*: The use of biochemical markers of bone turnover in osteoporosis. *Osteoporosis Int* 2000, 11(Suppl 6):S2–S17.

2. Rogers A, Hannon R, Eastell R: Biochemical markers as predictors of rates of bone loss after menopause. *J Bone Miner Res* 2000, 15:1398–1404.

3. Garnero P, Dargent-Molina P, Hans D, *et al.*: Do markers of bone resorption add to bone mineral density and ultrasonographic heel measurement for the prediction of hip fracture in elderly women? The EPIDOS prospective study. *Osteoporosis Int* 1998, 8:563–569.

4. Kanis JA, Johnell O, Oden A, *et al.*: Ten-year probabilities of osteoporotic fractures according to BMD and diagnostic thresholds. *Osteoporosis Int* 2001, 12:989–995.

5. Arlot M, Meunier PJ, Boivin G, *et al.*: Differential effects of teriparatide and alendronate on bone remodeling in postmenopausal women assessed by histomorphometric parameters. *J Bone Miner Res* 2005, 20:1244–1253.

6. Sahota O, Mundey MK, San P, *et al.*: The relationship between vitamin D and parathyroid hormone: calcium homeostasis, bone turnover, and bone mineral density in postmenopausal women with established osteoporosis. *Bone* 2004, 35:312–319.

7. Eastell R, Bainbridge PR: Bone turnover markers: their place in the investigation of osteoporosis. In *Osteoporosis: Pathophysiology and Clinical Management.* Edited by Orwoll ES, Bliziotes M. Totowa, NJ: Humana Press; 2003:185–198.

8. Tannenbaum C, Clark J, Schwartzman K, *et al.*: Yield of laboratory testing to identify secondary contributors to osteoporosis in otherwise healthy women. *J Clin Endocrinol Metab* 2002, 87:4431–4437.

Bone Densitometry in Osteoporosis Care

15

Neil Binkley

A bone density measurement is an integral part of osteoporosis prevention and treatment. The original methods for measuring bone density were developed several decades ago. Transitioning these technologies from research settings to clinical care began as the relationships between bone density and fracture risk were defined and when a definition of postmenopausal osteoporosis, based on bone density values, was provided. The subsequent widespread availability of instruments to measure bone mass, coupled with an increasing armamentarium of agents with proven efficacy at reducing fracture risk combined with an increasing number of older adults, has led to the increased clinical use of bone mass measurement. The International Society for Clinical Densitometry now exists to address the needs of the clinical bone density community and to advance excellence in skeletal health assessment. Additionally, an expanding number of technologies to evaluate fracture risk exist, with each providing different types of information. Although not clinically used at this time, such technologies may soon provide important information regarding "bone quality."

This chapter provides an overview of some important applications of devices for bone density testing that are used in clinical practice, including the assessment of fracture risk, osteoporosis diagnosis, and monitoring bone density over time. Principles of some technologies are briefly reviewed and current recommendations for interpretation are provided. In addition, some of the pitfalls and challenges encountered in applying these techniques are discussed, including lessons from three case examples.

Technology

Bone Density Technologies

Technology	Sites Measured
X-ray photon absorptiometry	
DXA	Spine, proximal femur, forearm, total body, fingers
SXA	Forearm, heel
QCT	
Central	Spine, proximal femur
Peripheral	Forearm
QUS	
Transmission	Heel
Reflective	Forearm, lower leg, fingers

Figure 15-1. Bone mass measurement technologies. Bone mass can be clinically evaluated using various technologies including x-ray absorptiometry, quantitative computed tomography (QCT), and quantitative ultrasound (QUS). X-ray absorptiometry techniques are based on the principle that the passage of photons through the body is inhibited (*ie*, photons are absorbed) by the mineral component of bone. The most widely used technology currently, dual-energy x-ray absorptiometry (DXA), uses x-ray photons of two different energies to factor out photon absorption by soft tissue. With this technique, bone mineral content (BMC) can be measured in central skeletal sites (the spine and hip), in peripheral sites (the heel and forearm), or in the total skeleton. Single-energy x-ray absorptiometry (SXA) devices require immersing the measured site (forearm or heel) in a water bath to factor out the soft tissue contribution to photon absorption. DXA has largely supplanted SXA devices. At this time, DXA has advantages over the other technologies, including its applicability to the World Health Organization (WHO) classification system, a proven fracture risk assessment utility, and documented effectiveness at targeting medical therapy to reduce fracture risk [1].

Both the DXA and SXA report "areal" rather than true volumetric density. Specifically, the BMC of a skeletal region is determined and these results are expressed as grams of mineral [2]. The area of the two-dimensional image is computed in units of centimeters squared (cm^2). Areal bone mineral density (BMD) is then derived by dividing the BMC of the measured region by the area of that region. As larger bones have greater depth, they will have a greater density as measured by these techniques. Thus, individuals with larger bones (*eg*, men compared to women) will have higher areal BMD even if the true volumetric density is identical. This is often alluded to as a weakness of these technologies; however, as bone size contributes importantly to bone strength (and therefore fracture risk), this attribute of absorptiometry methods likely contributes to their clinical utility as fracture risk prediction tools. Lumbar spine and hip DXA measurements are the most useful techniques in the clinical care of adults due to extensive experience with their use in observational and treatment studies.

QCT measures true tissue (volumetric) density, with the results expressed in grams per cubic centimeter (g/cm^3). When appropriately calibrated, standard CT scanners can measure bone density in the central portion of vertebral bodies, which is composed solely of trabecular bone or in the proximal femur. Peripheral CT scanners can measure bone in other skeletal sites such as the forearm. CT distinguishes between the cortical and trabecular compartments of bone and also evaluates bone geometric parameters. CT technology currently is less widely used clinically than is DXA, as few osteoporosis treatment trials enrolled patients on the basis of CT measurements and the WHO T-score classification system does not directly apply. However, the role of QCT in clinical practice continues to evolve.

Two types of QUS exist for the assessment of skeletal status [3,4]. Transmission ultrasound techniques determine the speed of sound waves or changes in the properties of these waves as they pass through a bone. The calcaneus is the site most commonly measured with this technique. It was hoped that ultrasound measurements would provide information about bone architecture in addition to measuring the amount of bone present. However, at the time of this writing, it appears that ultrasound techniques are influenced predominantly by bone mass. Reflective ultrasound techniques measure the speed of sound transmission along the surface of long bones, such as the tibia, radius, or phalanges. The results of these tests are likely influenced primarily by the amount and nature of the cortical shell of these long bones.

Other technologies including microcomputed tomography, magnetic resonance, texture analysis, and finite element analysis seem likely to enhance the ability to predict fracture risk [4]. Currently, these emerging approaches are not clinically applicable and remain limited to the research venue.

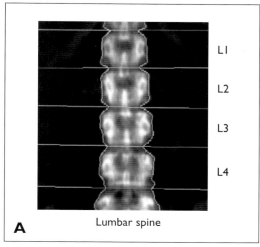

A   Lumbar spine

L1

L2

L3

L4

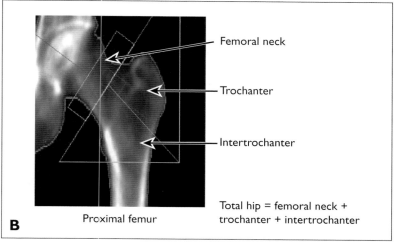

Femoral neck

Trochanter

Intertrochanter

B   Proximal femur

Total hip = femoral neck + trochanter + intertrochanter

Figure 15-2. Dual-energy x-ray absorptiometry (DXA) measurements of the lumbar spine and proximal femur. DXA images of the lumbar spine (**A**) and proximal femur (**B**) are shown. Bone mineral density (BMD) measurement of the thoracic spine is not possible because the sternum and ribs overlie the "soft tissue" regions. As the reproducibility of DXA measurements is enhanced with the measurement of larger amounts of bone, it is recommended that the L1–4 mean BMD be utilized clinically. Proximal femur measurement is a compilation of the femur neck, trochanter, and proximal shaft regions. DXA machines often report a value for Ward's region; however, this measurement is not useful in clinical practice because of this site's very small size and the fact that the World Health Organization classification does not apply to Ward's area [5].

The critical role of the DXA technologist in acquiring quality DXA data is often underappreciated [6]. Correct, clinically meaningful measurements require consistent patient positioning on the scanning table. Moreover, although the computer software initially locates bone edges, the DXA technologist must carefully verify and, if necessary, adjust bone edges and positioning of appropriate regions of measurement.

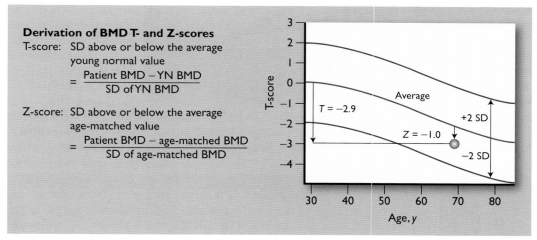

Derivation of BMD T- and Z-scores

T-score: SD above or below the average young normal value

$$= \frac{\text{Patient BMD} - \text{YN BMD}}{\text{SD of YN BMD}}$$

Z-score: SD above or below the average age-matched value

$$= \frac{\text{Patient BMD} - \text{age-matched BMD}}{\text{SD of age-matched BMD}}$$

T = −2.9

Average

+2 SD

Z = −1.0

−2 SD

Figure 15-3. Reporting of dual-energy x-ray absorptiometry bone mineral density (BMD) results. Bone density values are reported in grams per centimeter squared (g/cm²) and are usually expressed in relation to reference populations in SD units. This figure depicts the average bone density values in women of different ages (*green line*) and the values 2 SD above or below that average value (*purple lines*). The T-score is the number of SD above (a positive number) or below (a negative number) the average value in young adults. BMD, and therefore T-score values, commonly declines with age. When an individual's BMD is compared with that of average age-matched values, the results are described as Z-scores. In this example, a 69-year-old woman (results shown at the *circle*) has a T-score of −2.9 (2.9 SD below the average value of young women) and a Z-score of −1.0 (1 SD below the average for a 79-year-old woman.

T-scores are currently used to diagnose osteoporosis prior to the occurrence of a fragility fracture. In the past, T-scores were quite dependent on the reference database used for their derivation, in that the differences in the average young normal values or SD resulted in large T-score differences in patients with the same BMD values. Fortunately, widespread use of the NHANES database for the proximal femur (as currently recommended by the International Society for Clinical Densitometry) [7] appears to have resolved many of these differences. Though controversial, it is currently recommended that T-scores be derived for all individuals using Caucasian normative data [7]. YN—young normal

Diagnosing Osteoporosis

Figure 15-9. Diagnostic categorization of bone mineral density (BMD) values. The World Health Organization (WHO) proposed an epidemiologic classification system in which osteoporosis in postmenopausal women is defined as a T-score of –2.5 or lower and that the values between –1 and –2.5 are defined as low bone mass or osteopenia [20]. Values of –1.0 and higher were considered normal. This classification was initially proposed for epidemiologic purposes (comparing BMD values among different populations), not for clinical diagnosis or decision-making. However, numerous clinical trials have confirmed the usefulness of this diagnostic approach for osteoporosis and the value of –2.5 or lower in the lumbar spine or proximal femur is widely accepted as a definition of osteoporosis. However, it is important to recognize that an individual with "osteopenia" and a fragility fracture has osteoporosis clinically.

Use of the term osteopenia based on BMD values is widespread in clinical medicine. However, it must be recognized that this does not necessarily imply bone loss or increased short-term fracture risk and should not be applied to healthy premenopausal women. Furthermore, as the WHO classification system compares BMD with that of the average young normal adult, it is apparent that 50% of 30-year-old adults will have a below-average BMD value. Thus, a 30-year-old healthy adult with a BMD value that is 1.2 SD below average is not "diseased" any more than one whose height is 1.2 SD below average. Such an individual is not at high fracture risk

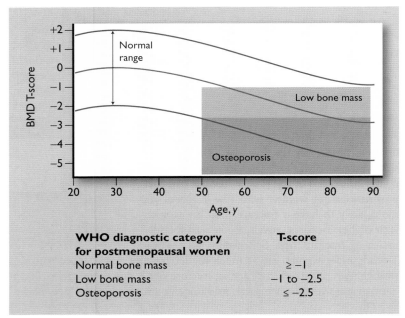

WHO diagnostic category for postmenopausal women	T-score
Normal bone mass	≥ –1
Low bone mass	–1 to –2.5
Osteoporosis	≤ –2.5

[11], should not receive a "disease" diagnosis (ie, osteopenia), and does not require therapy to reduce her fracture risk. This lower value is likely indicative of genetic lower than average peak bone mass.

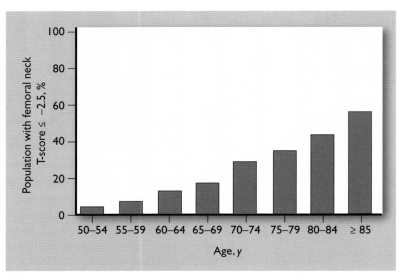

Figure 15-10. Prevalence of osteoporosis in women based on bone mineral density values. Bone density in the proximal femur was measured in a large population-based survey in the United States (NHANES III) [21]. The proportion of this population with femoral neck T-score values at or below –2.5 increased exponentially with advancing age, from 4% at age 55 years to about 50% at age 85. This NHANES database is now recommended for calculating T-score values in the proximal femur [7].

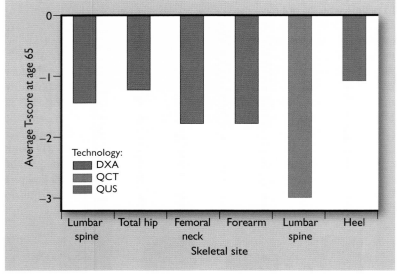

Figure 15-11. Disparity in T-score values among different bone mineral density (BMD) tests. T-scores measured at different skeletal sites, or with different techniques, are not identical due to differences in normative databases, variable rates at which bone is lost from different skeletal sites, and marked differences in the SD of BMD values in young adult populations depending on the technology used. As such, T-scores from different technologies cannot be used interchangeably and the International Society for Clinical Densitometry recommends that the World Health Organization classification only be applied to dual-energy x-ray absorptiometry (DXA) of the lumbar spine, femur neck, total proximal femoral, and mid-radius [7]. This difference between technologies is demonstrated here as the average T-scores calculated with different techniques in healthy 65-year-old women vary greatly [22]. QCT—quantitative computed tomography; QUS—quantitative ultrasound.

Reasons for Low Bone Density

Advanced age
Accelerated bone loss
Low–normal peak bone mass
Failure to acquire optimal peak bone mass because of:
    Small size
    Heredity
    Late or missed puberty

A

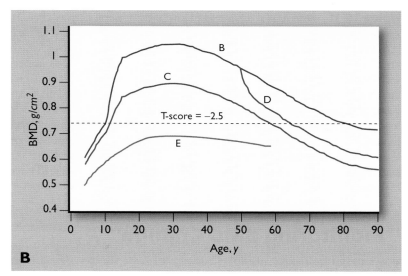

B

Figure 15-12. Mechanisms of developing low bone mineral density (BMD). Individuals may have low bone mass for various reasons (**A**). Since bone loss occurs in women after menopause and with advancing age in both men and women, simply becoming older increases the probability of having osteoporosis. **B,** As shown by *line B* depicting female average BMD, the average 85-year-old woman will have a T-score of –2.5. Women who attained a lower peak bone mass (*line C*) and thus have lower values at menopause will have values in the osteoporosis range in their late 50s or early 60s. Individuals with accelerated bone loss due to various medical or metabolic problems will develop osteoporosis more quickly (*line D*). A small number of people will never develop normal amounts of bone due to genetic reasons or impaired bone growth during childhood or adolescence (*line E*). These people will have values consistent with osteoporosis without ever sustaining bone loss. It is apparent from the above that low BMD does not always mean that bone loss has occurred and a single dual-energy x-ray absorptiometry report (without a prior study for comparison) should not state that bone has been "lost."

Interpretation of Bone Density Results

Premenopausal women
    Z-scores, not T-scores, are preferred
    A Z-score of –2.0 or lower is defined as "below the expected range for age" and a Z-score above –2.0 is "within the expected range for age"
Children and adolescents
    T-scores should not be used in children; Z-scores should be used instead
    T-scores should not appear in reports or on DXA printouts in children
    The diagnosis of osteoporosis in children should not be made on the basis of densitometric criteria alone
    Terminology such as "low bone density for chronologic age" or "below the expected range for age" may be used if the Z-score is below –2.0

Figure 15-13. Interpreting bone mineral density (BMD) values in children, adolescents, and premenopausal women. The World Health Organization criteria for the diagnosis of osteoporosis strictly apply only to healthy postmenopausal women. For healthy premenopausal women, or men under age 50, the use of Z-scores is recommended. In these individuals, the normal range includes Z-score values between –2 and +2. Z-scores below –2 are best described as "low bone density for age" [23].

Importantly, in children, T-scores should never be used to describe BMD values, as such individuals have not yet attained skeletal maturity and their BMD is less than that of an average 30-year-old adult. For example, the expected BMD value in a healthy 10-year-old boy would be equivalent to a T-score of –4, but this boy would not have osteoporosis; he simply has not yet reached his peak bone mass. In children or adolescents, BMD values are compared with age- and gender-specific reference ranges, ideally adjusted for body size. Thus, Z-score use is appropriate in children. Children with low bone mass do not have "osteoporosis" or "osteopenia." Recommended verbiage for BMD in children with a Z-score below –2 is "below the expected range for age" [23]. DXA—dual-energy x-ray absorptiometry.

Bone Density Diagnosis of Osteoporosis in Men

The World Health Organization densitometric classification is applicable
T-scores are preferred
In men younger than age 50, Z-scores are preferred
In some studies, fracture risk in men and women is the same as the BMD values. This suggests that the same (ie, female) database should be used for T-score calculation in both genders. However, using a male database to calculate T-scores provides a more realistic estimate of osteoporosis prevalence and fractures in men

Figure 15-14. Diagnosing osteoporosis in men. There is controversy about the appropriate bone mineral density (BMD) value for diagnosing osteoporosis in men. Because men, in general, have larger bones than do women, male BMD as measured by dual-energy x-ray absorptiometry is higher. Thus, young adult normal BMD is higher in men than in women. It follows that for any given BMD value (in g/cm²), a T-score derived using a male database will be lower than a T-score calculated with a female database. Some studies demonstrate that fracture risk in men and women are equal at the same BMD value, suggesting that the same (ie, female) database should be used to calculate T-scores in both genders [24]. However, using a male database to calculate T-scores provides a more realistic estimate of the prevalence of osteoporosis and fractures in men in the general population. European experts and societies suggest using a T-score threshold of –2.5, based on a female database to diagnose osteoporosis in men [8], while the International Society for Clinical Densitometry recommends using T-scores calculated with a male database [25].

Figure 15-24. Indications for bone mineral density (BMD) testing in women. Several national societies and organizations have made recommendations about when BMD measurement is appropriate [5,12,13]. Recently, the United States Preventative Services Task Force made recommendations based on a careful review of the evidence of clinical usefulness of BMD testing [32]. Each of the guidelines suggest that routine testing for women aged 65 years and older is appropriate. Although the specific recommendations differ somewhat among the guidelines, all recommend measuring BMD in younger postmenopausal women with other important risk factors for bone loss or fragility fracture. Testing postmenopausal women and older men who have experienced low-trauma fractures is generally recommended, as having such a fracture is a risk factor for subsequent fracture. None of the guidelines suggest routine measurement for all perimenopausal or premenopausal women; although some organizations recommend screening in men, no agreement has yet been reached on the indications for testing in men.

Indications for Bone Density Testing

Postmenopausal women with fragility fractures

All women older than 65 y of age

Younger postmenopausal women with risk factors for fracture or bone density, especially:

  Thinness

  Family history of hip or spine fracture

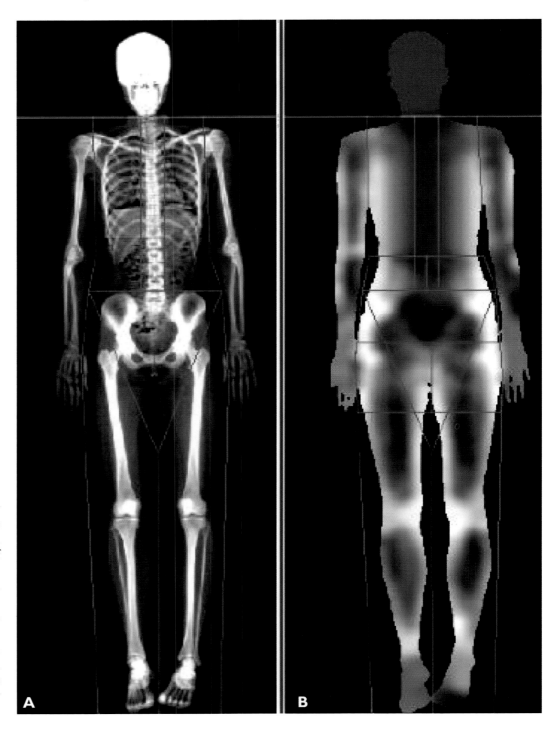

A

B

Figure 15-25. Other uses of dual-energy x-ray absorptiometry (DXA). **A,** DXA testing can be used to measure total body mineral content and bone density. Currently, the measurement of total body bone mass has a limited utility in osteoporosis management; however, it is often helpful in assessing the skeletal status of children.

B, Total body measurement is an accurate tool for measuring body composition and distinguishing body fat, lean tissue, and bone. These values are reported in grams of tissue and percent of total body composition. As is the case for total body bone mass, the clinical use of body composition is more common in children.

Case Examples

Figure 15-26. *Case Study 1.* This 67-year-old woman took estrogen for 5 years immediately following menopause. She has not experienced a fracture and has no evidence of medical causes of bone loss. Her intake of calcium and vitamin D is adequate. She weighs 148 pounds, is 5 feet 6 inches tall, and has not lost height. Her mother experienced vertebral fractures beginning at age 65.

This patient's spine bone mineral density (BMD) values are consistent with the diagnosis of osteoporosis, while the value in the total hip is in the lower portion of the normal range for young women. She should not receive different BMD diagnoses based on the measurement of two skeletal sites; rather, the value in the spine makes her a candidate for osteoporosis therapy. Although these values are not unexpected for her age, it is appropriate that the clinician exclude medical disorders that may cause low BMD before beginning osteoporosis treatment.

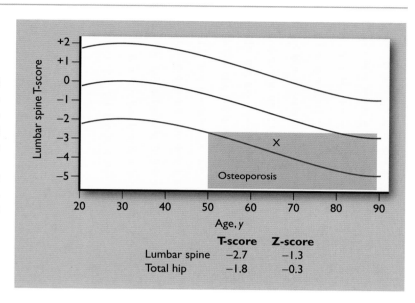

	T-score	Z-score
Lumbar spine	−2.7	−1.3
Total hip	−1.8	−0.3

Figure 15-27. *Case Study 2.* This 38-year-old woman had heel bone density measured at a health fair and subsequently obtained a dual-energy x-ray absorptiometry examination. She feels well, takes no medications, weighs 115 pounds, and is 5 feet 2 inches tall. She has not had fractures, but her mother experienced a hip fracture at 75 years of age. She is healthy, does not smoke, exercises regularly, and takes appropriate amounts of calcium and vitamin D. She was told that she has "moderate osteopenia," has lost 30% of her bone density, has the bones of a 67-year-old woman, and is at high risk for fracture.

This patient has bone mineral density (BMD) values in the low–normal range for young women. Note that reporting T-scores and applying the World Health Organization classification is inappropriate for healthy premenopausal women [23]. Given her family history and small stature, it is extremely likely that her "low" BMD simply reflects the genetic acquisition of less than average peak bone mass. Without knowing her peak bone mass, no statement about bone loss occurrence can be made on the basis of a single BMD test. Although her BMD values are the same as that of an average 67-year-old woman, her fracture risk is much lower than that of the older woman, who, on average,

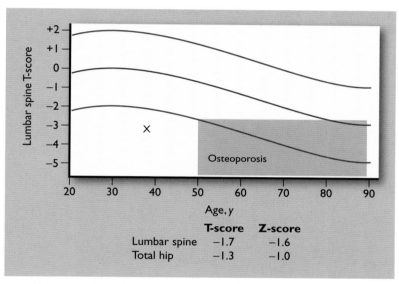

	T-score	Z-score
Lumbar spine	−1.7	−1.6
Total hip	−1.3	−1.0

would have experienced loss of bone mass and bone structure to arrive at this BMD. Given her low fracture risk and premenopausal status, no pharmacologic "osteoporosis" treatment is indicated.

Case Study 3

Bone density T-scores:
  Lumbar spine −3.5
  Total hip −2.8
Laboratory values:
  Serum calcium, 9.0 mg/dL
  Albumin, 4.0 g/dL
  High normal alkaline phosphatase
  24-h urinary calcium, 22 mg
  Serum total testosterone, 680 ng/mL

Figure 15-28. *Case Study 3.* This 55-year-old man experienced a metatarsal fracture while running. The x-ray report indicates "osteopenia." He is healthy, with no change in weight, no gastrointestinal symptoms, and normal sexual function. His calcium intake is approximately 1200 mg daily.

He has unusually low bone mineral density (BMD) for a man his age and the evaluation for secondary causes of bone loss is appropriate. His serum chemistry and serum testosterone values are normal, but his urinary calcium excretion is surprisingly low. Further evaluation included a measurement of serum 25-hydroxyvitamin D, which was less than 9 ng/mL (ideal > 30). The intact parathyroid level was 115 pg/mL (the normal range is 10–65 pg/mL). Anti-endomysial antibodies were positive and a duodenal biopsy demonstrated findings that are consistent with celiac disease. He was treated with a gluten-free diet, calcium, and high doses of vitamin D. One year later, his BMD T-score values were −2.0 in the spine and −1.8 in the total proximal femur. At the time of his initial evaluation, the BMD values were quite low. However, he did not

have osteoporosis and treatment with drugs for osteoporosis would not have been appropriate. It is important to exclude other causes of low BMD before concluding that a patient with a low T-score has osteoporosis.

Summary

Bone density testing is an important tool for assessing skeletal status and fracture risk in patients at risk for osteoporosis

T-score values must be combined with other risk factors to assess fracture risk

Only DXA of hip, spine, or one-third radius can be used to diagnose osteoporisis

Exquisite quality control is required for adequate interpretation, especially when serial studies are being evaluated

Figure 15-29. Summary. Bone mineral density measurement is a valuable tool for evaluating patients who are at risk for osteoporosis. When combined with other risk factors, BMD values are strongly correlated with fracture risk in untreated older adults. While a variety of bone density technologies may predict fracture risk, the World Health Organization classification system only applies to dual-energy x-ray absorptiometry (DXA) values of the lumbar spine, proximal femur, and mid-radius. Following the changes in bone density over time is both a technical and a clinical challenge and excellent quality control is required for adequate interpretation of serial studies. Understanding both the technical aspects of bone density tests and the clinical relevance of the results optimizes the application of these technologies to patient care.

References

1. Blake GM, Fogelman I: Role of dual-energy x-ray absorptiometry in the diagnosis and treatment of osteoporosis. *J Clin Densitom* 2007, 10:102–110.

2. Blake GM, Fogelman I: Technical principles of dual energy x-ray absorptiometry. *Semin Nucl Med* 1997, 27:210–228.

3. Njeh CF, Boivin CM, Langton CM: The role of ultrasound in the assessment of osteoporosis: a review. *Osteoporos Int* 1997, 7:7–22.

4. Kazakia GJ, Majumdar S: New imaging technologies in the diagnosis of osteoporosis. *Rev Endocr Metab Disord* 2006, 7:67–74.

5. Binkley N, Bilezikian JP, Kendler DL, *et al.*: Official positions of the International Society for Clinical Densitometry and executive summary of the 2005 Position Development Conference. *J Clin Densitom* 2006, 9:4–14.

6. Lewiecki EM, Binkley N, Petak SM: DXA quality matters. *J Clin Densitom* 2006, 9:388–392.

7. Hans PDD, Downs RW, Duboeuf F, *et al.*: Skeletal sites for osteoporosis diagnosis: the 2005 ISCD official positions. *J Clin Densitom* 2006, 9:15–21.

8. Kanis J: Diagnosis of osteoporosis and assessment of fracture risk. *Lancet* 2002, 359:1929–1936.

9. Cummings SR, Black DM, Nevitt MC, *et al.*: Bone density at various sites for prediction of hip fractures. The study of osteoporotic fractures research group. *Lancet* 1993, 341:72–75.

10. Marshall D, Johnell O, Wedel H: Meta-analysis of how well measures of bone mineral density predict occurrence of osteoporotic fractures. *Br Med J* 1996, 312:1254–1259.

11. Kanis JA, Johnell O, Oden A, *et al.*: Ten year probabilities of osteoporotic fractures according to BMD and diagnostic thresholds. *Osteoporos Int* 2001, 12:989–995.

12. National Osteoporosis Foundation: *Physician's Guide to Prevention and Treatment of Osteoporosis.* Washington, DC: National Osteoporosis Foundation; 2003.

13. Hodgson SF, Watts NB, Bilezikian JP, *et al.*: American Association of Clinical Endocrinologists medical guidelines for clinical practice for the prevention and treatment of postmenopausal osteoporosis: 2001 edition, with selected updates for 2003. *Endocr Pract* 2003, 9:544–564.

14. Schuit SCE, van der Klift M, Weel AEAM, *et al.*: Fracture incidence and association with bone mineral density in elderly men and women: the Rotterdam study. *Bone* 2004, 34:195–202.

15. Ross PD, Davis JW, Epstein RS, Wasnich RD: Pre-existing fractures and bone mass predict vertebral fracture incidence in women. *Ann Intern Med* 1991, 114:919–923.

16. Colon-Emeric CS, Sloane R, Hawkes WG, *et al.*: The risk of subsequent fractures in community-dwelling men and male veterans with hip fracture. *Am J Med* 2000, 109:324–328.

17. Delmas PD, Genant HK, Crans GG, *et al.*: Severity of prevalent vertebral fractures and the risk of subsequent vertebral and nonvertebral fractures: results from the MORE trial. *Bone* 2003, 33:522–532.

18. McClung MR: Do current management strategies and guidelines adequately address fracture risk? *Bone* 2006, 38:S13–S17.

19. Kanis JA, Johnell O, Oden A, *et al.*: Intervention thresholds for osteoporosis in men and women: a study based on data from Sweden. *Osteoporos Int* 2005, 16:6–14.

20. World Health Organization: Assessment of fracture risk and its application to screening for postmenopausal osteoporosis. *World Health Organ Tech Rep Ser* 1994, 843:1–129.

21. Looker AC, Wahner HW, Dunn WL, *et al.*: Updated data on proximal femur bone mineral levels of U.S. adults. *Osteoporos Int* 1998, 8:468–489.

22. Faulkner KG, von Stetten E, Miller P: Discordance in patient classification using T-scores. *J Clin Densitom* 1999, 2:343–350.

23. Leslie WD, Adler RA, Fuleihan GE, *et al.*: Application of the 1994 WHO classification to populations other than postmenopausal Caucasian women: the 2005 ISCD official positions. *J Clin Densitom* 2006, 9:22–30.

24. De Laet CEDH, Van Hout BA, Burger H, *et al.*: Hip fracture prediction in elderly men and women: validation in the Rotterdam study. *J Bone Miner Res* 1998, 13:1587–1593.

25. Binkley N, Schmeer P, Wasnich R, Lenchik L: What are the criteria by which a densitometric diagnosis of osteoporosis can be made in males and non-Caucasians? *J Clin Densitom* 2002, 5(Suppl):S19–S27.

26. Gluer CC: Monitoring skeletal changes by radiological techniques. *J Bone Miner Res* 1999, 14:1952–1962.

27. Lenchik L, Kiebzak GM, Blunt BA: What is the role of serial bone mineral density measurements in patient management? *J Clin Densitom* 2002(Suppl), 5:S29–S38.

28. Shepherd JA, Lu Y, Wilson K, *et al.*: Cross-calibration and minimum precisions standards for dual-energy x-ray absorptiometry: the 2005 ISCD official positions. *J Clin Densitom* 2006, 9:31–36.

29. Liberman UA, Weiss SR, Broll J, *et al.*: Effect of oral alendronate on bone mineral density and the incidence of fractures in postmenopausal osteoporosis. The Alendronate Phase III Osteoporosis Treatment Study Group. *N Engl J Med* 1995, 333:1437–1443.

30. Miller PD, Njeh CF, Jankowski LG, Lenchik L: What are the standards by which bone mass measurement at peripheral skeletal sites should be used in the diagnosis of osteoporosis? *J Clin Densitom* 2002, 5(Suppl):S39-S45.

31. Watts NB: Understanding the bone mass measurement act. *J Clin Densitom* 1999, 2:211–217.

32. US Preventive Services Task Force: Screening for osteoporosis in postmenopausal women: recommendations and rationale. *Ann Intern Med* 2002, 137:526–528.

33. Genant HK, Wu CY, Van Kuijk C, Nevitt MC: Vertebral fracture assessment using a semiquantitative technique. *J Bone Miner Res* 1993, 8:1137–1148.

34. Vokes T, Bachman D, Baim S, *et al.*: Vertebral fracture assessment: the 2005 ISCD official positions. *J Clin Densitom* 2006, 9:37–46.

Bisphosphonate Therapy for Osteoporosis

16

Jeffrey Curtis

Bisphosphonate treatment of osteoporosis began with the off-label use of etidronate in the 1980s. Alendronate (1995) and risedronate (1999) have been joined by ibandronate (2003) and are approved by the United States Food and Drug Administration (FDA) for the prevention and treatment of postmenopausal osteoporosis and for patients with osteoporosis due to glucocorticoid treatment. The newest of these agents, zoledronate, was approved in 2007 and shows great promise as an effective treatment option.

These compounds increase bone mineral density and reduce the risk of vertebral and nonvertebral fractures. The body of evidence for both the safety and efficacy of bisphosphonate treatment for osteoporosis is greater than for any other agents. Longer term data, and head-to-head and combination trials, now serve to expand the evidence base regarding reducing the risk for fractures with these agents. Bisphosphonates are safe, well tolerated, and the preferred drug of choice for most patients with osteoporosis.

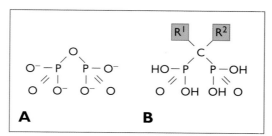

Figure 16-1. General structure of pyrophosphate (**A**) and bisphosphonates (**B**). Bisphosphonates are analogues of pyrophosphates. Pyrophosphates are ubiquitous compounds characterized by two phosphonic acid groups bound to a central oxygen molecule. The phosphate–oxygen bonds undergo rapid enzymatic degradation. Bisphosphonates consist of two phosphonic acids linked to a carbon, with two side chains (R^1 and R^2) that determine the avidity of binding to bone, antiresorptive potency, and side effects. (*Adapted from* Watts [1].)

Figure 16-2. Characteristics of bisphosphonates. Bisphosphonates can be administered either orally or intravenously, but they are poorly absorbed when given by mouth. Under ideal circumstances, only about 1% of an oral dose is absorbed; absorption is completely blocked if the drug is taken with calcium, magnesium, or other divalent cations. Bisphosphonates bind avidly to hydroxyapatite crystals on bone surfaces. Between 20% and 50% is absorbed on bone and the rest is excreted in urine over the next 12 to 24 hours. There is no systemic metabolism. Although the drug remains in bone for years, after remodeling is complete it is buried in bone and is no longer pharmacologically active. Bisphosphonates have little or no long-term toxicity. The main side effects are gastrointestinal (esophageal irritation), most likely with nitrogen-containing bisphosphonates given orally, and acute-phase reactions, hypocalcemia, and acute renal failure when

Characteristics of Bisphosphonates

Effective orally or intravenously

Absorption is poor when given by mouth and completely blocked by divalent cations

Bind avidly to hydroxyapatite crystals on bone surfaces

No systemic metabolism

Excreted by the kidney

Long retention in the skeleton

given intravenously. Etidronate, given continuously and in high doses, may impair bone mineralization, but this is rarely seen with the doses of other bisphosphonates used to treat osteoporosis.

Mechanisms of Antiresorptive Action of Bisphosphonates

Reduce activity of individual osteoclasts
  Inhibit lactate production
  Inhibit lysosomal enzymes
Reduce activiation frequency
  Inhibit recruitment of osteoclast precursors
  Inhibit differentiation of osteoclast precursors
Accelerate osteoclast apoptosis

Figure 16-3. Mechanisms of antiresorptive action of bisphosphonates. After being adsorbed onto hydroxyapatite crystals at sites of active bone remodeling, bisphosphonates decrease bone turnover through several different actions: 1) they reduce the activity of individual osteoclasts by inhibiting the production of lactate and lysosomal enzymes; 2) they reduce activation frequency by inhibiting the recruitment and differentiation of osteoclast precursors; and 3) they accelerate osteoclast apoptosis (programmed cell death).

Types of Bisphosphonates

Non–nitrogen-containing	Nitrogen-containing
Etidronate	Pamidronate
Clodronate	Alendronate
Tiludronate	Risedronate
	Ibandronate
	Zoledronate

Figure 16-4. Different types of bisphosphonates. Altering the R^2 side chain on bisphosphonates changes the antiresorptive potency. The antiresorptive potency differs 10- to 10,000-fold between compounds based on in vitro testing; for in vivo, there is less difference in potency between compounds. Early bisphosphonates in clinical use (etidronate, clodronate, and tiludronate) are rather simple compounds. Newer bisphosphonates (pamidronate, alendronate, risedronate, ibandronate, and zoledronate) have greater antiresorptive potency than the older compounds, in part because they contain at least one nitrogen in the R^2 side chain. Although sometimes classified in "generations," most authorities now classify bisphosphonates on the basis of whether or not a nitrogen is contained in the R^2 side chain.

Figure 16-5. Intracellular mechanism of action of nitrogen-containing bisphosphonates. Protein prenelation (the addition of 15- and 20-carbon lipid side chains) is essential for the optimal action of a number of GTPases that are critical for cellular function and integrity. Nitrogen-containing bisphosphonates interfere with protein prenelation by inhibiting the action of farnesyl pyrophosphate synthase, an enzyme in the mevalonate pathway. The end result of the decreased action of these GTPases is apoptosis (programmed cell death) of osteoclasts and, therefore, reduced bone resorption [2]. Non–nitrogen-containing bisphosphonates exert their action by causing the accumulation of toxic analogues of adenosine triphosphate within cells (not shown).

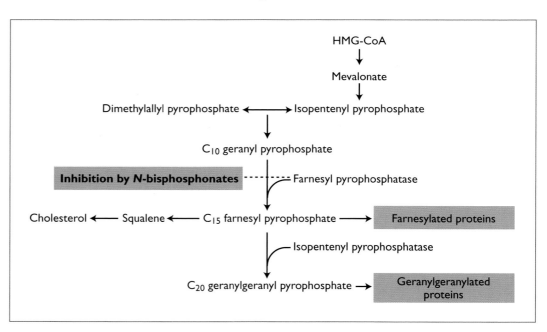

Potential Medical Uses for Bisphosphonates

Osteoporosis
Hypercalcemia
Paget's disease
Fibrous dysplasia
Osteogenesis imperfecta
Multiple myeloma
Bone metastases
Myositis ossificans
Heterotopic ossification
Periodontal disease
Neuropathic arthropathy (Charcot's joint)
Delay to collapse of the femoral head for osteonecrosis of the hip
Reflex sympathetic dystrophy

Figure 16-6. Potential medical uses for bisphosphonates. Bisphosphonates appear to be beneficial in almost any condition characterized by increased bone remodeling, including osteoporosis, hypercalcemia, and Paget's disease.

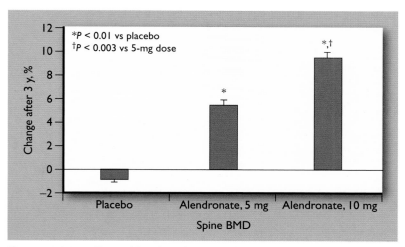

Figure 16-7. Effect of bisphosphonates on spine bone mineral density (BMD). In women with postmenopausal osteoporosis, bisphosphonates increase BMD in a dose-dependent manner. In this 3-year study of 478 women with postmenopausal osteoporosis, the optimal dose of alendronate for increasing bone density in the spine was 10 mg daily. (*Data from* Tucci *et al.* [3].)

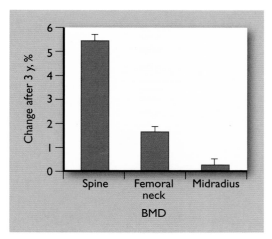

Figure 16-8. Effects of bisphosphonates on bone mineral density (BMD) at different skeletal sites. Although treatment with bisphosphonates produces significant gains in BMD in the spine in women with postmenopausal osteoporosis, treatment is less effective at the hip and the effect is negligible at the forearm, as shown in this 3-year study of 2458 women with osteoporosis receiving a 5-mg daily dose of risedronate [4].

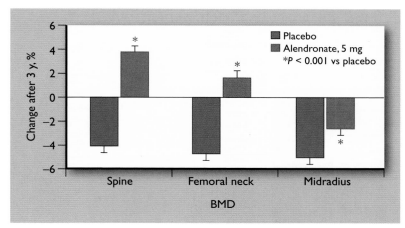

Figure 16-9. Bisphosphonates prevent the loss of bone mineral density (BMD) in recently menopausal women. Bisphosphonates have been shown to prevent or reduce the accelerated bone loss that occurs with menopause, as illustrated in this study of 1174 women in early menopause treated with a 5-mg daily dose of alendronate or placebo [5].

Figure 16-10. Bisphosphonates have positive effects on bone mineral density (BMD) in patients receiving corticosteroid therapy. Bisphosphonates prevent bone loss in patients beginning corticosteroid therapy and increase BMD in patients who have been on long-term corticosteroid therapy. In this 12-month study of 290 men and women who had received a daily dose of 7.5 mg or more of prednisone for an average of about 5 years, treatment with 5 mg daily of risedronate resulted in significantly better BMD in the spine and hip compared with placebo [6].

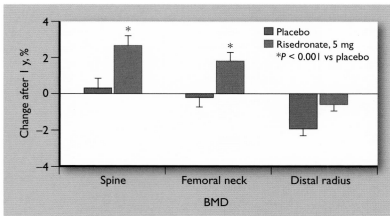

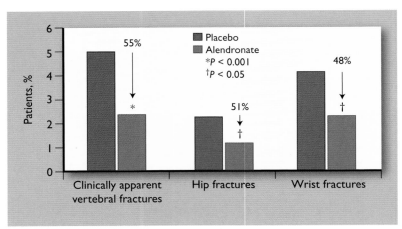

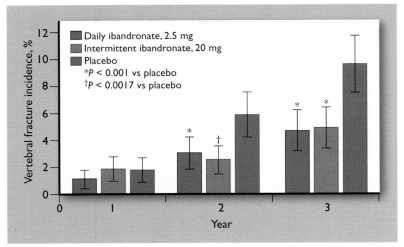

Figure 16-11. Bisphosphonates reduce fracture risk in women with postmenopausal osteoporosis. The main value of any treatment for osteoporosis is a reduction in fracture risk. The first prospective, randomized, double-blind, placebo-controlled trial to demonstrate an antifracture effect with any agent was the Fracture Intervention Trial, a 3-year study of 2027 women with postmenopausal osteoporosis (all with prevalent vertebral fractures) who received either alendronate (5 mg daily for 2 years, then 10 mg daily) or placebo. Rates of vertebral fractures, hip fractures, and wrist fractures were significantly decreased with alendronate treatment compared with placebo [7]. Of interest, in this study, fracture rates were reduced to a similar degree at these three skeletal sites, despite different effects on bone density at these sites.

Figure 16-12. Once-daily ibandronate at a dose of 2.5 mg orally was approved by the United States Food and Drug Administration for postmenopausal osteoporosis in 2003. In this 3-year study of 2946 osteoporotic women with prevalent vertebral fractures, ibandronate reduced the risk for a new vertebral fracture by 62%. In a post-hoc analysis, the reduction of nonvertebral fractures was seen only in women with a femoral neck T-score lower than –3.0.

The daily dose of ibandronate was never marketed in the United States, but was used as a comparator dose for other ibandronate formulations. A subsequent study established the noninferiority (using a bone mineral density endpoint) of an orally administered ibandronate dose of 150 mg once monthly [8] compared to the once-daily 2.5-mg daily dose and it was approved for use in the United States in 2005. (*Adapted from* Chesnut [9].)

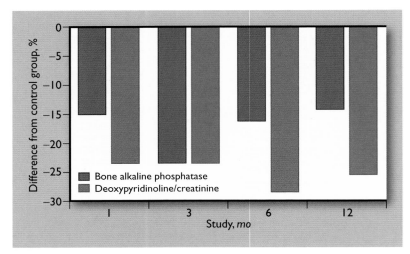

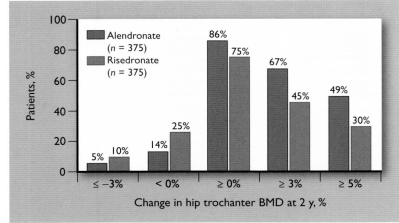

Figure 16-13. Effects of bisphosphonates on bone turnover markers. Bisphosphonates exert an antiresorptive effect that is reflected in a rapid reduction in bone turnover markers, such as bone alkaline phosphatase and deoxypyridinoline, as shown in this study during 12 months' treatment with risedronate, 5 mg daily [4]. The reduction in bone turnover markers is rapid (usually maximal after 3 to 6 months of treatment) and maintained for as long as treatment is continued. The timing of maximal reduction in bone turnover markers is concordant with the early fracture reduction. The degree of reduction in bone turnover correlates better with fracture reduction than does change in bone mineral density.

Figure 16-14. A 1-year head-to-head study of alendronate versus risedronate enrolled 1053 women and examined comparative changes in bone mineral density (BMD) and bone turnover markers. In a 1-year extension study of 833 of the originally enrolled women, alendronate increased BMD at the hip trochanter (the primary endpoint) by a mean of 4.6% compared to 2.5% among the risedronate users (P < 0.001). Examining these data in a different way, as shown in this figure, more alendronate-treated women gained more than 3% and fewer lost less than 3% compared to the risedronate-treated women; ± 3% is approximately the boundary of least significant change that reflects a true difference beyond measurement error. Of note, however, is that approximately one-quarter to one-half of women did not increase or decrease BMD greater or less than 3%, which is so-called "stable" BMD. Some have hypothesized that a lack of significant improvement in BMD may retard long-term patient compliance with bisphosphonate therapy if the patients' perception is that the medicine is not working (to significantly increase BMD). (*Adapted from* Bonnick [10].)

Figure 16-15. Although different osteoporosis medications yield differing changes in bone mineral density (BMD), changes in BMD explain only a minority of fracture risk reduction. In this post-hoc analysis of three pivotal risedronate fracture risk reduction trials that included 2561 risedronate-treated women, changes in lumbar spine and femoral neck BMD (shown) were not significantly correlated with fracture risk reduction. For this reason, it is controversial as to whether or not greater improvements in BMD following bisphosphonate therapy translate into greater reductions in either nonvertebral or vertebral [11] fracture risk. For this reason, BMD that is stable or increasing over time is likely an adequate goal for treatment. (*Adapted from* Watts *et al.* [12].)

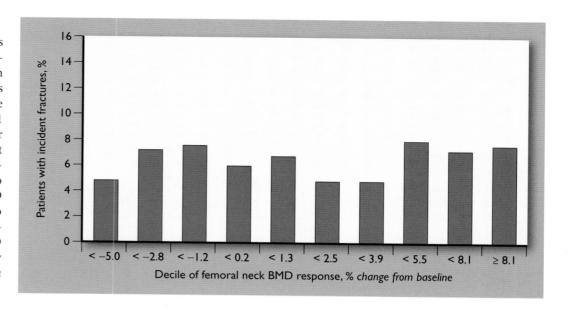

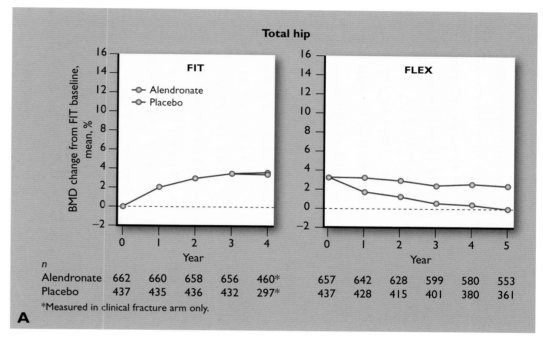

Figure 16-16. Given the long skeletal retention of bisphosphonates, the possibility of a drug holiday after a prolonged period of treatment has been a subject of high interest. **A,** A 5-year extension study to the Fracture Intervention Trial (FIT) randomized 1099 of the originally treated patients (mean duration of therapy = 5 years) to 5 additional years of alendronate or placebo. As shown, women who received placebo after 5 years of alendronate treatment had significant declines in bone mineral density (BMD) over the next 5 years and returned to their original baseline. Women who continued to receive therapy had stable BMD at the hip. However, as shown in **B,** the risk for all fracture types were similar between the placebo and the alendronate-treated patients except for clinical vertebral fractures, which were significantly reduced (relative risk 0.45, 95% CI 0.24–0.85) among those who received ongoing alendronate treatment rather than placebo. FLEX—Fracture Intervention Trial Long-Term Extension. (*Adapted from* Black *et al.* [13].)

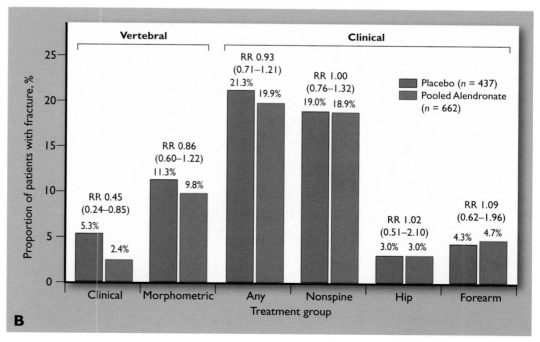

Proper Dosing of Daily or Weekly Bisphosphonates

Instruction	Reason
Take on an empty stomach first thing in the morning, with water only, and nothing else for 30 min	Avoiding binding with divalent cations to ensure adequate absorption
Take with 8 oz of water	Minimizes the risk of the tablet lodging in the esophagus
Remain upright until food or calcium is consumed to bind the drug	Minimizes the risk of reflux of the drug into the esophagus

Figure 16-17. Proper oral administration of bisphosphonates. Bisphosphonates are poorly absorbed when given by mouth and must be taken on an empty stomach, with water, but nothing else for at least 30 minutes. Alendronate may irritate the esophagus, so the tablet should be washed down with water (to avoid sticking) and the patient should remain upright (seated or standing) until they have taken some food or calcium to bind the drug. Bisphosphonates should not be given to patients with active upper gastrointestinal disease and should be stopped if upper gastrointestinal symptoms develop.

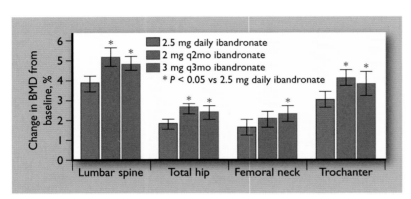

Figure 16-18. Intravenous (IV) ibandronate was approved by the Food and Drug Administration in 2006 for IV use for the treatment of postmenopausal osteoporosis. In this 1-year study of 1395 postmenopausal osteoporotic women, the intravenous form of ibandronate was shown to be superior ($P < 0.001$) to once-daily oral ibandronate using a bone mineral density endpoint. (*Adapted from* Delmas *et al.* [14].)

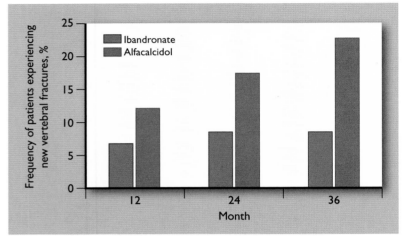

Figure 16-19. Although not approved for the treatment of glucocorticoid-induced osteoporosis, intravenous (IV) ibandronate has demonstrated significant efficacy in the reduction of vertebral fractures as compared to alfacalcidol. In this 3-year study of 115 patients receiving prednisone at a mean dose of 10–11 mg/d, the proportion of patients treated with ibandronate 3 mg IV every 3 months that experienced a vertebral fracture was significantly lower than those that were treated with alfacalcidol 1 ug daily (8.6 vs 22.8% at 36 mo, $P = 0.04$). This study is among the first to demonstrate fracture risk reduction with the use of an IV bisphosphonate in glucocorticoid-treated patients. (*Adapted from* Ringe *et al.* [15].)

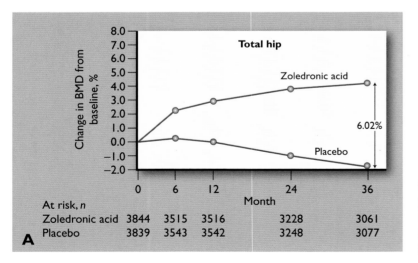

At risk, n	0	6	12	24	36
Zoledronic acid	3844	3515	3516	3228	3061
Placebo	3839	3543	3542	3248	3077

A

Figure 16-20. A and B, Intravenous zoledronate is the newest bisphosphonate to be studied for the treatment of postmenopausal osteoporosis. Given as a 5-mg, once-annual infusion over approximately 20 minutes, zoledronate demonstrated effectiveness in increasing bone mineral density in this 3-year study of 7865 postmenopausal women.

Continued on the next page

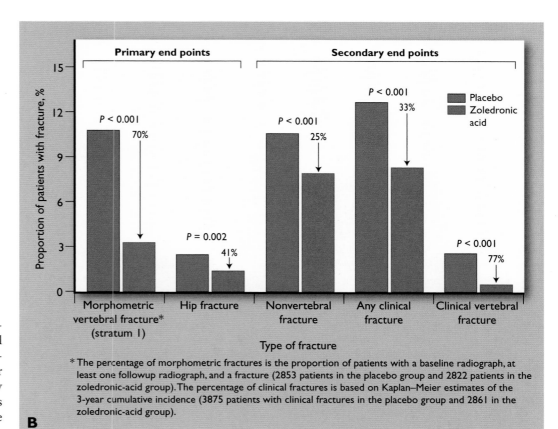

Figure 16-20. *(Continued)* Even more importantly, zoledronate demonstrated substantial effectiveness in reducing the risk for morphometric vertebral, clinical vertebral, hip, and other nonvertebral fractures. Zoledronate may be a very useful option for the treatment of osteoporosis given its unique dosing schedule. RR—relative risk. *(Adapted from* Black et al. [16].)

* The percentage of morphometric fractures is the proportion of patients with a baseline radiograph, at least one followup radiograph, and a fracture (2853 patients in the placebo group and 2822 patients in the zoledronic-acid group). The percentage of clinical fractures is based on Kaplan–Meier estimates of the 3-year cumulative incidence (3875 patients with clinical fractures in the placebo group and 2861 in the zoledronic-acid group).

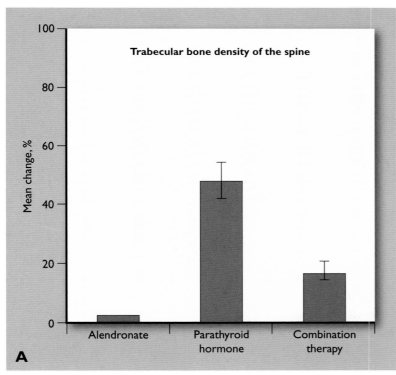

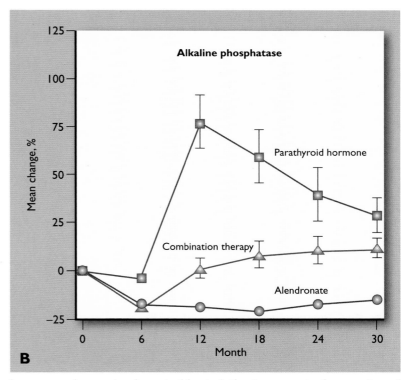

Figure 16-21. A and **B,** Given the anti-resorptive nature of bisphosphonates, the possibility of combining an anti-resorptive with an anabolic agent such as parathyroid hormone is very attractive in theory. However, in this 30-month study of 83 men treated with alendronate, parathyroid hormone, or both, the gain in trabecular bone density of the spine was significantly greater in the group receiving parathyroid hormone alone; alendronate blunted the increase in bone mineral density and serum alkaline phosphatase (a marker of bone formation) that resulted from parathyroid hormone therapy alone. For this reason, concurrent therapy with an anabolic agent and a potent anti-resorptive such as alendronate is not recommended. *(Adapted from* Finkelstein et al. [17].)

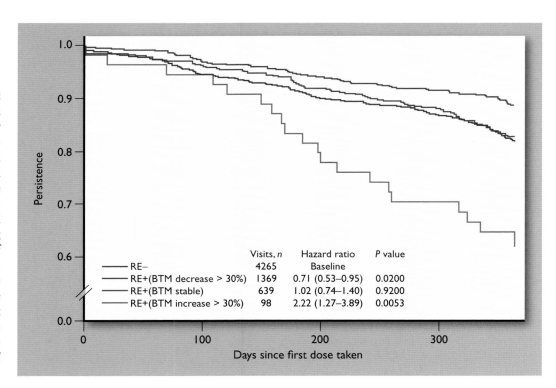

Figure 16-22. As in many chronic, asymptomatic diseases, long-term adherence with therapy is a major problem in osteoporosis. Approximately one-half of patients newly initiating bisphosphonate therapy discontinue its use between 12 and 18 months. In this study of 2383 postmenopausal women, participants were randomized to receive reinforcement with information regarding reduction in bone turnover markers, which were assessed at approximately 3 and 6 months after starting therapy. As shown, persons who had a reduction of greater than 30% (BTM decrease > 30%) in turnover markers and were given this information were significantly less likely to discontinue risedronate therapy than those who received no reinforcement or who were notified that their markers were stable or increased (BTM increase > 30%). BTM—bone turnover marker; RE—reinforcement. (*Adapted from* Delmas *et al.* [18].)

References

1. Watts NB: Bisphosphonate treatment for osteoporosis. In *The Osteoporotic Syndrome.* Edited by Avioli LV. San Diego: Academic; 2000:121–132.

2. Rogers MJ, Gordon S, Benford HL, *et al.*: Cellular and molecular mechanisms of action of bisphosphonates [review]. *Cancer* 2000, 88(Suppl 12):2961–2978.

3. Tucci JR, Tonino RP, Emkey RD, *et al.*: Effect of three years of oral alendronate treatment in postmenopausal women with osteoporosis. *Am J Med* 1996, 101:488–501.

4. Harris ST, Watts NB, Genant HK, *et al.*: Effects of risedronate treatment on vertebral and nonvertebral fractures in women with postmenopausal osteoporosis—a randomized controlled trial. *JAMA* 1999, 282:1344–1352.

5. Hosking D, Chilvers CED, Christiansen C, *et al.*: Prevention of bone loss with alendronate in postmenopausal women under 60 years of age: Early Postmenopausal Intervention Cohort Study Group. *N Engl J Med* 1998, 338:485–492.

6. Reid DM, Hughes R, Laan RF, *et al.*: Efficacy and safety of daily risedronate in the treatment of corticosteroid-induced osteoporosis in men and women: a randomized trial. *J Bone Miner Res* 2000, 15:1006–1013.

7. Black DM, Cummings SR, Karpf DB, *et al.*: Randomised trial of effect of alendronate on risk of fracture in women with existing vertebral fractures. *Lancet* 1996, 348:1535–1541.

8. Reginster, JY: Efficacy and tolerability of once-monthly oral ibandronate in postmenopausal osteoporosis: 2 year results from the MOBILE study. *Ann Rheum Dis* 2006, 65:654–661.

9. Chesnut CH III, Skag A, Christiansen C, *et al.*: Effects of oral ibandronate administered daily or intermittently on fracture risk in postmenopausal osteoporosis. *J Bone Miner Res* 2004, 19:1241–1249.

10. Bonnick S, Saag KG, Kiel DP, *et al.*: Comparison of weekly treatment of postmenopausal osteoporosis with alendronate versus risedronate over two years. *J Clin Endocrin Metab* 2006, 91:2631–2637.

11. Chapurlat RD: Risk of fracture among women who lose bone density during treatment with alendronate. The Fracture Intervention Trial. *Osteoporos Int* 2005, 16:842–848.

12. Watts NB, Geusens P, Barton IP, Felsenberg D: Relationship between changes in BMD and nonvertebral fracture incidence associated with risedronate: reduction in risk of nonvertebral racture is not related to change in BMD. *J Bone Miner Res* 2005, 20:2097–2104.

13. Black DM, Schwartz AV, Ensrud KE, *et al.*: Effects of continuing or stopping alendronate after 5 years of treatment. The Fracture Intervention Trial Long-Term Extension (FLEX): a randomized trial. *JAMA* 2006, 296:2927–2938.

14. Delmas PD, Adami S, Strugala C, *et al.*: Intravenous ibandronate injections in postmenopausal women with osteoporosis. *Arthritis Rheum* 2006, 54:1838–1846.

15. Ringe JD, Dorst A, Faber H, *et al.*: Intermittent intravenous ibandronate injections reduce vertebral fracture risk in corticosteroid-induced osteoporosis: results from a long-term comparative study. *Osteoporos Int* 2003, 14:801–807.

16. Black DM, Delmas PD, Eastell R, *et al.*: Once-yearly zoledronic acid for treatment of postmenopausal osteoporosis. *N Engl J Med* 2007, 356:1809–1822.

17. Finkelstein JS, Hayes A, Hunzelman JL, *et al.*: The effects of parathyroid hormone, alendronate, or both in men with osteoporosis. *N Engl J Med* 2003, 349:1216–1226.

18. Delmas PD, Vrijens B, Eastell R, *et al.*: Effects of monitoring bone turnover markers on persistence with risedronate treatment of postmenopausal osteoporosis. *J Clin Endocrinol Metab* 2007, 92:1296–1304.

Bone Anabolic Agents

17

David L. Kendler

Bone remodeling is a coupled process in which old bone is resorbed and new bone is formed at the site of resorption. In the past, little has been understood about the molecular processes governing this linkage and its control. In particular, there has been a lack of understanding of how bone can remodel adaptively in response to fracture or mechanical load. Each of these circumstances requires "uncoupling" the linked processes of bone resorption and bone formation. Discovering the regulatory pathways for these physiologic processes could shed light on new molecular targets for intervention in patients with severe osteoporosis who require more than just the stabilization of bone tissue, but who require a true anabolic response. The contributions of molecular biology in unravelling bone anabolic pathways cannot be underestimated and, through this understanding, a wide range of new therapeutic targets is being identified. Parallel developments in bone imaging including micro-CT and micro-MRI imaging of bone hold the promise of noninvasively following bone anabolic changes in individual patients on therapy.

Antiresorptive agents have been the mainstay of osteoporosis therapy and they have made a valuable contribution to bone tissue stabilization and fracture reduction. By reducing bone turnover to premenopausal levels, these agents allow the repair of bone microarchitecture. In time, however, the linkage of resorption and formation leads to reduced bone-formation activity and a new steady state of low bone turnover. Long-term increases in bone density are likely related to the passive mineralization of bone resulting from this slowed bone turnover. Therefore, significant further reductions in fracture risk in patients who are on long-term antiresorptive therapy are not likely to occur. There is a need for therapies that can sequentially or in combination stimulate new bone formation, which are the bone anabolic agents.

Sodium fluoride was the first anabolic drug trialed in osteoporosis patients and was used extensively "off label." High-dose fluoride therapy is difficult for patients to tolerate and can produce structurally unstable "woven bone," which may cause a predisposition to fracture [1].

Parathyroid hormone (PTH) and its analogues have been investigated for over 20 years as bone anabolic agents. Recently, clinical trials of both full-length PTH 1-84 and teriparatide (PTH 1-34) have shown fracture risk reduction [2,3]. Both trials demonstrated vertebral fracture efficacy but only the teriparatide trial was able to demonstrate nonvertebral fracture risk reduction.

Subsequent research with PTH 1-84 sought to clarify the role of concomitant therapy with alendronate versus sequential bone anabolic therapy then antiresorptive therapy. Bone density increases were greatest with monotherapy alendronate or monotherapy PTH 1-84 and, at all sites, an inferior effect was seen with combination therapy [4].

PTH therapy has its limitations. It is rapidly degraded in the stomach and must currently be administered by injection. New methods of drug administration are desirable. There is a variable incidence of hypercalcemia and hypercalciuria in patients on therapy. Treatment is limited to 18 to 24 months due to the dose-dependent incidence of osteosarcoma in rats treated with lifelong high-dose PTH therapy. Other modalities of generating a pulse of PTH endogenously are being investigated through novel calcium-sensing receptor-blocking peptides.

Other anabolic agents under investigation include growth hormone and insulin-like growth factor-I (IGF-I). Recombinant human growth hormone may be useful in patients with growth hormone (GH) deficiency and can increase total body bone density when administered for 1 year [5,6]. In catabolic states such as burns, hip fractures, and major surgery, the short-term use of IGF-I, GH, and GH-releasing peptides has been investigated with promising results [7].

Strontium ranelate has been shown in animal trials to have bone anabolic properties as well as antiresorptive effects. The exact mechanism of its bone anabolic activity is not yet known. Both vertebral and nonvertebral fracture efficacy has been demonstrated in postmenopausal women [8]. Bone density increases in part due to the strontium artifact in bone and in part due to the formation of new bone tissue. However, the fracture risk reduction attributable to increases in bone mineral density is greater than with any other agent [9].

Perhaps most promising in the area of bone anabolic agents is the elucidation of the Wnt/β-catenin pathway and its role in the regulation of bone formation in the adult skeleton [10]. Several promising targets for pharmaceutical therapy have been identified and clinical trials have begun. Sclerostin is an osteocyte protein product of the SOST gene with inhibitory effects on osteoblast function. Congenital absence of this gene leads to sclerosteosis, where patients have high bone density and a fracture-resistant phenotype [11]. Clinical trials with sclerostin monoclonal antibody therapy have begun with a goal of developing a potent specific anabolic agent acting by neutralizing sclerostin and permitting anabolic effects on bone.

The effects of vibration of the adult skeleton in stimulating bone formation are being investigated as a bone anabolic therapy [12]. Mechanical stimulation may offer an interesting alternative to pharmaceutical approaches. This chapter examines the relevant pathways that control bone formation and highlights possible areas for therapeutic manipulation. Where available, the results of clinical trials using these agents are illustrated.

Anabolic Agents That Stimulate Bone Formation

Pharmacologic agents that are undergoing clinical trials but have not yet been approved in the United States for primary or secondary osteoporosis

Growth hormone

IGF-1

Sodium fluoride

BMPs

Strontium ranelate

Sclerostin mAb

PTH 1-84

Anabolic agents that have been approved in the United States for postmenopausal osteoporosis

PTH (1-34) administered daily for 18–24 mo

Agents with potential utility as anabolic factors in osteoporosis and currently under investigation

BMPs

IGF-1/IGFBP-3 (IGF-1 complexed to IGFBP-3)

PTH-related peptide

IGFBP-5

Transforming growth factor-beta

BMP-2

Figure 17-1. Anabolic agents that stimulate bone formation. BMPs—bone morphogenetic proteins; IGF-1—insulin-like growth factor-1; PTH—parathyroid hormone.

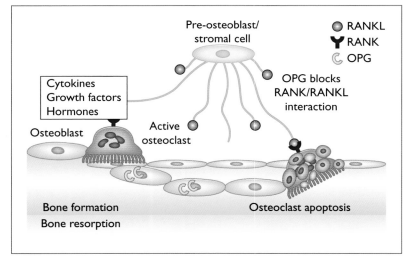

Figure 17-2. The receptor activator for nuclear factor κ (RANK)/RANK B ligand (RANKL)/osteoprotegerin (OPG) pathway: a key regulator of osteoclast formation. Hormonal regulation of bone remodeling is shown. The bone-remodeling unit tightly couples the processes of bone formation and resorption. In postmenopausal women, remodeling increases with estrogen withdrawal. Similar increases in bone remodeling occur with excess thyroxine, continuously elevated parathyroid hormone, and other cytokines. These agents interact directly with specific receptors in osteoblasts . Release from osteoblasts of various cytokines then modulate the maturation, proliferation, and differentiation of osteoclasts, the primary bone-resorbing cell. The most important pathway regulating the commitment of pre-osteoclast to osteoclast and their differentiation is the RANK/RANKL/OPG pathway. Interleukins 1, 6, and 11 are also mediators of osteoclast activation. With osteoclastic bone resorption, insulin-like growth factors I and II are released from the bone matrix complexed to matrix-binding proteins. These proteins likely participate in the recruitment, proliferation, and activation of new osteoblasts, which replace the resorbed bone [13].

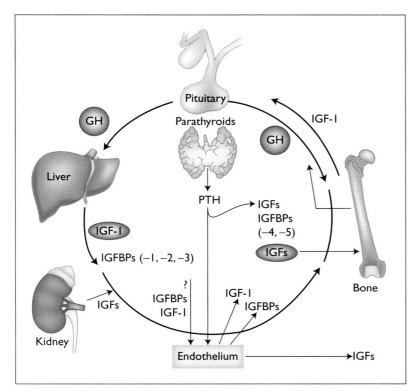

Figure 17-3. The circulating insulin-like growth factor (IGF) regulatory system is shown. This system is complex and redundant, and is composed of the same elements as the skeletal IGF system. IGF-I is produced by many cells and constantly shuttles in and out of the circulation. Most circulating IGF exists bound to one of several specific binding proteins (BPs). At least six IGFBPs are known to exist and are produced independently by separate genes. The dominant circulating BP is IGFBP3, which depends on growth hormone (GH) for its production. IGF-I, IGF-II, and BP3 are also bound in the circulation to a 70-kd protein called the acid-labile subunit, giving rise to a stable ternary complex. PTH—parathyroid hormone.

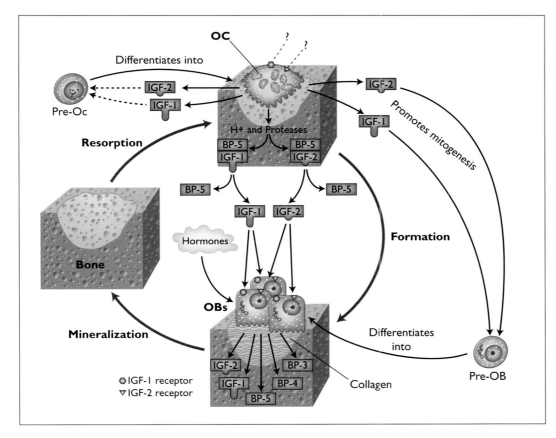

Figure 17-4. Balanced bone formation and resorption in healthy individuals. Osteoblasts (OBs) synthesize insulin-like growth factors (IGFs). IGF-II is more abundant than IGF-I in the skeleton and in the circulation. Circulating IGF-I concentrations decline with age; the skeletal IGF-I content of cortical and trabecular bone is lower in specimens from elderly persons than from younger individuals. IGF binding protein (BP)-5 anchors IGF to the hydroxyapatite crystal. OC—osteoclast. (*Adapted from* Yvonne Walston, CMI, ©1997.)

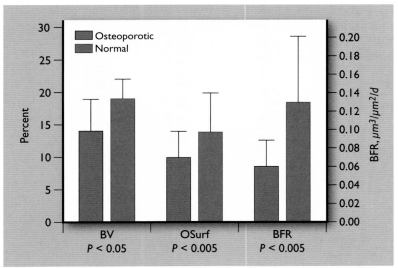

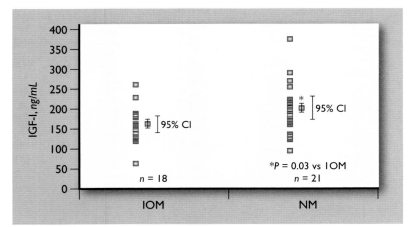

Figure 17-8. Role of insulin-like growth factor (IGF)-1 in idiopathic osteoporosis in males (IOM). Several reports of postmenopausal women have been unable to show a significant correlation between IGF-I concentrations and bone mineral density [15,16]. This contrasts with findings in IOM, a condition associated with normal biochemical evidence of bone turnover but reduced bone formation defined on bone biopsy [17]. This graph shows bone volume (BV), an index of trabecular bone mass; osteoid surfaces (OSurf), the fraction (%) of bone surfaces undergoing bone-formation activity; and bone-formation rate (BFR) expressed in μm³ per μm² of bone area per day. Trabecular bone mass and formation characteristics are lower in osteoporotic men than in normal controls.

Figure 17-9. Serum insulin-like growth factor (IGF)-1 concentrations in men with and without osteoporosis. Although there is considerable overlap, average IGF-I concentrations are lower in osteoporotic men. IOM—idiopathic osteoporosis in males; NM—normal men.

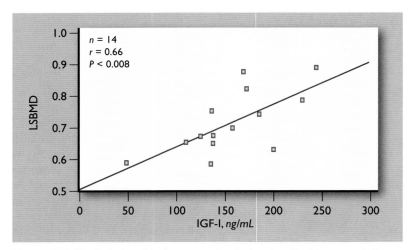

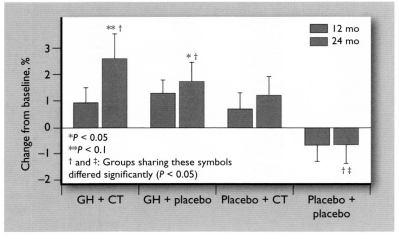

Figure 17-10. Relationship between circulating insulin-like growth factor (IGF)-1 concentrations and lumbar spine bone mass density (LSBMD) in osteoporotic men. In this series of idiopathic osteoporosis in males (IOM), a highly significant relationship was found between circulating IGF-I and bone mineral density, as opposed to that in normal men and women. It is likely that the designation IOM applies to a group of heterogeneous disorders. IGF-I may not be an important factor for all of them, accounting for the substantial degree of overlap shown in Figure 17-9. However, it appears that diminished IGF-I status contributes to low bone mass for at least some, or even most, affected men. Whether this effect represents a failure of adequate peak bone mass acquisition or of adult bone maintenance is unknown.

Figure 17-11. Effect of cyclic growth hormone (GH) with or without calcitonin on bone mineral density (BMD) in osteopenic older women. GH administration increases both resorption and formation marker activity; thus, it is likely that GH promotes an increase in new bone remodeling units, with a concomitant increase in the remodeling space. This hypothesis was tested that administration of recombinant human GH (rhGH) together with the antiresorptive hormone, salmon calcitonin, might permit a greater rise in BMD than would rhGH alone. This figure illustrates the effect on lumbar spine BMD of a 2-year program of GH with or without calcitonin (CT) given every 2 months for 24 months. rhGH stimulated modest increases in BMD, but these were not magnified by CT. The achieved rise in BMD resembles those observed with approved antiresorptive medications. Thus, it appears there is little, if any, therapeutic role for GH in the treatment of osteoporosis [18].

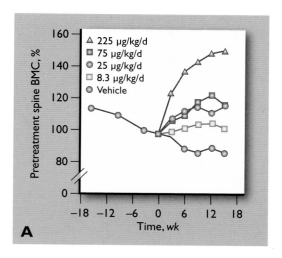

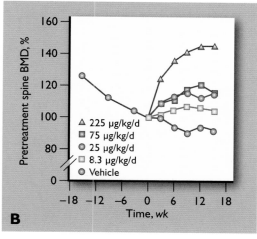

Figure 17-12. Lineage of mesenchymal cells. Skeletal effects of exogenous parathyroid hormone (PTH) are shown. Although continuously high serum PTH levels have been associated with bone disease in patients suffering severe primary hyperparathyroidism, intermittent elevation of PTH increases bone mass by increasing bone turnover, particularly in the spine. This figure shows the effects of daily PTH treatment on spine bone mineral content (BMC) (**A**) and bone mineral density (BMD) (**B**) in ovariectomized rats. A dose-dependent response is observed [19,20].

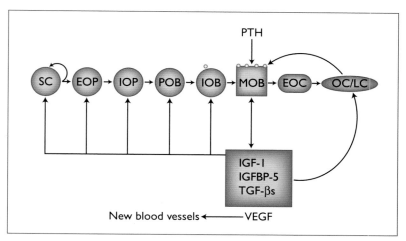

Figure 17-13. Anabolic actions of parathyroid hormone (PTH) on bone. One mechanism of action by which PTH affects bone is thought to be through the insulin-like growth factor (IGF) regulatory system, with direct induction of IGF-I and several IGF binding proteins (IGFBPs) in osteoblasts [21]. TGF-β—transforming growth factor-β; VEGF—vascular endothelial growth factor.

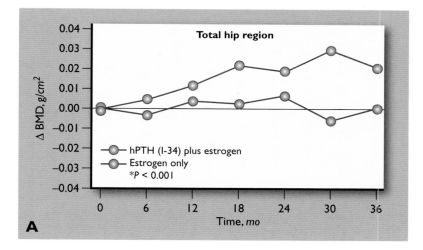

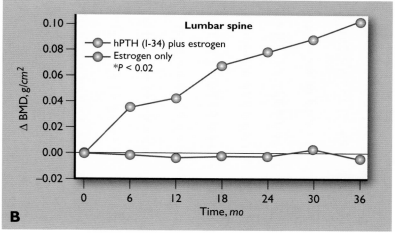

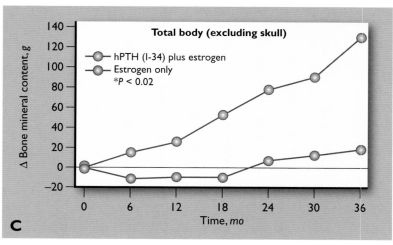

Figure 17-14. Effects of parathyroid hormone (PTH) (1-34) on bone mineral density (BMD) of postmenopausal women. **A,** Connections between osteoclast formation and the immune system [22]. **B,** Receptor activator for nuclear factor κ ligand (RANKL) inhibitors prevent osteoclast formation. In this randomized trial, human PTH (hPTH) increased bone mass in postmenopausal women who had been receiving hormone replacement therapy for at least 1 year [23]. **C,** RANKL inhibitors induce osteoclast apoptosis and stop resorption. Results were particularly dramatic at the lumbar spine. Although PTH 1-34 alone might predictably decrease cortical BMD, the rise in total body bone mineral content in these estrogen-replete women was reassuring. No deleterious effect on bone formation is seen.

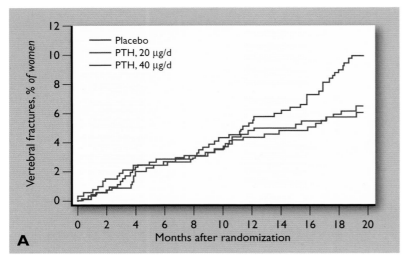
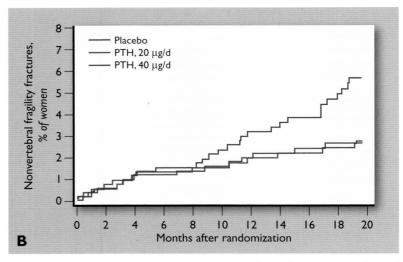

Figure 17-15. Vertebral and nonvertebral fracture prevention was demonstrated with parathyroid hormone (PTH) 1-34 over approximately 20 months of followup. Illustrated here are the cumulative proportion of women assigned to receive either placebo or PTH 1-34 at a daily dose of 20 or 40 µg who had one or more vertebral fractures (**A**) and the cumulative proportion who had one or more nonvertebral fragility fractures (**B**) during the study [2].

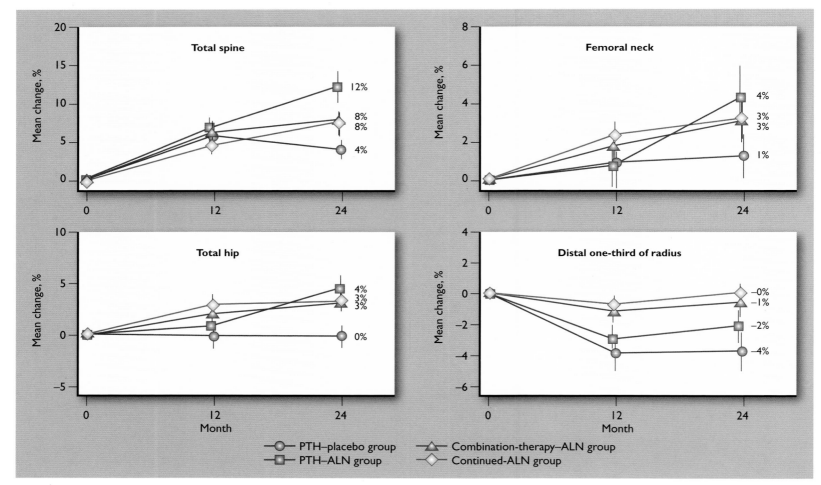

Figure 17-16. Treatment in the Parathyroid Hormone and Alendronate Therapy for Osteoporosis (PATH) study was for 1 year with either parathyroid hormone (PTH) 1-84, alendronate (ALN), or both. The bone mineral density (BMD) response was greater with monotherapy than with combination therapy. In the second year, PTH-treated patients were either crossed over to ALN or placebo. Increases in BMD were maintained if ALN was subsequently administered, but lost if patients were switched to placebo. Percent changes from baseline in areal BMD at the spine, hip, and distal radius, according to treatment group, are shown [4].

Strontium

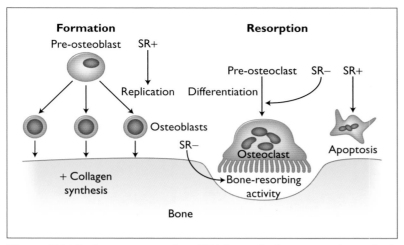

Figure 17-17. Strontium ranelate (SR) has a dual action on bone, both reducing bone resorption and increasing bone formation. The exact molecular mechanism for these effects remains unclear [24].

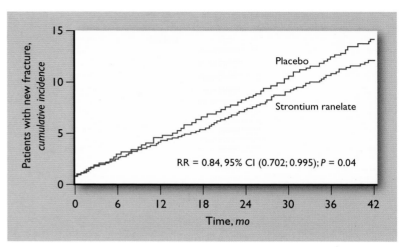

Figure 17-18. In a large clinical trial of postmenopausal women with osteoporosis (TROPOS), a 2-g daily dose of strontium ranelate led to significant reductions in nonvertebral fracture risk in association [25].

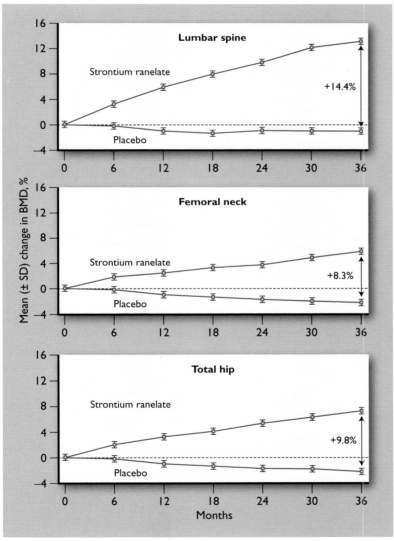

Figure 17-19. Patients who took strontium ranelate for 3 years experienced dramatic increases in bone mineral density (BMD) partially related to artifactual increases in BMD related to the strontium substitution for calcium in bone and partly related to the bone anabolic effects of strontium [26].

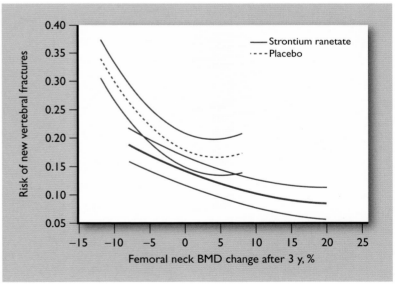

Figure 17-20. Logistic regression analysis curves (95% CI) of the percentage changes in femoral neck bone mineral density (BMD) at 3 years and the new vertebral fractures rates at 3 years in the placebo and strontium ranelate groups are shown. Increases in bone density on strontium ranelate therapy account for about 75% of the reduction of risk of fracture, which is much greater that the risk reduction attributable to increases in BMD with other therapies [8].

Sodium Fluoride

Fracture Studies Using Fluoride: Randomized Double-Blind Placebo Trials

Study	Reduction in vertebral fractures	Fluoride dose
Riggs, 1990	No	High dose—NIH
Kleerekoper, 1991	No	High dose—NIH
Pak, 1994, 1995	Yes	With moderate doses—mild–low BMD
Riggs, 1994	Yes	Moderate dose
Ringe, 1998	Yes	Males with IOM
Favos, 1998	No	High dose

Figure 17-21. Summary of the trials of sodium fluoride for both sustained-release and monosodium fluoride in relation to vertebral fracture reduction efficacy [27,28]. Fluoride salts remain without regulatory approval for the treatment of osteoporosis in the United States due to undocumented fracture efficacy. BMD—bone mineral density; IOM—idiopathic osteoporosis in males; NIH—National Institute of Health.

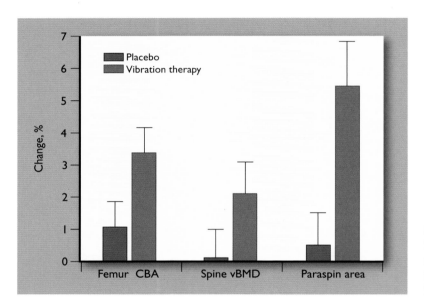

Figure 17-22. Adults treated with low-level vibration therapy or placebo for 10 minutes daily over a 12-month period. Significant increases in CT-measured femur cortical bone area, the cancellous bone mineral density of the spine, and the total paraspinous musculature [12]. vBMD—volumetric bone mineral density.

References

1. Riggs BL: Effect of fluoride treatment on the fracture rate in postmenopausal women with osteoporosis. *N Engl J Med* 1990, 322:802–809.

2. Neer RM, Arnaud CD, Zanchetta JR, *et al.*: Effect of parathyroid hormone (1-34) on fractures and bone mineral density in postmenopausal women with osteoporosis. *N Engl J Med* 2001, 344:1434–1441.

3. Greenspan SL, Bone HG, Ettinger MP, *et al.*: Treatment of osteoporosis with parathyroid hormone study group. Effect of recombinant human parathyroid hormone (1-84) on vertebral fracture and bone mineral density in postmenopausal women with osteoporosis: a randomized trial. *Ann Intern Med* 2007, 146:326–339.

4. Black DM, Bilezikian JP, Ensrud KE, *et al.*: PATH Study Investigators. One year of alendronate after one year of parathyroid hormone (1-84) for osteoporosis. *N Engl J Med* 2005, 353:555–565.

5. Finkenstedt G, Gasser RW, Hofle G, *et al.*: Effects of GH replacement on bone metabolism and bone mineral density in adult onset of GH deficiency: results of a double-blind placebo controlled study with open follow-up. *Eur J Endocrinol* 1997, 136:282–289.

6. Boonen S, Rosen C, Bouillon R, *et al.*: Musculoskeletal effects of the recombinant human IGF-I/IGF binding protein-3 complex in osteoporotic patients with proximal femoral fracture: a double-blind, placebo controlled pilot study. *J Clin Endocrinol Metab* 2002, 87:1593–1599.

7. Kendler DL: Strontium ranelate—data on vertebral and nonvertebral fracture efficacy and safety: mechanism of action. *Curr Osteoporos Rep* 2006, 4:34–39.

8. Bruyere O, Roux C, Detilleux J, *et al.*: Relationship between bone mineral density changes and fracture risk reduction in patients treated with strontium ranelate. *J Clin Endocrinol Metab* 2007, 92:3076–3081.

9. Baron R, Rawadi G: Minireview: targeting the Wnt/β-catenin pathway to regulate bone formation in the adult skeleton endocrinology. *Endocrinology* 2007, 148:2635–2643.

10. Gardner JC, van Bezooijen RL, Mervis B, *et al.*: Bone mineral density in sclerosteosis: affected individuals and gene carriers. *J Clin Endocrinol Metab* 2005, 90:6392–6395.

11. Krishnan V, Bryant HU, Macdougald OA: Regulation of bone by Wnt signaling. *J Clin Invest* 2006, 116:1202–1209.

12. Gilsanz V, Wren TAL, Sanchez M, *et al.*: Low-level, high-frequency mechanical signals enhance musculoskeletal development of young women with low BMD. *J Bone Miner Res* 2006, 21:1464–1474.

13. Rosen CJ, Donahue LR, Hunter SJ: IGFs and bone: the osteoporosis connection. *Proc Soc Exp Biol Med* 1994, 206:83–101.

14. Kiel DP, Puhl J, Rosen CJ, *et al.*: Lack of an association between IGF-I and body composition,muscle strength, physical performance, or self-reported mobility among older persons with functional limitations. *J Am Geriatr Soc* 1998, 46:822–828.

15. Beamer WG, Donahue LR, Rosen CJ, Baylink DJ: Genetic variability in adult bone density among inbred strains of mice. *Bone* 1996, 18:397–405.

16. Harris TB, Kiel DP, Roubenoff R, *et al.*: Association of IGF-I with body composition, weight history and past health behaviors in the very old. *J Am Geriatr Soc* 1997, 45:133–139.

17. Kurland E, Rosen CJ, Cosman F, *et al.*: Osteoporosis in men: abnormalities in the IGF-I axis. *J Clin Endocrinol Metab* 1997, 82:2799–2805.

18. Holloway L, Kohlmeier L, Kent K, Marcus R: Skeletal effects of cyclic recombinant human growth hormone and salmon calcitonin in osteopenic postmenopausal women. *J Clin Endocrinol Metab* 1997, 82:1111–1117.

19. Mitlak BH, Burdette-Miller P, Schoenfeld D, Neer RM: Sequential effects of chronic human PTH treatment of estrogen deficiency osteopenia in the rat. *J Bone Miner Res* 1996, 11:430–439.

20. Reeve J: PTH: a future role in the management of osteoporosis. *J Bone Miner Res* 1996, 11:440–445.

21. Watson P, Lazowski D, Han V, Hodsman AH: PTH restores bone mass and enhances osteoblast IGF-I gene expression in ovariectomized rats. *Bone* 1995, 16:357–365.

22. Xing L, Schwarz EM, Boyce BF: Osteoclast precursors, RANKL/RANK, and immunology. *Immunol Rev* 2005, 208:19–29.

23. Lindsay R, Nieves J, Formica C, *et al.*: Randomised controlled study of effect of parathyroid hormone on vertebral-bone mass and fracture incidence among postmenopausal women on oestrogen with osteoporosis. *Lancet* 1997, 350:550–555.

24. Marie PJ: Strontium ranelate: a physiological approach for optimizing bone formation and resorption. *Bone* 2006, 38(Suppl 1):S10–S14.

25. Reginster J-Y, Seeman E, De Vernejoul MC, *et al.*: Strontium ranelate reduces the risk of nonvertebral fractures in postmenopausal women with osteoporosis: treatment of peripheral osteoporosis (TROPOS) study. *J Clin Endocrinol Metab* 2005, 90:2816–2822.

26. Meunier PJ, Roux C, Seeman E, *et al.*: The effects of strontium ranelate on the risk of vertebral fracture in women with postmenopausal osteoporosis. *N Engl J Med* 2004, 350:459–468.

27. Zerwekh JE, Padalino P, Pak CYC:The effect of intermittent slow release NaF and continuous calcium citrate therapy on calciotropic hormones, biochemical markers of bone metabolism, and blood chemistry in postmenopausal osteoporosis. *Calcif Tissue Int* 1997, 61:272–278.

28. Meunier PJ, Sebert JL, Reginster JY, *et al.*: Fluoride salts are no better at preventing new vertebral fractures than calcium-vitamin D in postmenopausal osteoporosis. The FAVO study. *Osteoporos Int* 1998, 8:4–12.

Recommended Reading

Baron R, Rawadi G: Minireview: targeting the Wnt/β-catenin pathway to regulate bone formation in the adult skeleton endocrinology. *Endocrinology* 2007, 148:2635–2643.

Black DM, Bilezikian JP, Ensrud KE, *et al.*: PATH Study Investigators. One year of alendronate after one year of parathyroid hormone (1-84) for osteoporosis. *N Engl J Med* 2005, 353:555–565.

Bondy CA: Clinical uses of IGF-I. *Ann Intern Med* 1994, 120:593–601.

Ebeling PR, Jones JD, O' Fallon WM, *et al.*: Short-term effects of recombinant human IGF-I on bone turnover in normal women. *J Clin Endocrinol Metab* 1993, 77:1384–1391.

Ghiron LJ, Thomspon JL, Holloway L, *et al.*: Effects of recombinant IGF-I and GH on bone turnover in elderly women. *J Bone Miner Res* 1995, 10:1844–1854.

Johansson AJ, Rosen CJ: The IGFs: potential anabolic agents for the skeleton. In *Anabolic Treatments for Osteoporosis*. Edited by Whitfield JF, Morley P. New York: CRC; 1998:185–201

Neer RM, Arnaud CD, Zanchetta JR, *et al.*: Effect of parathyroid hormone (1-34) on fractures and bone mineral density in postmenopausal women with osteoporosis. *N Engl J Med* 2001, 344:1434–1441.

Nicholas V, Prewett A, Bettica P, *et al.*: Age-related decreases in IGF-I and TGF-beta in femoral cortical bone from both men and women: implications for bone loss with aging. *J Clin Endocrinol Metab* 1994, 78:1011–1020.

Rosen CJ: Insulin-like growth factor-I and PTH: potential new therapeutic agents for the treatment of osteoporosis. *Exp Opin Invest Drugs* 1997, 9:1193–1198.

Rubin J, Ackert-Bicknell CL, Zhu L, *et al.*: IGF-I regulates osteoprotegerin (OPG) and receptor activator of nuclear factor-kappaB ligand in vitro and OPG in vivo. *J Clin Endocrinol Metab* 2002, 87:4273–4279.

Tritos NA, Mantzoros CS: Recombinant human growth hormone: old and novel uses. *Am J Med* 1998, 105:44–57.

New Therapeutic Agents 18

Michael R. McClung

Multiple treatment options are now available that have been documented to substantially reduce the incidence of fracture in postmenopausal women with osteoporosis, men with low bone mass, and patients who are receiving glucocorticoid therapy [1]. In general, these drugs are well tolerated. However, several factors limit the acceptance and usefulness of these therapies. Each of the currently available drugs is associated with documented or perceived intolerance and there are concerns about the long-term safety of bisphosphonate therapy. Most importantly, poor adherence to all current treatments significantly limits their effectiveness [2]. These factors provide the opportunity for new drugs.

Several unique pharmaceutical agents are in various stages of development as potential treatments for osteoporosis. This review will be confined to agents that are already in clinical trials. Members of currently available classes of drugs are being developed and these agents are potentially more effective than current drugs or are being developed in different dosing regimens. Additionally, new classes of agents are in development. These new classes exploit specific biological pathways and mechanisms, leading us away from the era of serendipitous pharmacology for osteoporosis treatment.

Current Osteoporosis Treatments	
Benefits	Reduce vertebral fracture incidence by 30%–70%
	Some drugs reduce hip fracture incidence by 40%–50%
	Are well tolerated in most patients
Limitations	Real or perceived intolerance
	Concerns about long-term safety
	Inconvenient dosing regimens
	Poor adherence to therapy
	Do not restore skeleton to normal
	Expense

Figure 18-1. Current osteoporosis treatments. Our current therapies (bisphosphonates, selective estrogen receptor modulators, nasal calcitonin, and teriparatide) are effective treatments for osteoporosis in postmenopausal women. Bisphosphonates and teriparatide are also useful for treating men with osteoporosis and for patients receiving glucocorticoid therapy. Important issues, most importantly concerns about safety, tolerability, and poor compliance with all drugs, limit the potential effectiveness of these agents.

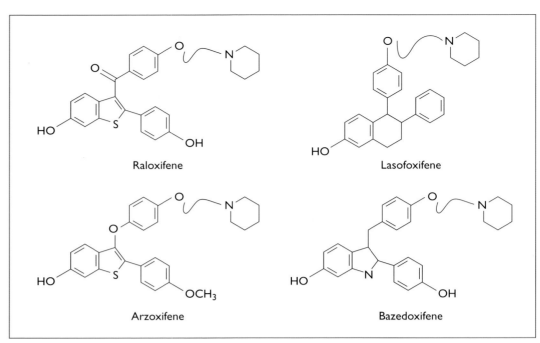

Figure 18-2. New drugs in clinical development. These new drugs or new delivery routes for current drugs have completed phase I clinical studies. PTH—parathyroid hormone; RANKL—receptor activator of nuclear factor κ B ligand; SERMs—selective estrogen receptor modulators.

New Drugs in Clinical Development

New forms of current drugs	New SERMs
	Oral calcitonin
	New forms or analogues of PTH
New antiresorptive agents	RANKL inhibitors
	Cathepsin K inhibitors
New anabolic agents	Calcilytic agents
	Sclerostin inhibitors

Figure 18-3. Selective estrogen receptor modulators (SERMs) in clinical development. The molecular structures of raloxifene (our current SERM and the three new SERMs undergoing late-phase clinical trials) are depicted. SERMs are structurally different compounds that interact with intracellular estrogen receptors in target organs as estrogen agonists and antagonists [3]. In bone, these drugs are weak estrogen-like agonists whereas the drugs inhibit estrogen-dependent responses in reproductive tissues including the breast and uterus. Arzoxifene and bazedoxifene are structural analogues of raloxifene while lasofoxifene, a derivative of the nonsteroidal anti-estrogen nafoxidine, differs structurally.

New Forms of Current Drugs

Figure 18-4. Selective estrogen receptor modulators (SERMs) in clinical development. Each of the three new SERMs has been demonstrated to have salutary effects on bone mineral density (BMD) in postmenopausal women. The phase III fracture data from two of the agents, bazedoxifene and lasofoxifene, have been reported recently [4,5]. The phase III study of arzoxifene, evaluating its effect on fracture incidence and breast cancer, is scheduled to be completed in 2010.

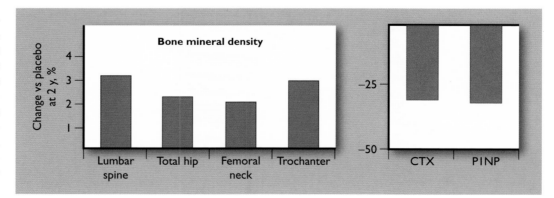

SERMs in Clinical Development

Drug	
Arzoxifene	Increases BMD and reduces bone turnover
	In late phase III trials
Bazedoxifene	Increases BMD similarly to raloxifene
	Reduces the risk of spine fracture in postmenopausal women with osteoporosis
	Reduces nonvertebral fracture in the high-risk subgroup
Lasofoxifene	Increases BMD slightly more than raloxifene
	Reduces the risk of spine and nonspine fractures

Figure 18-5. Arzoxifene therapy in young postmenopausal women. In a 24-month, phase III, placebo-controlled multicenter trial, arzoxifene 20 mg daily was demonstrated, compared to placebo, to increase bone density and to reduce biochemical indices of bone resorption (C-terminal peptide of type I collagen [CTX]) and bone formation (N-terminal propeptide of type 1 procollagen [P1NP]) in 331 young postmenopausal women (mean age 55) [6]. Treatment was well tolerated and the incidence of hot flushes was similar between the treatment and placebo groups.

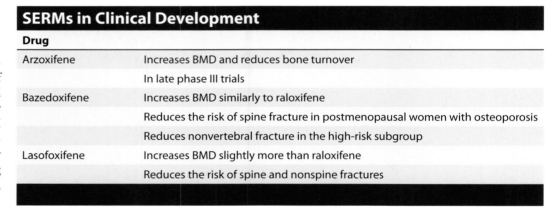

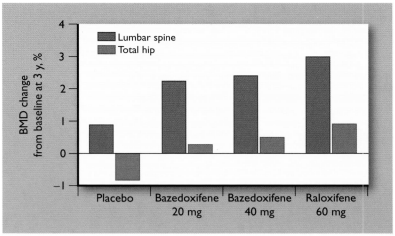

Figure 18-6. Bazedoxifene and bone mineral density (BMD) in a phase III study. Bazedoxifene prevented bone loss without stimulating the endometrium in healthy postmenopausal women with normal or low BMD [7]. The data depicted are from the phase III, randomized, double-blind fracture end-point trial in which 6847 postmenopausal women 55 to 85 years old received bazedoxifene in doses of 20 or 40 mg daily, raloxifene 60 mg daily, or placebo. Therapy with both doses of bazedoxifene and raloxifene significantly increased BMD in the lumbar spine and total hip regions [4]. In addition to being developed as a treatment for the prevention and treatment of postmenopausal osteoporosis, bazedoxifene is being studied in combination with oral conjugated equine estrogen as a treatment for menopausal symptoms [8].

Basedoxifene and Fracture Risk

Therapy	Vertebral fracture, %	Hazard ratio (95% CI)	Nonvertebral fracture, %
Placebo	4.1	—	6.3
Bazedoxifene 20 mg	2.3	0.58 (0.38, 0.89)	5.7
Bazedoxifene 40 mg	2.5	0.63 (0.42, 0.96)	5.6
Raloxifene 60 mg	2.3	0.58 (0.38, 0.89)	5.9

Figure 18-7. Bazedoxifene and fractures in women with osteoporosis. The effects of bazedoxifene on vertebral and nonvertebral fracture risk are shown. In the phase III fracture study in women with postmenopausal osteoporosis, therapy with both doses of bazedoxifene (20 and 40 mg daily) significantly reduced the incidence of vertebral fracture compared to placebo and was similar in effectiveness to a 60-mg daily dose of raloxifene [4]. Overall, no effect was observed on the risk of nonvertebral fracture. A high-risk subgroup ($N = 1772$) was defined post hoc as those subjects with a femoral neck T score of –3.0 or lower and/or the presence of one or more moderate or severe vertebral fractures or multiple mild vertebral fractures at baseline. In the combined bazedoxifene treatment groups, nonvertebral fracture risk was significantly reduced whereas no effect was observed in the small group of subjects who received raloxifene. The tolerability profile of bazedoxifene treatment was similar to raloxifene and included an increased incidence of vasomotor symptoms, venous thrombotic events, and leg cramps compared to placebo.

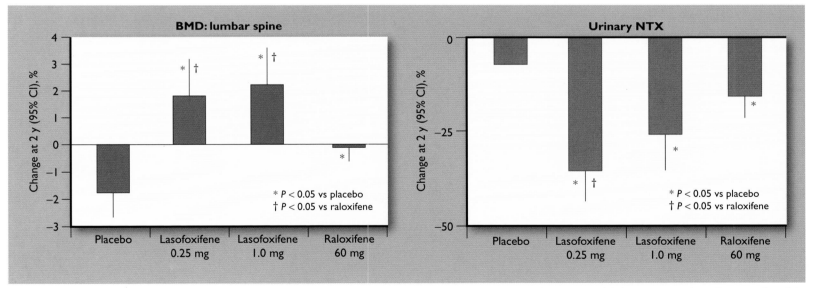

Figure 18-8. Lasofoxifene and bone mineral density (BMD). In a 24-month, phase III, placebo-controlled multicenter trial, lasofoxifene in doses of 0.25 and 1.0 mg daily increased bone density and decreased the urinary N-terminal peptide of type I collagen (NTX) in postmenopausal women between 47 and 74 years old (mean age 57) with normal or low bone mass [9]. The effects of both doses of lasofoxifene on lumbar spine bone density were significantly greater than was the response to a daily dose of raloxifene 60 mg.

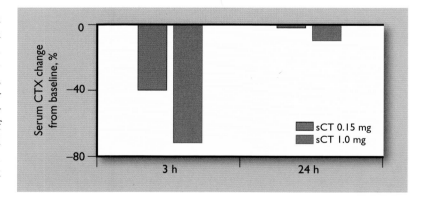

Figure 18-9. Lasofoxifene and fractures in women with osteoporosis. In a phase III trial (PEARL) involving 8556 postmenopausal women with osteoporosis, lasofoxifene in doses of 0.25 and 0.5 mg daily significantly reduced vertebral fracture risk compared to placebo by 31% and 42%, respectively [5]. The higher dose also significantly reduced the incidence of nonvertebral fractures by 22%. HR—hazard ratio.

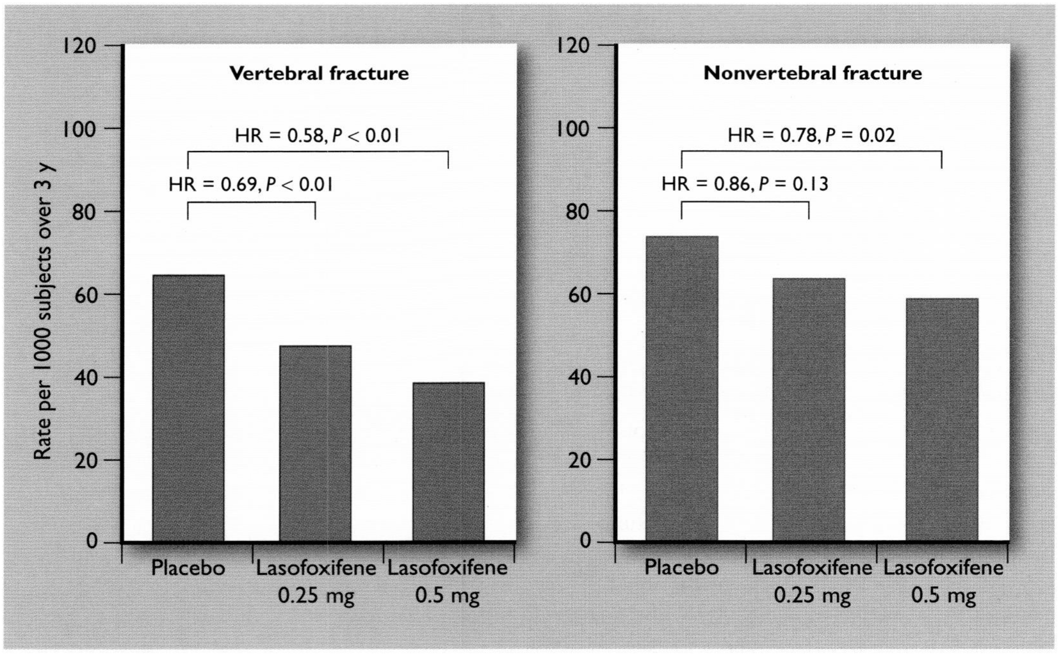

Lasofoxifene: Other Clinical Outcomes

Outcome	Placebo	Lasofoxifene 0.25 mg	Hazard ratio (95% CI)	P value	Lasofoxifene 0.5 mg	Hazard ratio (95% CI)	P value
ER+ breast cancer	4.4	0.7	0.16 (0.04, 0.73)	0.01	1.5	0.33 (0.11, 1.02)	0.04
VTE	3.5	9.1	2.60 (1.26, 5.40)	0.01	7.7	2.20 (1.04, 4.64)	0.03
Stroke	7.0	4.9	0.70 (0.35, 1.38)	0.30	6.0	0.85 (0.44, 1.62)	0.62
Coronary heart disease	19.3	16.1	0.83 (0.56, 1.23)	0.36	15.1	0.78 (0.52, 1.16)	0.21

Figure 18-10. Lasofoxifene and other clinical outcomes. In the PEARL study, lasofoxifene significantly decreased the incidence of estrogen receptor-positive (ER+) breast cancer [5]. The incidence of venous thrombotic events was increased with both doses of therapy, similar to the effects seen with estrogen, raloxifene, tamoxifen, and bazedoxifene. No significant treatment effects were observed on the incidence of stroke or coronary heart disease, although the estimates of risk reduction trended lower with lasofoxifene therapy than with placebo. VTE—venous thrombotic event.

Figure 18-11. Oral calcitonin. The effects of an oral preparation of salmon calcitonin for oral administration on serum levels of the bone resorption marker C-terminal peptide of type I collagen (CTX) are demonstrated. Salmon calcitonin is a potent inhibitor of bone resorption in vitro. Subcutaneous administration is associated with significant side effects (nausea, flushes). Nasal administration has variable and generally poor bioavailability and has only weak antiresorptive effects. New oral preparations significantly inhibit bone resorption. One of the oral calcitonin preparations, in doses of 0.15 and 1.0 mg per day, reduced serum levels of CTX at 3 hours by 40% and 73%, respectively [10]. Values returned almost to baseline for the next dose. A large phase III study evaluating the effect of oral calcitonin on fracture risk is underway. sCT—salmon calcitonin.

New Forms of PTH	
PTH analogue	**Route of administration**
PTH 1-34	Subcutaneous
	Oral
	Transdermal
	Intranasal
PTH 1-31	Subcutaneous
	Intranasal
PTHrP	Subcutaneous

Figure 18-12. New parathyroid hormone (PTH) preparations and analogues. Intermittent administration of bioactive forms of PTH stimulate osteoblast activity and bone formation, increasing bone mass, restoring trabecular architecture, and increasing the thickness of cortical bone [11]. Parathyroid hormone (PTH 1-84) and teriparatide (PTH 1-34) reduce the fracture risk in women with postmenopausal osteoporosis [12,13]. Both forms of PTH are administered by daily subcutaneous injection. With the approved dose of PTH 1-84 and with higher doses of teriparatide, hyper-calcemia and hypercalciuria have been observed. Alternate dosing forms of these two molecules have been developed (oral, transdermal, intranasal) that might provide more convenient dosing options, assuming that efficacy can be demonstrated [14]. Other analogues of PTH including PTH 1-31 and PTH-related peptide stimulate the biochemical indices of bone formation and increase bone mineral density in small early clinical studies [15,16]. Whether these alternate molecular forms of PTH have a better benefit/safety profile awaits further studies. PTHrP—PTH-related protein.

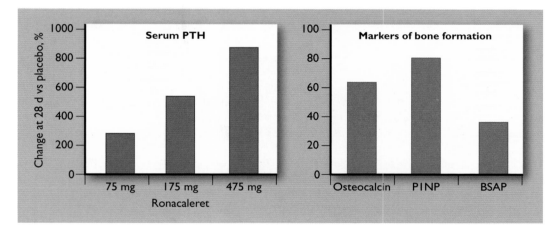

Figure 18-13. Ronacaleret treatment of healthy women. The effects of a calcilytic agent (ronacaleret) on serum levels of parathyroid hormone (PTH) and markers of bone formation are shown. Calcilytic compounds are calcium receptor antagonists that increase the secretion of PTH by inhibiting a negative feedback signal of serum calcium [17]. Several agents have been developed that have pharmacodynamic profiles similar to that of teriparatide injection. Such compounds could be orally administered and be less-expensive alternatives to the use of exogenous PTH or its peptide fragments in treating osteoporosis.

Ronacaleret in doses from 75 to 475 mg daily for 28 days increased endogenous levels of circulating intact PTH levels by 200% to 800% and increased biochemical indices of bone formation in healthy postmenopausal women [18]. A phase II bone mineral density (BMD) study with this agent was terminated prematurely due to its lack of effect on BMD in women with osteoporosis [19]. Other calcilytic agents are still in development. BSAP—bone-specific alkaline phosphatase; P1NP—propeptide of type 1 procollagen.

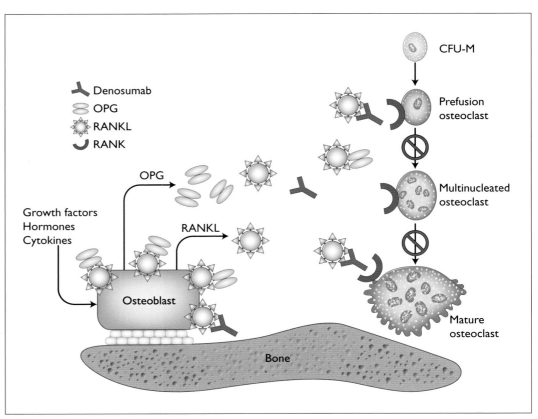

Figure 18-14. Inhibition of receptor activator of nuclear factor κ B ligand (RANKL)–receptor activator for nuclear factor κ B (RANK) pathway by denosumab. This schematic depicts the pathway whereby the interaction between RANKL and RANK regulate bone metabolism and the role of denosumab in effecting that pathway. Osteoclasts and osteoblasts function in a coordinated fashion, requiring communication between cell types [20]. The discovery of the RANKL–RANK pathway provided the explanation for how that communication occurs [21]. RANKL is a member of the tumor necrosis factor superfamily and is expressed on the surface of osteoblasts. RANKL binding to its receptor RANK on the surface of an osteoclast precursor promotes the proliferation and differentiation of osteoclasts. Upregulation of the RANKL–RANK pathway is involved in many skeletal disorders characterized by focal (Paget's disease, bone metastases) or systemic (osteoporosis) bone loss. Osteoprotegerin (OPG) is a soluble form of RANK secreted into the local environment by osteoblasts that, by binding RANKL, serves as a natural inhibitor of this osteoclast activation pathway. OPG administration to humans inhibits bone resorption.

Denosumab is a fully human monoclonal antibody to RANKL that is being developed as a treatment for various forms of osteoporosis and for the management of skeletal complications of malignancy [22]. It is the pharmacological equivalent of OPG but with more favorable pharmacokinetics and, since it is not the endogenous regulator of the pathway, it does not carry the risk of autoimmunization against OPG that would have detrimental skeletal effects. CFU-M—colony-forming unit macrophage.

Figure 18-15. Denosumab and bone resorption. The effects of denosumab every 6 months (Q6M) on serum C-terminal peptide of type I collagen (CTX) are compared with the effects of open-label weekly alendronate therapy. In this phase II study of postmenopausal women with low bone mineral density (BMD), denosumab was administered by subcutaneous injection every 3 to 6 months. Within 3 days, serum CTX was reduced to levels lower than those achieved with alendronate [23]. The duration of the inhibition of bone resorption with denosumab was dose dependent. The BMD response was at least as great with 60 mg denosumab Q6M as was seen with alendronate. An extension of this study to 4 years demonstrated persistent effectiveness with an increase in lumbar spine of 10.3% with the 60-mg Q6M dose while BMD in the placebo group decreased by 2.3% [24]. Upon discontinuation of therapy after 2 years, biochemical indices of bone turnover returned to baseline within a few months and BMD decreased toward the baseline as predicted by the pharmacokinetics of the drug. Retreatment 1 year after stopping denosumab therapy restored BMD to the levels present before therapy had been stopped.

The 60-mg Q6M dose of denosumab was evaluated in a phase III randomized, double-blind study involving 7808 women with postmenopausal osteoporosis [25]. After 3 years, denosumab 60 mg Q6M significantly reduced the incidence of vertebral, hip, and other nonvertebral fractures as compared to placebo. The semi-annual injections were well tolerated and no major safety concerns were identified. The simple, infrequent dosing regimen and its targeted, fully reversible mechanism of action are attractive features of this therapy. It will be important to determine whether such a potent inhibitor on bone turnover has adverse long-term skeletal effects or offtarget (nonbone) actions. (*Adapted from* McClung *et al.* [23].)

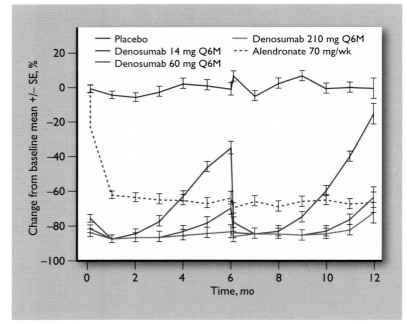

Figure 18-16. Cathepsin K and osteoclast function. The multiple steps involved in the activation and function of osteoclasts to resorb bone are shown. Receptor activator of nuclear factor κ B ligand (RANKL)–receptor activator of nuclear factor κ B (RANK) interaction is required for cellular activation. Integrins anchor the cell to the surface of bone so that a specialized, sequestered microenvironment is created beneath the osteoclast in which bone resorption occurs. Acid secreted into that space dissolves the mineral component of bone. Cathepsin K and other proteolytic enzymes are released and hydrolyze the protein matrix of bone tissue.

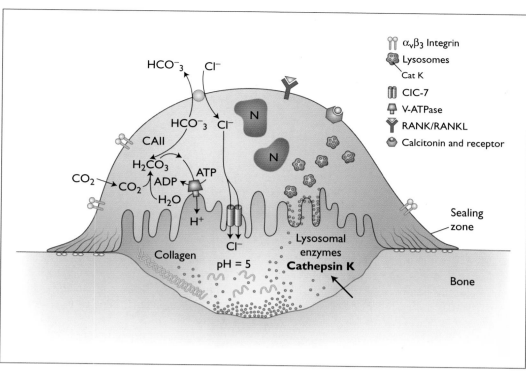

Cathepsin K is one of 11 lysosomal cysteine proteases (cathepsins) expressed in the human genome [26]. The enzyme is located intracellularly in lysosomes and extracellularly in bone resorption lacunae, where it is required for the hydrolysis proteins of bone matrix including type 1 collagen. Mice that are deficient in cathepsin K developed a form of osteopetrosis, but with normal bone quality and increased bone formation. In humans, pycnodysostosis, a high bone mass disorder, is the clinical expression of cathepsin K deficiency [27].

At least two inhibitors of cathepsin K have progressed to clinical trials. Balicatib treatment of women with osteoporosis increased bone mineral density by 4% to 5% in the lumbar spine at 12 months, reduced serum C-terminal peptide of type I collagen by 70%, and reduced bone formation markers by 10% to 20% [28]. A small proportion of subjects developed morphea-like skin lesions and further development was halted. ADP—adenosine diphosphate; ATP—adenosine triphosphate; CAII—carbonic anhydrase II. (*Adapted from* Rodan and Duong [26].)

Figure 18-17. Odanacatib therapy in women with low bone mass. The effect of odanacatib, a potent, reversible, and highly selective inhibitor of cathepsin K, on bone mineral density (BMD) and bone remodeling is demonstrated. In a 24-month phase II dose-ranging study of postmenopausal women with low bone density, once-weekly treatment with 10, 25, and 50 mg of odanacatib increased bone density in the lumbar spine and proximal femur in a dose-dependent manner [29]. A smaller dose resulted in bone loss. At the highest dose, urinary N-terminal peptide of type I collagen (NTX) was reduced to levels seen with other potent antiresorptive agents. As was observed with balicatib, biochemical indices of bone formation were only modestly reduced. Because the osteoclast number appears not to be decreased in response to odanacatib therapy, it is possible that cathepsin K inhibition results in a preferential reduction in bone resorption without the concomitant and significant decrease in bone formation observed with other potent antiresorptive agents. Important

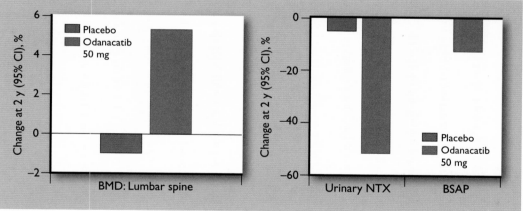

safety issues including skin and pulmonary problems were not observed in the study involving 399 subjects. A large phase III study has begun to evaluate the effect of odanacatib on fracture risk and its tolerability in a much larger cohort of study subjects with osteoporosis. In this large trial, it will be important to assess whether nonbone effects of this cathepsin inhibitor occur. BSAP—bone-specific alkaline phosphatase.

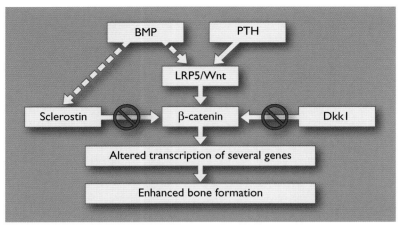

Figure 18-18. Inhibition of the LRP5/Wnt signaling pathway by sclerostin. This diagram outlines the role of the LRP5/Wnt signaling pathway in osteoblast function [30]. The pathway is activated by bone-forming agents including parathyroid hormone (PTH) and bone morphogenic protein (BMP), increasing bone formation. Sclerostin, an osteocyte-derived protein, and Dkk are endogenous inhibitors of the Wnt pathway. Through their actions, bone formation is inhibited. Sclerostin appears to be a tonic inhibitor of osteoblast function in healthy adults, keeping bone forming activity at rest until it is needed in response to a fracture or other stimulus. Activating mutations in this pathway results in high bone mass, while inactivating mutations cause forms of osteoporosis [31]. A genetic deficiency of sclerostin results in sclerosing bone dysplasias (sclerostiosis and Van Buchem disease) [32]. Antisclerostin antibody therapy in animal models of osteoporosis results in the restoration of bone mass, bone structure, and bone strength. A phase I study demonstrated that a single dose of antisclerostin antibody increased the biochemical indices of bone formation in healthy volunteers [33]. Phase II studies are planned to evaluate the effect of sclerostin in addition to bone density. This therapy has the potential to restore skeletal structure in patients with severe osteoporosis. The fact that sclerostin appears to be uniquely expressed in bone tissue could be an important attribute of this treatment strategy.

New Classes of Drugs

Antiresorptive agents	
GLP-2	Inhibits bone resorption
	No apparent effect on bone formation
	Increases BMD
Inhibitor of integrin in osteoclasts	Reduces bone resorption
	Increases BMD
Anabolic agents	
Inhibitor of activin	Increases bone formation
	Decreases bone resorption

Figure 18-19. Other new therapies in early development. Several other molecular mechanisms and pathways have been identified as potential targets for treating osteoporosis and have been studied in early clinical trials.

Inhibition of integrin: In bone tissue, integrins anchor the osteoclast to the bone surface, a process that is required for osteoclast activity. An antagonist of $\alpha_v\beta_3$ integrin (L-000845704) reduced bone resorption and increased bone mineral density (BMD) in postmenopausal women with osteoporosis [34].

Inhibition of bone resorption by glucagon-like peptide-2 (GLP-2): GLP-2 is a 33-amino acid peptide formed by the specific posttranslational proteolytic cleavage of proglucagon. GLP-2 is produced by the intestinal endocrine L cell and is co-secreted along with GLP-1 (involved in glucose homeostasis) upon nutrient ingestion. When administered to humans, GLP-2 reduced bone resorption without inhibiting bone formation and caused dose-dependent increases in BMD [35]. This peptide may effect intestinal function and other tissues, which could limit its utility in the treatment of osteoporosis.

Stimulation of bone formation by inhibiting activin: Activin is a member of the growth and differentiation factor protein family. It inhibits bone formation and stimulates bone resorption, resulting in a bone loss. ACE-011 is the human type II activin receptor IIA linked to the Fc portion of human IgG1. This agent interferes with activin interaction with its receptor. In animal models of bone loss, ACE-011 increased BMD and improved bone architecture and mechanical strength. In a phase I study, ACE-011 increased the biochemical indices of bone formation and reduced markers of bone resorption [36]. As with other biological agents, careful evaluation of offtarget (nonbone) effects of this therapy will be necessary.

References

1. Papapoulos S, Makras P: Selection of antiresorptive or anabolic treatments for postmenopausal osteoporosis. *Nat Clin Pract Endocrinol Metab* 2008, 4:514–523.

2. Siris ES, Harris ST, Rosen C, *et al.*: Adherence to bisphosphonate therapy and fracture rates in osteoporotic women: relationship to vertebral and nonvertebral fractures from 2 US claims databases. *Mayo Clin Proc* 2006, 81:1013–1022.

3. Shelly W, Draper MW, Krishnan V, *et al.*: Selective estrogen receptor modulators: an update on recent clinical findings. *Obstet Gynecol Surv* 2008, 63:163–181.

4. Silverman SL, Christiansen C, Genant HK, *et al.*: Efficacy of bazedoxifene in reducing new vertebral fracture risk in postmenopausal women with osteoporosis: results from a 3-year, randomized, placebo- and active-controlled clinical trial. *J Bone Miner Res* 2008, 23:1923–1934.

5. Cummings SR, Eastell R, Ensrud K, *et al.*: The effects of lasofoxifene on fractures and breast cancer: 3-year results from the PEARL trial. *J Bone Miner Res* 2008, 23(Suppl 1):S81.

6. Bolognese M, Krege J, Utian WH, *et al.*: Arzoxifene in postmenopausal women with normal or low bone mass. *J Bone Miner Res* 2008, 23(Suppl 1):S211.

7. Miller PD, Chines AA, Christiansen C, *et al.*: Effects of bazedoxifene on BMD and bone turnover in postmenopausal women: 2-yr results of a randomized, double-blind, placebo- and active-controlled study. *J Bone Miner Res* 2008, 23:525–535.

8. Lewiecki EM: Bazedoxifene and bazedoxifene combined with conjugated estrogens for the management of postmenopausal osteoporosis. *Expert Opin Investig Drugs* 2007, 16:1663–1672.

9. McClung MR, Siris E, Cummings S, *et al.*: Prevention of bone loss in postmenopausal women treated with lasofoxifene compared with raloxifene. *Menopause* 2006, 13:377–386.

10. Tankó LB, Bagger YZ, Alexandersen P, *et al.*: Safety and efficacy of a novel salmon calcitonin (sCT) technology-based oral formulation in healthy postmenopausal women: acute and 3-month effects on biomarkers of bone turnover. *J Bone Miner Res* 2004, 19:1531–1538.

11. Girotra M, Rubin MR, Bilezikian JP: The use of parathyroid hormone in the treatment of osteoporosis. *Rev Endocr Metab Disord* 2006, 7:113–121.

12. Greenspan SL, Bone HG, Ettinger MP, *et al.*: Effect of recombinant human parathyroid hormone (1-84) on vertebral fracture and bone mineral density in postmenopausal women with osteoporosis: a randomized trial. *Ann Intern Med* 2007, 146:326–339.

13. Neer RM, Arnaud CD, Zanchetta JR, *et al.*: Effect of parathyroid hormone (1-34) on fractures and bone mineral density in postmenopausal women with osteoporosis. *N Engl J Med* 2001, 344:1434–1441.

14. Lane NE, Cosman F, Bolognese M, *et al.*: Transdermal delivery of hPTH (1-34) (zp-PTH) is effective in increasing bone mineral density of the lumbar spine and hip in postmenopausal women with osteoporosis. Presented at the 2008 American College of Rheumatology Annual Scientific Meeting. San Francisco, CA; October 24–29, 2008. Abstract LB-5383.

15. Hodsman A, Bone H, Gallagher C, *et al.*: Ostabolin-C™ increases lumbar spine and hip BMD after 1 year of therapy: results of a Phase II clinical trial. *J Bone Miner Res* 2007, 22(Suppl 1):S38.

16. Horwitz MJ, Tedesco MB, Gundberg C, *et al.*: Short-term, high-dose parathyroid hormone-related protein as a skeletal anabolic agent for the treatment of post-menopausal osteoporosis. *J Clin Endocrino Metab* 2003, 88:569–575.

17. Nemeth EF: Anabolic therapy for osteoporosis: calcilytics. *IBMS BoneKey* 2008, 5:196–208.

18. Ethgen D, Phillips J, Baidoo C, *et al.*: Dose-dependent increases in endogenous parathyroid hormone concentrations after administration of a calcium sensing receptor antagonist to normal volunteers: potential for an oral Bone forming agent. *J Bone Miner Res* 2007, 22(Suppl 1):S38.

19. GSK terminates development of NPS' ronacaleret. Available at http://pharma-times.co.uk/Forums/forums/t/2404.aspx. Accessed September 2008.

20. Boyle WJ, Simonet WS, Lacey DL: Osteoclast differentiation and activation. *Nature* 2003, 423:337–342.

21. Kearns AE, Khosla S, Kostenuik P: Receptor activator of nuclear factor-κB ligand and osteoprotegerin regulation of bone remodeling in health and disease. *Endocr Rev* 2008, 29:155–192.

22. McClung MR: Inhibition of RANKL as a treatment for osteoporosis: preclinical and early clinical studies. *Curr Osteoporos Rep* 2006, 4:28–33.

23. McClung MR, Lewiecki EM, Cohen SB, *et al.*: Denosumab in postmenopausal women with low bone mineral density. *N Engl J Med* 2006, 354:821–831.

24. Miller PD, Bolognese MA, Lewiecki EM, *et al.*: Effect of denosumab on bone density and turnover in postmenopausal women with low bone mass after long-term continued, discontinued, and restarting of therapy: a randomized blinded phase 2 clinical trial. *Bone* 2008, 43:222–2229.

25. Cummings SR, McClung MR, Christiansen C, *et al.*: A phase III study of the effects of denosumab on vertebral, nonvertebral, and hip fracture in women with osteoporosis: results from the FREEDOM Trial. *J Bone Miner Res* 2008, 23 (Suppl 1):S80.

26. Rodan SB, Duong LT: Cathepsin K—a new molecular target for osteoporosis. *IBMS BoneKey* 2008, 5:16–24.

27. Schilling AF, Mülhausen C, Lehmann W, *et al.*: High bone mineral density in pycnodysostotic patients with a novel mutation in the propeptide of cathepsin K. *Osteoporos Int* 2007, 18:659–669.

28. Adami S, Supronik J, Hala T, *et al.*: Effect of one year treatment with the cathepsin-K inhibitor, balicatib, on bone mineral density (BMD) in postmenopausal women with osteopenia/osteoporosis. *J Bone Miner Res* 2006, 21(Suppl 1):S24.

29. McClung M, Bone H, Cosman F, *et al.*: A randomized, double-blind, placebo-controlled study of odanacatib (MK-822) in the treatment of postmenopausal women with low bone mineral density: 24-month results. *J Bone Miner Res* 2008, 23(Suppl 1):S82.

30. Krishnan V, Bryant HU, Macdougald OA: Regulation of bone mass by Wnt signaling. *J Clin Invest* 2006, 116:1202–1209.

31. Baron R, Rawadi G: Wnt signaling and the regulation of bone mass. *Curr Osteoporos Rep* 2007, 5:73–80.

32. Gardner JC, van Bezooijen RL, Mervis B, *et al.*: Bone mineral density in scler-osteosis: affected individuals and gene carriers. *J Clin Endocrinol Metab* 2005, 90:6392–6395.

33. Padhi D, Stouch B, Jang G, *et al.*: Anti-sclerostin antibody increases markers of bone formation in healthy postmenopausal women. *J Bone Miner Res* 2007, 22(Suppl 1):S37.

34. Henriksen D, Alexandersen P, Hartmann B, *et al.*: GLP-2 significantly increases hip BMD in postmenopausal women: a 120-day study. *J Bone Miner Res* 2007, 22(Suppl 1):S37.

35. Murphy MG, Cerchio K, Stoch SA, *et al.*: Effect of L-000845704, an $alpha_v beta_3$ integrin antagonist, on markers of bone turnover and bone mineral density in postmenopausal osteoporotic women. *J Clin Endocrinol Metab* 2005, 90:2022–2028.

36. Ruckle J, Jacobs M, Kramer W, *et al.*: A single dose of ACE-011 is associated with increases in bone formation and decreases in bone resorption markers in healthy, postmenopausal women. *J Bone Miner Res* 2007, 22(Suppl 1):S38.

Index

Cardiac transplantation, 103–104
Castration in men, 126
Cathepsin K, 207
Cement lines, 5
Childhood
  bone mass genetics in, 26
  disorders with low bone mass in, 32–34
  dual-energy x-ray absorptiometry in, 32
  fracture incidence in, 26
  glucocorticoid-induced fractures in, 95
Chronic kidney disease, 137–141
Cigarette smoking, 81, 86
Collagen type I bone markers, 162
Colles' fracture, 155
Compression fractures
  vertebral, 148–152
Computed tomography, 56, 152, 168
Contraceptive agents, 81, 88
Corticosteroids. *See* Glucocorticoids
Cyclosporine, 102, 139–140
Cystic fibrosis, 33

D

Denosumab, 206
Densitometry, 167–180
Dual-energy x-ray absorptiometry, 3–4, 168–169, 174–176.
  See also Bone densitometry
  indications for, 177–178
  pediatric, 32

E

Economic costs
  by fracture type, 79
  of osteoporosis, 22
Epidemiology
  of fractures, 63, 68–72
  of osteoporosis, 63–68, 119–122, 172
Estrogen
  epiphyseal fusion and, 27
Estrogen deficiency, 107–109
Estrogen replacement therapy
  bone mineral density and, 107, 110–112
  fracture risk and, 113–115
Ethnicity
  hip fractures and, 69–70
Exercise, 21–22, 31–32

F

Femoral neck bone mineral density, 68
Fractures
  age, 4, 157
  bone biopsy in, 13–19
  bone geometry and, 6–7
  bone mineral density and, 4, 74, 121–122
  bone turnover markers and, 162–163
  childhood, 26
  costs of, 79
  epidemiology of, 2, 63, 68–72
  estrogen deficiency and, 109
  estrogen replacement therapy and, 113–115
  falls and trauma in, 77–78
  glucocorticoid-induced, 91–96, 100–101
  in men, 119–120
  new therapies and, 203–204
  overview of, 147
  posttransplant, 100
  radiology of, 147–157
  risk factors for, 72–76, 86–87, 162–163
  survival after, 78, 121

G

Gender
  age-related bone loss and, 82, 123
  bone size and density and, 123
  calcium intake and, 29
Genes, 42, 45
Genetic linkage, 43
Genetics, 37–49
  investigative methods in, 41–44
  metabolic bone disease and, 45–49
  overview of, 37
  peak bone mass and, 21, 25–26, 39
  skeletal characteristics and, 39–41
  terminology in, 38
Genotyping assays, 44
Glucocorticoids, 91–97, 145
  apoptosis induced by, 17, 19
  bisphosphonates and, 183
  bone mass in men and, 128
  fractures induced by, 91–96
  management of osteoporosis from, 97, 101–102
  in organ transplantation, 100–101
Growth hormone therapy, 189, 194

H

Hip axial length, 6
Hip fractures
  estrogen replacement therapy and, 113–115
  femoral neck bone mineral density and, 68
  glucocorticoid-induced, 92–94, 96
  hip axial length and, 6
  radiologic imaging of, 153–154
  risk factors for, 72–74, 76–77, 216
  survival after, 121
  total hip bone mineral density and, 69
Histomorphometry, 13–19
  confusing terms in, 15
  in glucocorticoid-induced osteoporosis, 101
Humeral fractures, 156
Hyperparathyroidism, 137–138
Hypogonadism
  male, 127

I

Ibandronate, 184, 186
Inhaled glucocorticoids, 91, 95–96
Insulin-like growth factor, 191, 194
International Osteoporosis Foundation
  diagnostic criteria of, 64

K

Kyphosis, 1

L

Laboratory skeletal status assessment, 161–165
Lactation, 81, 87–88
Lasofoxifene, 203
Lifestyle factors, 21–22, 31–32, 81, 86–87
Liver transplantation, 103–104
Low bone mass
  causes of, 173
  differential diagnosis of, 174
  in men, 130–131
  pediatric, 32–34
  prevalence of, 66
Low turnover renal bone disease, 144
LRP5/Wnt signaling pathway, 208

M

Magnetic resonance imaging, 150–151, 155
Male osteoporosis, 119–132
Mechanics.
  See Biomechanics of bone
Medicare reimbursement
  for bone densitometry, 177
Men
  fracture risk in, 83
  hip fractures in, 68–70, 122
  importance of estrogen in, 116
  osteoporosis in, 65–66, 173
  postcastration bone changes in, 126
  smoking in, 86
Menarchal age, 28
Menopause, 108–109
Metabolic bone disease, 45–49
Microarrays, 49
Mortality
  fracture-related, 78
Multifactorial disorders, 39
Mutinucleated osteoclasts, 17–19

N

Nano-indentation, 58
Nonsteroid immune modulators, 102
Nutrition, 84–86

O

Odanacatib, 207
Organ transplantation, 99–105
Osteitis fibrosa cystica, 137–138
Osteoblast production, 192
Osteoclasts
  multinucleated, 17–19
Osteocytes, 9
Osteoid, 16–17
Osteomalacia, 17, 142
Osteopenia
  acquisitional, 8
  in men, 124
  prevalence of, 66

Osteoporosis
  adolescent calcium intake and, 21–22
  anabolic therapy in, 189–198
  bisphosphonate therapy in, 132, 181–188
  bone densitometry in, 167–180
  diagnostic approach to, 129–130, 164–165
  economic costs of, 22
  epidemiology of, 2, 4, 10, 22, 63–79, 119–122, 172
  from estrogen deficiency, 107–116
  genetics of, 37–49
  glucocorticoid-induced, 91–97
  histomorphometry in, 13–19
  in men, 119–132, 173
  micrography of, 3, 5–6
  nature of, 1–10
  new therapeutic agents in, 201–208
  organ transplantation and, 99–105
  parathyroid hormone therapy in, 132
  pathogenesis of, 38, 46
  pros and cons of current treatments of, 201
  qualitative bone abnormalities in, 5
  radiology of fractures in, 147–157
  in renal disease, 135–146
  risk factors for, 64, 124
  secondary, 164–165
  spinal, 1–3
  treatment algorithm for, 131

P

Paget's disease, 18
Parathyroid hormone
  bisphosphonates and, 187
  excess, 137–138
  therapeutic use of, 132, 189, 195–196, 205
Peak bone mass
  acquisitional osteopenia and, 8
  bone acquisition and, 21–34
  bone geometry changes and, 24
  calcium and, 21–22, 28–32
  genetics and, 21, 25–26, 39, 45
  hormonal regulation of, 27
  in men, 123
  race and, 21–22, 25

Pediatric disorders.
  See also Childhood
  bone mass in, 32–34
Pelvic insufficiency fractures, 154–155
Pharmacotherapy
  bisphosphonate, 181–188
  bone anabolic agents in, 189–198
  new agents in, 201–208
Polykaryons, 17–18
Polymorphisms, 44, 46
Prednisone, 17
Pregnancy, 81, 87–88
Protein intake, 84–85
Puberty, 21–23

Q

Quantitative computed tomography, 168
Quantitative trait loci analysis, 48–49
Quantitative ultrasound, 168

R

Race
  age-related bone loss and, 82
  calcium intake and, 29
  fracture risk and, 75
  hip fractures and, 70
  osteopenia and, 67
  osteoporosis and, 67
  peak bone mass and, 21–22, 25
Radiology
  of bone morphology, 55
  of fractures, 147–157
  of kyphosis, 1
RANK/RANK B ligand/osteoprotegerin pathway, 190
Remodeling.
  See Bone remodeling
Renal bone disease, 135–146
  pretransplant, 103
Renal transplantation, 103–104
Restriction fragment length polymorphism, 44
Risedronate, 184
Risk factors
  for fracture, 72–76, 86–87
  for osteoporosis, 64
Ronacaleret, 205

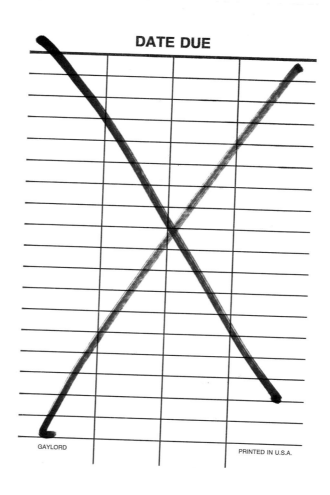